Practice Handbook of
Acupuncture

Commissioning Editors: *Karen Morley, Mary Law*
Development Editor: *Kerry McGechie, Natalie Meylan*
Project Manager: *Jane Dingwall, Jess Thompson*
Designer: *Charles Gray*
Illustrator: *Henriette Rintelen, Gerda Raichle*

Practice Handbook of
Acupuncture

Edited by

Gertrude Kubiena
Boris Sommer

3rd, completely revised edition

With contributions from:

Dorothee Bergfeld, Gertrude Kubiena, Alexander Meng, Johannes Nepp, Heidi Rausch, Ansgar Römer, Birgit Seybold, Boris Sommer, Ursula Völkel

Translated by
Johanna Schuster

Foreword by
Adrian White
Editor, *Acupuncture in Medicine*
Clinical Research Fellow, Peninsula Medical School,
Universities of Exeter and Plymouth, UK

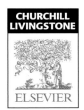

Edinburgh   London   New York   Oxford   Philadelphia   St Louis   Sydney   Toronto 2010

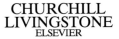

CHURCHILL LIVINGSTONE
An imprint of Elsevier Limited

First, second and third editions published in German.
First and second editions published under the title: *Therapiehandbuch Akupunktur, Praxisorientiertes Lehr – und Arbeitsbuch* **and third edition published under the title** *Praxishandbuch Akupunktur,*
ISBN: 978-3437551178

First edition 1997
Second edition 1999
Third edition 2004
English translation of third edition 2010
© **Elsevier GmbH, Munich**
First edition published in English.
© 2010, Elsevier Limited. All rights reserved.
This is a translation of *Praxishandbuch Akupunktur*, **3rd edition** © **Elsevier GmbH, Urban & Fischer Verlag, Munich, 978-3437551178**

The right of Gertrude Kubiena and Boris Sommer to be identified as editors of this work has been asserted by them in accordance with the Copyright, Designs and Patents Act 1988
Translation from German edition by Johanna Schuster on behalf of Elsevier Ltd, 2008

ISBN-13: 9780443102653

British Library Cataloguing in Publication Data
A catalogue record for this book is available from the British Library

Library of Congress Cataloging in Publication Data
A catalog record for this book is available from the Library of Congress.

Important user information
Knowledge and best practice in this field are constantly changing. As new research and experience broaden our knowledge, changes in practice, treatment and drug therapy may become necessary or appropriate. Readers are advised to check the most current information provided (i) on procedures featured or (ii) by the manufacturer of each product to be administered, to verify the recommended dose or formula, the method and duration of administration, and contraindications. It is the responsibility of the practitioner, relying on their own experience and knowledge of the patient, to make diagnoses, to determine dosages and the best treatment for each individual patient, and to take all appropriate safety precautions. To the fullest extent of the law, neither the Publisher nor the Editors assumes any liability for any injury and/or damage to persons or property arising out or related to any use of the material contained in this book.

The Publisher

ELSEVIER your source for books, journals and multimedia in the health sciences
www.elsevierhealth.com

Working together to grow libraries in developing countries
www.elsevier.com | www.bookaid.org | www.sabre.org
ELSEVIER   BOOK AID International   Sabre Foundation

The publisher's policy is to use **paper manufactured from sustainable forests**

Printed in China

Contents

Contents

Contents

Contributors

Dr. Dorothee Bergfeld
Heinrich-Delp-Straße 201
64297 Darmstadt

Professor Gertrude Kubiena
Weimarer Straße 41
A-1180 Wien – Österreich

Professor Alexander Meng
Schmerzakupunktur/TCM-Ambulanz der
Neurologischen Abteilung, Krankenhaus Lainz
der Stadt Wien
A-1130 Wien – Österreich

Dr. Johannes Nepp
Abteilung für Augenheilkunde der
Universität Wien
Währinger Gürtel 18–20
A-1090 Wien – Österreich

Dr. Heidi Rausch
Steinbrinkstraße 96
46145 Oberhausen

Dr. Ansgar Römer
Spreyer Straße 137
67112 Mutterstadt

Dr. Birgit Seybold
Türkenstraße 54
80799 München

Dr. Boris Sommer
Heinrich-Delp-Straße 201
64297 Darmstadt

Dr. Ursula Völkel-Petricek
Anton-Bruckner-Gasse 3
A-3400 Kloster Neuburg – Österreich

Preface

In 1972 – now 36–37 years ago – I started to study and at the same time to practise acupuncture. The literature available at that time was poor, and so was my education in and knowledge of acupuncture at that time. Since then, I have learned that acupuncture is only a small part of Traditional Chinese Medicine, and that it can be performed far better if the laws of TCM theory of science are also taken into account.

In 1997 the first edition of this book was published in German. Now – 12 years later – the fourth German edition is already on the German-speaking market and the book has enjoyed many alterations. These changes were not just of a cosmetic nature: they were essential. Consequently, the English-reading community will be able to enjoy a mature work, fitting for any practitioner of TCM.

This *Practice Handbook of Acupuncture* will enable you to find the ideal acupuncture point combination for your patient from both the Western and the Chinese points of view. Without needing to turn over the page, it will give you a basic treatment protocol as well as an introduction to the Chinese way of thinking: you will come to understand what it is that you are actually doing. The description and TCM actions of any given acupuncture point, together with the suggested treatment protocol and associated illustrations guiding you to the region of the point's location, make it easy to design the ideal acupuncture point combination. The introduction is short but essential. It provides important information about what Traditional Chinese Medicine actually means.

The *Practice Handbook of Acupuncture* is, without doubt, the most user-friendly book on the market. It gives instructions on how to treat Western diagnoses without neglecting the Chinese background.

Having taught for several years in Manhattan, I know how useful this book will be for acupuncture practitioners in the English-speaking community. I hope it will help all readers to improve their practice and to increase their skills in TCM. For me, it has been a pure pleasure to create this book. May reading and using the book be a pure pleasure for you!

Gertrude Kubiena
Vienna

Foreword

This textbook represents the mature wisdom of one of the foremost acupuncture establishments in the western world, the Vienna School founded by Professor Bischko. Like the school, the book uses a traditional approach to acupuncture that is firmly based within a professional approach to western medicine. This text, already well established in the German-speaking world, is at last available in English translation.

Readers will be immediately struck by its thoroughness and attention to detail. The first one third of the book describes all the traditional approaches to treatment, including auricular and hand acupuncture, and the rest of the book contains detailed information on every condition that may be treated using acupuncture. The layout is very practical, and so perfect for both the student who is starting to discover acupuncture, and the busy clinician who wants a quick reference text and reminder. This book takes a firmly experience-based approach, so the text is not ornamented by references to research papers. It is full of practical advice, and yet succeeds in remaining very clear with excellent diagrams and illustrations showing essential bony structures and underlying muscles on a single figure.

Clinicians facing patients with many conditions will find information that is unsurpassed by any other text of this kind. One example is the detail given for dealing with different stages of stroke, from the acute stage starting about one week after onset, through post-stroke rehabilitation starting after 3 months with specific instructions for a range of symptoms and residual deficits, accompanied by another entire entry on treating the pain that may complicate rehabilitation.

Though basically traditional, the book contains innovations that experienced acupuncturists will welcome, ranging from treatments that Prof Bischko introduced in the Vienna School, through lists of the European master points, a description of puTENS which will be novel for many, and detailed information on formulae to use at full term pregnancy for softening and ripening the cervix in preparation for natural onset of labour. Another valuable reference feature is a list of all the Pinyin point names in alphabetical order.

The book emphasises the need for placing acupuncture in safe context, stressing that it should only be considered after making a careful western diagnosis, and deciding whether western medicine might be more appropriate. The authors recommend that Western trained practitioners should make themselves familiar with the main points for any indication, then adapt it according to the individual symptoms, and they note how often a treatment designed in this way using a western approach ends up similar if not identical to the traditional Chinese approach

Readers will find here a text that is authoritative, comprehensive and safe. This book will start off as a mentor for the young student, and then develop into a trusted companion throughout a professional life. And towards the end of their career, practitioners might turn to the pages to remind themselves of the treatments recommended here for the forgetfulness of old age!

Adrian White

1

Introduction

G. Kubiena, B. Sommer

Acupuncture, as part of Traditional Chinese Medicine (TCM), is considered to be a holistic form of medicine. It has therefore become fashionable to describe TCM as being the opposite of modern Western medicine, the latter being construed as 'purely symptomatic'. This is wrong, as there is no form of medicine that is more 'symptomatic' than TCM.

During the evolution of TCM and acupuncture, there were no laboratory tests or imaging techniques, so, for diagnosis, physicians had to rely on their sensory organs and the subjective sensations of the patient. The result was an **individual** diagnosis, leading to an individual therapy. It is this fact alone that justifies the description of acupuncture as holistic.

Inserting a needle into an acupuncture point has more than just a local effect: it causes the vital energy, Qi, to move, which, as a result of the complex network within the organism, may restore balance, drain Excess and eliminate stagnation.

Acupuncture may be combined with a number of conventional and complementary forms of therapy. In China, acupuncture and moxibustion are mentioned in the same breath. Moxibustion is the application of heat, which in some cases (Yang Deficiency or Exterior Cold) is necessary, but in other cases may be contraindicated (Yin Deficiency or Heat). In addition, acupuncture is often combined with massage, exercises, dietary advice and/or herbal therapy. For example, in the treatment of cervical syndrome the combination of analgesic and muscle-relaxing acupuncture, manual therapy and physiotherapy would be the treatment of choice.

Book versus course

It is self-evident that a book cannot replace a good training course in acupuncture – I mention this only for the sake of completeness. Use of the correct stimulation method of the correct acupuncture point is the logical prerequisite for successful therapy with acupuncture. This skill can be acquired only by means of personal instruction.

The position of acupuncture

Acupuncture is a highly effective and specific form of therapy. However, it is important for the patient to find a well qualified practitioner, as only good training will lead to good results. It is not recommended that acupuncture be dabbled in as a sideline just because it is known to be free from side-effects. Whether acupuncture is indicated depends on the patient and the diagnosis. The positive effect of acupuncture for disorders such as headaches, migraines and rheumatic disorders of the musculoskeletal system is well known. Colds and other ENT disorders such as sinusitis and (allergic) rhinitis also respond well to acupuncture.

A retrospective study of 599 patients at the Ludwig Boltzmann Institute for Acupuncture in Vienna (Kubiena 1986) demonstrated good results with asthma and, in particular, with disorders of the gastrointestinal tract (gastritis, ulcers, colitis). A pilot study (Wagner & Wolkenstein 1995) showed that Crohn's disease treated with acupuncture led to a reduction of bowel movement frequency, liquid stools became loose, and loose stools became formed. However, colonoscopy findings remained unchanged.

Acupuncture influences functional disorders: it regulates that which is disturbed, but cannot repair that which is destroyed. It is not suitable for the causal treatment of malignancies, organ damage, severe bacterial infections or psychoses (for inpatients, yes, but never for outpatients). Acute life-threatening disorders also belong in the realm of conventional medicine, if available (well proven indications → Ch. 6).

Contraindications

Acupuncture is contraindicated for coagulation disorders, and thus caution is necessary in patients taking anticoagulant medication (warfarin, acetylsalicylic acid [aspirin]). There should be no strong needle manipulation! However, in more than 30 years of practice, the author has not experienced any real complications in patients taking such medication (although there were complications when she was treating her husband, who is neither a haemophiliac nor is he taking anticoagulant medication – quite simply, his jugular vein was punctured).

During pregnancy, abdominal and lumbosacral points as well as hormonally active points should not be needled (→ 3.1). Also contraindicated is G.B.-21, which can lead to a miscarriage. Strong needle manipulations should be avoided as they move the *Qi* and therefore may induce labour (e.g. L.I.-4).

Frequently asked questions

What is acupuncture?

Acupuncture is the insertion of fine needles at specific points.

Does it hurt?

It hurts less than an injection, but needle acupuncture is not painless. Only laser acupuncture does not hurt at all. A strange sensation, different from the insertion pain, may be felt at some points. It can be described as a distending, heavy, sore or warm feeling (→ *De Qi*, 3.2).

How does acupuncture work?

According to TCM, the needles cause the omnipresent, vital energy *Qi* to move. Only through movement can a disturbed balanced be restored, unnecessary ballast be eliminated from the body, and painful stagnation resolved. Scientific research has proven that acupuncture may, for example, promote circulation and the production of analgesic substances (such as endorphins).

How long does a treatment take?

A body acupuncture treatment tends to take around 20 minutes. However, the whole session will take longer, because the practitioner will need to gather information about the current condition of the patient in order to perform an optimal treatment.

How often do I have to come for treatments?

This depends on the nature of the disorder. Acute musculoskeletal pain occurring for the first time may be resolved by only one treatment, whereas chronic pain usually requires 8 to 15 weekly treatments. Severe pain and acute disorders need to be treated several times per week until improvement sets in.

How long does it take for a disorder to improve?

Again, this depends on the nature of the disorder. Acute disorders tend to respond immediately, whereas in chronic disorders there should be a positive effect after four or five treatments. The author has also experienced a case of longstanding arthritis of the knee responding after only seven sessions.

Can acupuncture be harmful?

Acupuncture is not harmful if performed by a properly trained practitioner. In contrast to many drugs, acupuncture has no side-effects. However, a healing crisis may sometimes occur, as found with various other complementary therapies. This can be considered as a positive response as it indicates that the body is responding to the therapy.

Do I have to believe in acupuncture?

No! But a positive attitude never hurts. Nor does a negative one – at least in the author's experience.

Can I continue to take my medication?

Generally, yes. However, many patients would like to decrease their drug intake, and this has to be discussed with the treating physician. Some drugs should not be discontinued abruptly: the patient has to be 'weaned off' the drug (e.g. beta-blockers). Other drugs may block the effects of acupuncture, such as immunosuppressants, cortisone and very strong pain medication.

Can acupuncture treat several disorders at the same time?

This is the truly wonderful thing about acupuncture – it is a form of regulatory therapy and affects the whole body. Often, TCM will see a connection among symptoms that are unknown in Western medicine.

How much is an acupuncture treatment?

It is difficult to give precise information on the cost of acupuncture treatment as this will change over time. Rates charged will also depend on the location of the clinic and the experience and reputation of the practitioner. Established practitioners in major cities are likely to charge more than less experienced practitioners or those working in smaller centres of population. Specialist treatment, such as acupuncture alongside in-vitro fertilization treatment for infertility, may also cost more. Practitioners setting up a new practice are advised to check with their national professional organization for guidance on what is acceptable when setting their fees.

Patients may also check with the relevant professional organization, or with other practitioners in their area, to find the average fees they will be expected to pay. Generally there will be a slightly higher charge for the initial treatment. Subsequent treatment sessions will be shorter and cost less. In some countries, most fully accredited teaching institutions have low-cost teaching clinics attached to their courses. In these clinics the treatment is normally given by final-year students under the supervision of experienced practitioners. The charges for these treatments are generally considerably lower than for treatment in a private practitioner's clinic. Patients with private health insurance should also check their policy as some, but not all, will cover the cost of acupuncture treatments for certain conditions.

Non-responders

The fact that some patients do not respond to acupuncture therapy (as can also be observed with other balancing therapies) is expressed in various terms and theories (e.g. regulatory rigidity, block to therapy).

A short comment is required here: none of these theories is in itself definitive or final. A so-called 'regulatory rigidity' may be resolved by neural therapy (clearing an active focus, or finding the primary lesion or 'disturbance field'), provided the therapist has the preliminary knowledge.

If a patient is not responding to acupuncture, it is important to eliminate the following: wrong diagnosis (Western or Chinese), wrong point selection, wrong point location, wrong needle stimulation, or contrary effects of medication. Generally it is possible to determine the success or failure of acupuncture after four to six treatments. When treatment is unsuccessful, another form of complementary therapy could be tried instead, provided the therapist has the preliminary knowledge.

2

Principles of acupuncture within the framework of Traditional Chinese Medicine (TCM)

G. Kubiena

2.1 What is acupuncture?

Western definition

The term 'acupuncture' comes from the Latin:

- *acus* = needle, tip and
- *pungere* = to puncture.

Thus acupuncture refers to the insertion of needles at specific points for therapeutic purposes. The classical acupuncture points are located on channels, so-called meridians. Acupuncture may rectify that which is disturbed, but it cannot restore that which has been destroyed.

TCM definition

There is no separate term for acupuncture in the Chinese language. One can, of course, say that a patient has been treated with needles (*Gei Bing Ren Zha Zhen*), but the common expression for acupuncture is *Zhen Jiu*, which literally means 'needles and moxibustion':

- *Zhen* means 'needle'
- *Jiu* means 'burning moxa'.

This fact, that there is no separate term for 'acupuncture', but only the compound phrase 'to needle and to moxa', demonstrates that acupuncture is not considered a monotherapy. In China, acupuncture represents only one aspect of TCM, which is complemented not only by the specific application of heat (moxa), but also by a highly developed herbal therapy using plant, animal and mineral substances, as well as massage, exercises, dietary recommendations, etc.

2.2 Effects of acupuncture

Acupuncture research from the viewpoint of Western medicine

Scientific research has shown that acupuncture has an effect on the following systems:

- **Central and peripheral nervous system:** analgesic effects (Jellinger 1984, Kaada 1984, Pauser 1979, Pauser et al. 1977)
- **Humoral–endocrine system:** influence on the production of endorphins, serotonin and cortisone (Cheng et al. 1980, Pomeranz 1977, Pomeranz et al. 1977, Riederer et al. 1975, 1978)
- **Blood circulation** (Kaada 1984): direct effect on blood circulation; activation of vasoactive intestinal polypeptide (VIP)
- **Musculature:** effect on musculoactive substances (neurotransmitters); effect on the neurological control of movement
- **Immune system** (Wogralik et al. 1985)

Effects of acupuncture based on the principles of TCM

Acupuncture has the following effects:

- It restores any disturbances of the flow within the body by resolving stagnation; it drains and diverts Blood (*Xue*), Body Fluids, Heat and Energy.
- It restores the energetic balance between different areas of the body, both on the surface of the body (muscular system) as well as between the surface

(skin, connective tissue, muscular system) and the interior of the body (internal organs).

- It can directly influence the internal organs through the surface of the body.
- It can restore a disturbed balance according to the principles of TCM ($\rightarrow$ 2.6)

2.3 Acupuncture points

Acupuncture research from the viewpoint of Western medicine

Acupuncture points can be determined objectively by bioelectrical (by measuring the resistance of the skin) and histological methods.

Bioelectrical research

- Reduced skin resistance (Bischko's Introduction, in Maresch 1966)
- High electrical conductivity (Bischko's Introduction, in Maresch 1966)
- 'Transmitter and receiver' properties of acupuncture points: acupuncture points have the same properties as de-modulation diodes; they can act as both transmitter and receiver of electrical vibrations in the bioelectrical environment. Information in the form of electromagnetic impulses can be transformed into bioelectrical signals, to which the body can respond (Meng & Kokoschinegg 1980).

Histology

- **Receptors:** Meissner and Krause corpuscles, Hoyer–Grosser organs
- **Effectors:** smooth muscle fibres in contact with lymphatic vessels (Bischko's Introduction, in Kellner 1966)
- **'Specifically structured bundles':** a vessel–nerve bundle following the course of the perforating veins, 5–7 mm (Heine 1988, Heine & König 1994).

Effects of acupuncture based on the principles of TCM

What we refer to as 'points' are called *Xue* in Chinese. *Xue* does not really mean 'point', but rather 'cave', 'hole' or 'nest'. *Xue* refers to a point on the surface of the body that allows access to its deeper structures. An acupuncture point is thus considered as giving access to a complex branched channel system that connects the surface of the body and the internal organs.

2.4 The meridians

Western definition and interpretation

The Chinese term *Jing* can be interpreted in many ways. Unfortunately, in both English and German it is commonly translated as 'meridian', which from the beginning has led to many misunderstandings. A geographical meridian is an imaginary longitudinal line on the Earth's surface. However, within the framework of acupuncture, a meridian is much more than an imaginary line on the body's surface: it is part of a branched system of longitudinal channels, the *Jing* (meridians) and *Luo* (connections, collaterals), that connect all parts of the body with one another.

Only with this concept in mind does it become understandable that internal diseases can be projected on to the meridian points on the surface of the body. Acupuncture utilizes this fact in two ways:

- Diagnosis: changes at the surface of the body indicate disease of the internal organs
- Therapy: by treating the surface of the body (for example with plasters, neural therapy or, of course, acupuncture), internal areas of the body can be accessed.

It has not yet been possible to determine a material substrate for the meridians using histological methods. However, isotopes injected into acupuncture points spread along the course of the meridian – in contrast to isotopes injected into neutral points (Darras & de Vernejeul 1992). From a modern Western viewpoint, the meridians can be described as:

- the synthesis of several systems – cardiovascular, nervous, lymphatic
- linkages of muscle chains
- an electromagnetic field of force.

TCM definition and interpretation

Meridians and collaterals together are called *Jing Luo*:

- *Jing* means meridian, but also 'chain', 'warp', 'channels'; it refers to the superficial pathway of the meridians
- *Luo* means 'net' and is also translated as 'collaterals'; it refers to the connections between the meridians, and between the meridians and the internal organs.

Together they form a network of Energy and Blood channels. In Five Phase theory, each meridian on the surface of the body is part of an organ–channel whole, or Element (→ 2.6).

It is in the meridians that *Qi* (vital energy) circulates together with the Blood (*Xue*) in a daily and seasonal rhythm, supplying all regions, levels and organs of the body. Undisturbed circulation – the 'smooth flow' – of *Qi* and Blood (*Xue*) is the most important prerequisite for good health: only then will there be no pain.

2.5 What is Traditional Chinese Medicine?

The basic principles of TCM are a synthesis of several different, sometimes contradictory, schools of natural philosophy, reaching back to the second to fifth centuries BC. The founders of TCM are allegedly three of the five mythical emperors of the fourth millennium BC:

* *Huang Di*, the Yellow Emperor: the 'Classic of Internal Medicine' is attributed to *Huang Di*. It is composed of two parts, the *Nei Jing Su Wen* (Simple Questions) and the *Ling Shu* (The Spiritual Pivot). According to recent research this classic was compiled between the fifth and second century BC. There have been multiple later additions.
* *Shen Nong*, the Divine Ploughman: the *Shen Nong Ben Cao*, a classic about herbal medicine, is attributed to him.
* *Fu Xi*, also called Founder of the Empire, invented the eight trigrams (the basis of the 64 hexagrams) and writing. He (or his wife for that matter) also invented marriage.

2.6 Basic Principles of TCM

The basic principles of TCM have to be understood in the context of the time of their origin. They are the result of observations of nature and are clearly not based on scientific findings in the modern sense.

What is unique about TCM is that, from the beginning, the person was seen as part of an all-encompassing system – an insight that has regained popularity today under the heading 'holistic medicine'. In this sense TCM uses several working hypotheses that consider both material and immaterial aspects of the person:

Yin and Yang

The original meaning of *Yin* is 'the shady side of a mountain', whereas *Yang* refers to the 'sunny side of a mountain'. *Yin* and *Yang* represent a polar pair: on the one hand they

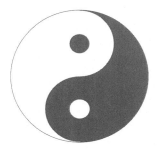

Fig. 2.1 *Yin–Yang* monad

exclude each other, and on the other hand they complement each other – even mutually create one another. The symbol of *Yin* and *Yang* is the monad: a circle that is divided by a sinus curve into a light half and a dark half. Each half contains a small circle of opposite shading to denote that *Yin* always contains some *Yang*, and vice versa (→ Fig. 2.1).

All natural phenomena and all manifestations of life can be explained by the interaction between *Yin* and *Yang* (→ Table 2.1).

Yin and *Yang*:

* are mutually dependent (e.g. light and shadow)
* oppose one another (e.g. exterior and interior)
* cannot exist without each other (e.g. substance and function)
* transform into one another (e.g. day and night).

When the *Yang* is at its lowest, *Yin* is at its peak (at midnight), but at this point the *Yang* will begin to increase (the new day dawns), and vice versa. After one peak has been reached, the decline begins, from the bottom of the valley there can only be ascension (→ Fig. 2.1).

Table 2.1 Aspects of *Yin* and *Yang*

YIN	*YANG*
Water	Fire
Feminine	Masculine
Interior	Exterior
Passive	Active
Right	Left
Earth	Heaven
Cold	Warm
Moon	Sun
Night	Day
Dark	Light
Body	Spirit
Slow	Fast
Colour: white	Colour: red, yellow

> TCM considers the balance between *Yin* and *Yang* as a major factor in good health. Restoring this balance is one of the aims of acupuncture therapy.

The interaction between *Yin* and *Yang* can also be transferred into a medical context (→ Table 2.2).

The Five Substances

The Five Substances are:
- *Qi* (vital energy, function)
- Blood (*Xue*)
- Essence, constitutional foundation (*Jing*)
- Body Fluids (*Jin Ye*)
- Spirit (*Shen*).

The Five Substances are important philosophical terms in TCM. However, they should not be confused with the Five Elements (→ see below).

Qi – vital energy

There exist a number of translations for the term *Qi*. In acupuncture we generally refer to the aspect of *Qi* that is energy, function, motivating force or vital life force – the moving agent that transforms dead into living matter. Examples of the different kinds of *Qi*:

Original *Qi*	Inherited constitution
Clear *Qi* (*Qing Qi*)	The air we breathe
Defensive *Qi* (*Wei Qi*)	Immune system
Nutritive *Qi* (*Ying Qi*)	Usable part of food
Organ *Qi*	Basis of the functioning of the internal organs
True *Qi* (*Zhen Qi*)	Sum of all biochemical and bioelectrical processes in the body, life energy

According to TCM, the 'true *Qi*' – the vital life energy – circulates in a 24-hour rhythm together with the Blood (*Xue*) through the body, organs and meridians. At the same time, the *Qi* itself keeps this cycle in motion. Any disturbance of this eternal *Qi* circulation will lead to disorders of health. Thus, one of the aims of acupuncture is to eliminate such *Qi* stagnations.

Blood (*Xue*)

While *Qi* is considered to be the moving agent, Blood (*Xue*) is the nourishing agent. Blood (*Xue*) nourishes the *Qi* and *Qi* moves the Blood (*Xue*). One is inconceivable without the other. In TCM the functions of Blood (*Xue*) include moistening and nourishing the skin, muscles, sinews, bones and internal organs.

Essence (*Jing*)

Essence (*Jing*) is a substance that forms the foundation of all organic life. It is the material substance, from which *Qi* is made (see above table, different kinds of *Qi*).

Prenatal *Jing*	Sum of all genetic factors
Postnatal *Jing*	Supplied to the body in order to maintain life – it is the 'Essence' derived from food and air

Body Fluids (*Jin Ye*)

According to TCM, the Body Fluids and Blood (*Xue*) derive from the same source.

Table 2.2 Significance of *Yin* and *Yang* in medicine

YIN	YANG
Topography	
Internal	External
Below	Above
Abdomen	Back
Physiology	
Substance	Function
Internal organs	Musculoskeletal system
Musculoskeletal system	
Flexor aspect	Extensor aspect
Internal organs	
Zang organs	*Fu* organs
Heart	Small Intestine
Kidney	Bladder
Liver	Gall Bladder
Lung	Large Intestine
Spleen	Stomach
Pathophysiology	
Too little (hypofunction)	Too much (hyperfunction)
Cold sensations	Heat sensations, fever
Atrophy	Inflammation
Arthrosis	Arthritis
Acupuncture: location of meridians and points	
Medial aspect of the extremity	Lateral aspect of the extremity

The term *Jin Ye* embraces all Fluids in the body. *Jin* (liquids) refers to the clear, thin Fluids, such as serous fluid; *Ye* (humours) refers to the thick Fluids, such as synovial fluid, the physiological mucus of the mucous membranes, etc.

Clear/thin Body Fluids – *Jin* (liquids)	Turbid/thick Body Fluids – *Ye* (humours)
Governed by the Large Intestine	Governed by the Small Intestine
Serous fluid, watery component of sweat	Synovial fluid, tears, urine, fatty component of sweat, sebum

TCM distinguishes five types of *Ye*:

Fluid	Secreted by
Sweat	Heart
Tears	Liver
Nasal discharge	Lungs
Parotid saliva	Spleen
Sublingual saliva	Kidneys

Both the thick and thin Fluids moisten the organs, muscles, skin and hair; they 'lubricate' the joints and 'nourish' the brain, marrow and bones.

The parenchymatous organs (*Zang*) produce and the hollow organs (*Fu*) store the Body Fluids.

According to another interpretation, the clear Fluids (*Jin*) are not excreted, whereas the turbid Fluids (*Ye*) are excreted.

Spirit (*Shen*)

Shen is the material base of the Spirit, which is unique to human beings. It corresponds to consciousness in Western thinking.

Five Element Theory

Although the philosophy of *Yin* and *Yang* is of Chinese origin, the Five Element Theory, in common with Buddhism, has its roots in India. It was adapted to the Chinese way of thinking and integrated into existing teachings. Each element is associated with a wide variety of correspondences (→ Table 2.3). Five Element Theory represents a model that describes the physiological and pathological relationships between the five elements and their many correspondences, for example between the internal organs and meridians. In Chinese, this model is

referred to as (*Xiang*) *Sheng Ke Cheng Wu*. The individual syllables have the following meaning:

- *Xiang*   mutual
- *Xiang Sheng*   to support one another, to generate, to give birth
- *Xiang Ke*   to have an effect on one another, working in two directions: control and resistance
- *Xiang Cheng*   to overact, to overcontrol
- *Xiang Wu*   to rebel against control, to insult

Xiang Sheng and *Xiang Ke* describe primarily physiological relationships, whereas *Xiang Cheng* and *Xiang Wu* refer exclusively to pathological conditions within the *Ke* cycle.

Primarily physiological cycles (→ Fig. 2.2)

Sheng cycle – *Xiang Sheng*

Generating, engendering or interpromoting cycle: each element, in its role as 'Mother', generates a further element, the 'Child'. The mother always promotes and strengthens its Child. At the same time, each element is engendered as a Child by the previous element, its Mother, who, through this process, becomes weakened – the Mother is 'consumed'. The order of the elements is as follows:

> Wood becomes Fire ➔ Fire becomes Earth ➔ Earth gives birth to Metal ➔ Metal gives birth to Water ➔ Water is necessary for the growth of Wood (a synonym for all plants).

This principle also forms the basis for the concept regarding tonification points (Mother) and sedation points (Child) (→ 5.2.2).

Examples: the Liver (Wood) stores the Blood (*Xue*) and thus supports the Heart. The element pertaining to the Heart (Fire) warms the Spleen (Earth), so that the latter is able to carry out its transporting and transforming functions, in order to be able to pass on pure *Qi* to its Child, the Lungs (Metal). The Lungs in turn have a purifying and descending function, thus supporting the Kidneys (Water) in elimination; Water, the element of the Kidneys, is an elixir necessary for all forms of plant life (Wood/Liver).

However, the *Sheng* cycle may also give rise to some pathological conditions:

- A disease can be transferred from the Mother to the Child: 'The Mother attacks the Child'.
  Example: an impairment of the transforming function of the Spleen (Earth) leads to the formation of Phlegm, which will be stored in the Lungs (Metal), resulting in chronic bronchitis.
- In the reverse scenario, the Child might turn against its Mother: 'The Child attacks the Mother'.

Table 2.3 The system of the Five Phases

MERIDIAN PAIR	G.B. YANG FU	LIV YIN ZANG	HE YIN ZANG	S.I. YANG FU	ST YANG FU	SP YIN ZANG	LU YIN ZANG	L.I. YANG FU	BL YANG FU	KID YIN ZANG
MACROCOSM, ENVIRONMENT										
Element	Wood		Fire		Earth		Metal		Water	
Exterior factors (environmental influences)	Wind		Summer-Heat (Fire)		Dampness		Dryness		Cold	
Season	Spring		Summer		Late summer		Autumn		Winter	
Time of day	11pm–1am	1–3am	11am–1pm	1–3pm	7–9am	9–11am	3–5am	5–7am	3–5pm	5–7 pm
Direction	East		South		Centre		West		North	
Colour	Blue-green		Red		Yellow		White		Black	
Taste	Sour		Bitter		Sweet		Pungent		Salty	
Tissue ('levels')	Sinews, muscles (function), nails		Subcutaneous tissue, perivascular tissue		Connective tissue, muscles ('flesh')		Skin, body hair		Bones, head hair	
Phase	Birth		Growth		Transformation		Gathering		Storage	
Opens into the…	Eyes		Tongue		Mouth		Nose		Ear	
Interior factors (emotions)	Anger		Joy, hectic pace		Sorrow (overthinking)		Grief, melancholy		Fear, shock	
MICROCOSM, INTERNAL FACTORS										
Zang function		Storage of Blood, smooth flow of Qi and Blood	• Vascular system • Circulation • Transport of Fluid contents			• Receiving and assimilating energy/food	• Breathing • Opening and closing the pores, defence			Water metabolism, urogenitary weakness, fertility
Zang reaction		• Emotional disorders • Pain with limited range of motion	• Palpitations • Disturbances of the mind and consciousness • Disturbed sleep			• Disorders affecting transport and transformation • Fluid-related disorders • Abnormal stools, e.g. chronic diarrhoea	• Cough • Weak immune system • Sweating			Urogenitary disorders/fertility/water metabolism, pain in the lumbar region
Fu function	Collects secretions of the liver (bile)			Governs Ye (turbid Fluids, humours); collects processed food for further transportation	Collects food and prepares it for further processing by Spleen			Governs Jin (thin Fluids, liquids); separates that which can be used from that which cannot	Collects urine processed by the kidneys	
Fu reaction	• Stagnation: pain and choleric behaviour • Deficiency: cowardly weakness			• Transport function: pain, colic • Separating function: urinary disorders	Belching, vomiting			• Dampness: diarrhoea • Dryness: constipation	Urinary disorders	

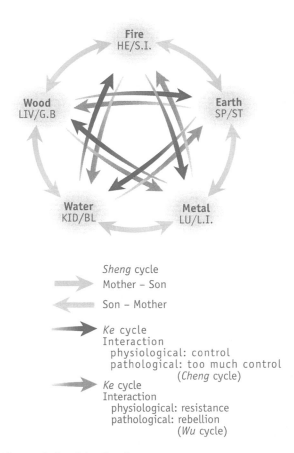

Sheng cycle
Mother – Son

Son – Mother

Ke cycle
Interaction
   physiological: control
   pathological: too much control
                    (*Cheng* cycle)
Ke cycle
Interaction
   physiological: resistance
   pathological: rebellion
                    (*Wu* cycle)

Fig. 2.2 Cycles of the Five Phases

Example: if the Lungs (metal) are affected, for example due to a cold or tuberculosis, this can have a negative effect on appetite and digestion, i.e. the Spleen (Earth).

Ke cycle – *Xiang Ke*

The interacting or controlling cycle is characterized by control (restraint) and healthy resistance against the control. In a physiological condition, the former is dominant. An important factor is the balance between the elements and their correspondences:

> Wood controls Earth ➜ Earth controls Water ➜ Water controls Fire ➜ Fire controls Metal ➜ Metal controls Wood.

Examples
- The purifying and descending function of the Lung *Qi* (Metal) acts against the ascending tendencies of Liver *Yang* (Wood).
- The smoothing function of the Liver (Wood) prevents tendencies towards stagnation of the lethargy-prone Spleen.

- The Spleen (Earth) governs the transportation and transformation of Fluids, preventing the Kidneys (Water) from becoming overburdened.
- The element of the Kidneys (Water) prevents the blazing of Heart Fire.
- Only the perfect functioning of the Heart (Fire) guarantees that the Lungs (Metal) will also function without complaint.

Pathological cycles (→ Fig. 2.2)

The pathological manifestations of the *Ke* cycle (infringing or encroaching actions) are described by the following two cycles.

Cheng cycle – *Xiang Cheng*

The overacting control described here follows the controlling sequence of the *Ke* cycle, but here the control is overwhelming, for example a disease shifting from the controlling organ to the controlled organ.
Example: emotions (Liver – Wood) lead to digestive disorders (Spleen – Earth); the Liver is overacting on the Spleen.

Wu cycle – *Xiang Wu*

The sequence of the insulting (or rebellious, counteracting) cycle corresponds to the sequence of resistance within the *Ke* cycle, but here the resistance is excessive. The controlled organ 'rebels' against the controlling organ.
Example: if the digestion (Spleen – Earth) is disturbed, for example due to poor diet (too many raw foods or too many dairy products) which leads to the accumulation of 'refuse', the Liver cannot fulfil its function of maintaining a smooth flow of *Qi* and Blood (*Xue*). The result is Liver *Qi* stagnation (for example in strict vegetarians).

This complex system of correspondences attributes to the Five Elements certain functions, descriptive terms as well as meridian pairs (→ Table 2.3). **Correspondences** are the terms that are associated with a particular element, whereas the term **Element** refers to the sum of all correspondences.

The meanings of the various correspondences in TCM are explained below:
- **Yin–Yang:** universal principle
- **Element:** the central concept; all correspondences have the same relationships between one another as the elements
- **Season:** seasonal adaptation of therapeutic strategies, depth of insertion, medication, diet. For example, needle insertions should be deeper in winter than in summer

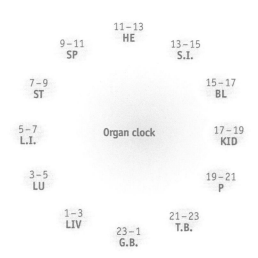

Fig. 2.3 Organ clock

- **Time of day:** organ disorders manifest at the time of day pertaining to the relevant organ (→ Fig. 2.3). As well as the 'standard' system with its approximately 361 meridian points, there are other, more specific, systems that calculate the factor 'time' in a minute way
- **Taste:** information about the taste of the appropriate herb, but also information on the organ affected. For example, a craving for a particular taste may give an indication about the organ or element that is affected: the desire for sweet foods points towards a disharmony of the Spleen and the Stomach; craving sour foods indicates a Liver irritation – just think of a 'hangover breakfast' with marinated herring!
- **Internal factors (emotions) and external factors (environmental influences):** these include, on the one hand, potential pathogens, especially regarding their corresponding organ; on the other hand, external pathogens are also used to describe symptoms. Whether a person becomes ill depends on which is stronger: the pathogenic influence or the person's immune system (TCM refers to this as defensive *Qi*)
- ***Zang* organs:** these pertain to *Yin*
- ***Fu* organs:** these pertain to *Yang*; each *Yin* organ is paired with a *Yang* organ, together forming an inseparable unit, which also includes their meridians.

'Health' and 'illness' in TCM

According to Western concepts, health 'is a state of complete physical, mental and social well-being' (World Health Organization definition).

TCM describes health as harmony and balance between the body and the environment, between *Yin* and *Yang*; it is the unimpaired flow of Blood (*Xue*) and *Qi* (Energy) within the body.

The causes of illness are:

- The five external and seven internal pathogenic factors, which primarily affect their corresponding organ, but secondarily may damage all organs (viscerovisceral reflex) (→ 2.7)
- Unhealthy lifestyle, for example alcohol abuse, drugs, eating too much or too little, wrong diet
- Injuries, insect bites, snake bites
- Obstruction of the *Qi* and Blood (*Xue*) flow
- Hereditary illnesses.

2.7 TCM diagnosis

Any therapeutic intervention has to be preceded by a modern Western diagnosis.

Based on this foundation, acupuncture treatment is then justified, beginning with proven point prescriptions. Should there be no significant improvement, the diagnosis has to be refined based on the Chinese way of thinking, so that point selection can be further differentiated according to the existing signs and symptoms.

In TCM, a 'syndrome' describes all aspects of a patient's condition, including his or her disorder, using TCM terms and phrases (Kubiena 1996).

The syndrome describes the disorder, and the disorder determines the therapy.

The syndrome describes:

- the cause of the disorder
- the location of the disorder
- the condition of the patient
- the stage, severity and course of the disorder
- the symptoms and functional condition (hyper/ hypofunctioning)
- information regarding the immune system and reaction of the body to pathogenic factors
- disturbances between the different regions of the body.

In TCM the diagnosis of a syndrome can be achieved using different methods, some of which are overlapping. These methods are described below.

2.7.1 Syndromes according to the Eight Principles

The Eight Principles are in essence four pairs of principles, which provide information about the location, type, severity and duration of the disease. They also inform us about the location, type and technique of therapy, as well as prognosis.

The Eight Principles (four pairs of principles)

Yang	Yin	(→ Table 2.3)
Exterior (*Biao*)	Interior (*Li*)	(→ Table 2.4)
Heat (*Re*)	Cold (*Han*)	(→ Table 2.5)
Excess (*Shi*)	Deficiency (*Xu*)	(→ Table 2.6)

The *Yin/Yang* principle is the most important principle; the other pairs of principles play a subordinate role in comparison. However, to arrive at a differential diagnosis, each pair has to be considered in its own right (→ Fig. 2.4).

Figure 2.4 illustrates how to obtain a diagnosis according to the Eight Principles, using the example of Heat/Cold and Excess/Deficiency.

As long as both *Yin* and *Yang* are sufficient and in balance, and as long as sufficient *Qi* (Energy) and Blood (*Xue*) are flowing without obstruction, a person will be healthy. In TCM, illness is seen as a lack of balance between *Yin* and *Yang*: either *Yin* or *Yang* has become predominant (→ Fig. 2.5).

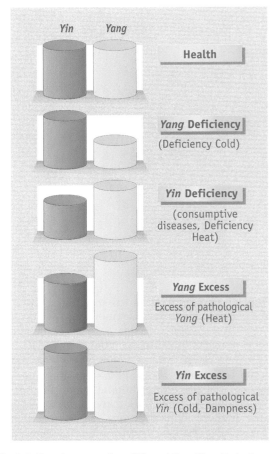

Fig. 2.5 Mutual consumption of *Yin* and *Yang* (from Focks & Hillenbrand 2003)

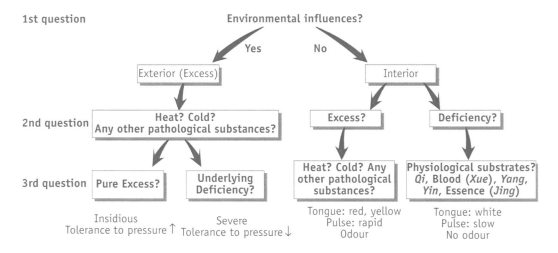

Fig. 2.4 Diagnostic procedure using the Eight Principles in the example of Heat–Cold and Excess–Deficiency

- A pure *Yin* syndrome will present with symptoms that are a combination of Interior, Cold and Deficiency.
- A pure *Yang* syndrome will present with symptoms that are a combination of Exterior, Heat and Excess.

However, only rarely will a case be as clearcut. Much more frequently there will be mixed *Yin* and *Yang* symptoms.

A disturbed balance between *Yin* and *Yang* will result in the following:

- When there is too much of one aspect, the other aspect will be relatively weaker.
- When there is too little of one aspect, the other factor will be relatively stronger. So-called 'Deficiency symptoms' are not always easily recognizable.
- When there is too little of both, then either *Yin* or *Yang* can still be relatively dominant. TCM refers to this scenario as a 'false' syndrome. These are generally difficult to treat!

Interpreting the diagnostic findings according to the Eight Principles allows a basic classification of the disorder. The following tables (→ Tables 2.4–2.6) help to provide an overview of how to differentiate the Eight Principles.

2.7.2 Syndromes according to the theory of Blood (Xue) and Qi

Qi and Blood (*Xue*) may stagnate so that they are no longer flowing smoothly. They may also be deficient (→ Table 2.7) or the direction of *Qi* flow may be disturbed.

2.7.3 Meridian syndromes

The following are summarized under the heading 'meridian syndromes':

- Symptoms on the surface of the body and along the path of the meridian
- Key symptoms that occur in addition to disorders of the organ in question (→ Table 2.8).

A meridian syndrome is considered to be an External syndrome, which might present with some symptoms typical of the organ in question. The symptoms occur mainly on the surface of the body, which, in the context of TCM, comprises the musculoskeletal system and the meridian pathway. They are therefore easily accessible by acupuncture.

Table 2.8 lists the symptoms typical of a particular meridian by differentiating between the location of the pain and further symptoms.

Table 2.4 Differentiation: Exterior–Interior (*Biao–Li*)

	YANG (EXTERIOR)	YIN (INTERIOR)
Location	Superficial parts of the body, meridians, head	Internal organs
Onset	Acute	Rarely acute, mostly insidious
Medical history	Short	Usually longer
Prognosis	Good, easy to treat	Not as good, more difficult to treat
General condition	Good	Impaired
Stools	Unchanged	Changed
Urine	Unchanged	Changed
Tongue body	Changed depending on pathogen	Changed
Tongue coating	Unchanged	Changed
Pulse	Superficial	Deep (in general)
Cause according to TCM	'Battle' between external pathogenic factors and body's defence system	External or internal pathogenic factors lead to internal disharmony
Diagnosis (examples)	Muscle pain, early stages of cold	Pneumonia following a cold, chronic diarrhoea
Therapeutic consequence	Focus on location and pathogenic factor; acupuncture	Focus on organ involved, strengthening the immune system; primarily herbal therapy, but also acupuncture
Acupuncture	Strong needle manipulation, frequent treatments; select points on affected meridians, distal points	Gentle needle manipulation and greater intervals between treatments
	Highly acute: points on corresponding, contralateral meridian and local points	*Fu* organs: front-*Mu* point and lower *He*-sea point
	Acute: corresponding, ipsilateral meridian and local points	*Zang* organs: *Yuan*-source point and back-*Shu* point
	Chronic: distal points on affected meridian, many local points	

Table 2.5 Differentiation: Heat–Cold *(Re–Han)*

	YANG-HEAT	*YIN*-COLD
Main colour	Red, yellow	White
Face	Red	Pale
Movement	Rapid	Slow
Behaviour	Extroverted	Introverted
Speech	Talkative, fast	Taciturn, slow
Body temperature	Fever	Chills, cold extremities
Aversion to	Heat	Cold
Better with	Cold	Warmth
Thirst	Yes	No
Desire to drink	Cold drink	Warm drink
Urine	Dark yellow	Pale
Stool	Constipated	Loose
Smell of stool	Foul smelling	Only slight odour
Tongue body	Red	Pale
Tongue coating	Yellow	White
Pulse	Rapid	Slow
Cause	Too much *Yang*-Heat or too little cooling *Yin*	Too much *Yin*-Cold or *Yang Qi* Deficiency
Diagnosis (examples)	Fully developed infection, arthritis, high fever	Beginning infection, arthrosis (worse with cold), chronic pain
Therapeutic consequence	No application of Heat, drain Heat	Apply heat, e.g. moxa
Acupuncture	Heat points, e.g. Du-14, L.I.-4, L.I.-11	Acupuncture and/or moxa, e.g. on L.I.-4

Table 2.6 Differentiation: Excess–Deficiency *(Shi–Xu)*

	EXCESS[a]	DEFICIENCY[a]
Note	Excess signs and symptoms tend to be quite pronounced; they signify an Excess of **pathological** energies (pathogenic factors) and are characterized by the pathogenic factor present (e.g. Summer-Heat, Fire, Cold, Dampness, Dryness, Wind) **Physiological** energies and substances that are in the wrong place: *Qi*/Blood stagnation, pain	Deficiency always refers to physiological energies and substances: *Qi*, Blood (*Xue*), *Yin*, *Yang*, Essence (*Jing*), Body Fluids
With pressure	Worse	Better
Stage	Acute, subacute	Chronic
Cause	Pathogenic factors or 'obstruction' lead to *Qi* and Blood (*Xue*) stagnation	Constitutional weakness or excessive consumption
Examples of diagnosis	Acute infection, biliary colic	Emphysema, congenital heart defect
Therapeutic consequence	Acupuncture	Mainly herbal therapy
Acupuncture	Reducing needling techniques, frequent treatments, shorter intervals between treatments; bloodletting	Tonifying needling techniques, longer intervals between treatments, fewer points per treatment, select tonifying points (e.g. BL-20, ST-36, SP-6, Ren-6) with slight manipulation; no bloodletting

[a]With Excess and Deficiency, the questions should always be: **Of what** is there too much? **Of what** is there too little?

Table 2.7 The four *Qi* and Blood (*Xue*) pathologies

PATHOLOGY	SYMPTOMS	THERAPY
Qi deficiency	• Tired, listless • Sweating upon exertion, dyspnoea	Ren-4+, Ren-6+, ST-36+, or Ren-12, BL-20 *Yang*-opening points[a]: S.I.-3, BL-62, T.B.-5, G.B.-41
Qi stagnation	• Distension • Pain that changes location	Course and spread the *Qi*: Ren-6, ST-36+/−
Counterflow *Qi*	Depend on organ affected: • Lung: cough • Stomach: vomiting, belching • Liver: headaches, dizziness, haemoptysis	Descend counterflow *Qi*: BL-17, Ren-22 Lung: LU-9, LU-7, BL-13 Stomach: P-6, Ren-12, ST-36 Liver: LIV-3
Qi sinking	Prolapse, descensus, ptosis	Strengthen the Spleen, raise the *Qi*:Ren-12, ST-36, SP-6, BL-20, Du-20
Blood (*Xue*) deficiency	• Lusterless, pale • Blurry vision • Self-esteem lowered	BL-17+, BL-20+, SP-6+, SP-10+; *Si Wu Tang*
Blood (*Xue*) stagnation	• Stabbing, localized pain • Swelling, haematoma, myogelosis	Resolve stagnation, regulate the Blood: BL-17+/−, SP-10− Move *Qi* and Blood: SP-6−, Ren-6−, ST-36; BL-54 [Bi] −, LU-5 with bloodletting Moxa locally In general: *Yue Ju Wan* Post-partum: *Sheng Hua Tang*
Blood (*Xue*) stasis/congealed Blood (*Xue*)	Hard tumours, masses	May hinder treatment progress! 'Blood breakers' Uterus: *Gui Zhi Fu Ling Wan*
Blood (*Xue*) Heat	Bleeding	SP-6, SP-10, BL-40, Ren-5, HE-3 Formulas with rhinoceros horn (today replaced by hair restorers)

[a]Feit and Zmiewski (1989)

Table 2.8 Symptoms by meridians

MERIDIAN	LOCATION OF PAIN	FURTHER SYMPTOMS
LU	• In shoulder, on anterior aspect of arm, in supraclavicular fossa • Sore throat • Chest tightness	• Cough, asthma • Haemoptysis
L.I.	• Along the course of the meridian (arm, shoulder, neck) • Tooth pain, sore throat	• Borborygmus, diarrhoea, abdominal pain • Epistaxis • Rhinitis with clear discharge
ST	• Pain or distension along the course of the meridian (leg, hypochondrium, neck)	• Facial paralysis with deviation of corners of mouth and eyes • Oedema • Borborgymus, abdominal distension, epigastric pain • Bloating • Vomiting, hunger sensations • Fever, malaria
SP	• In epigastrium • Swellings and cold sensations on medial aspect of thigh and leg	• Bloating, loose stools • Jaundice • Sensations of heaviness, fatigue • Belching, vomiting • Lethargy and pain of root of tongue

(Continued)

Table 2.8 Symptoms by meridians—cont'd

MERIDIAN	LOCATION OF PAIN	FURTHER SYMPTOMS
HE	• In heart region • In hypochondrium • On anterior aspect of upper arm	• Thirst, dry throat and tongue • Heat sensations in palms, night sweats • Insomnia
S.I.	• In lower abdomen • On posterior aspect of shoulder and upper arm	• Bloating • Polyuria • Raw throat • Swelling of cheeks • Yellow sclera • Deafness
BL	• (Lower) back pain • Head, occiput • On posterior aspect of legs	• Retention of urine, enuresis • Epistaxis, rhinitis, blocked nose • Tearing of eyes with exposure to wind • Mental confusion (bipolar disorder) • Malaria
KID	• Sciatica • Pain in the back and posteromedial aspect of leg	• Weakness of lower extremities, heat sensations on soles of feet • Polyuria, spermatorrhoea, enuresis, impotence • Menstrual disorders • Asthma-related dyspnoea • Haemoptysis • Dry tongue • Pain and distending sensations of throat • Oedema
P	• Spasms in upper extremities • Chest tightness • Heart pain	• Palpitations • Axillary swellings • Red face, hot flushes • Restlessness • Bipolar disorders • Heat in palm of hands
T.B.	• Retroauricular • Outer canthus of eye • Shoulder and lateral aspect of arm • Elbow	• Pain and distending sensations of throat • Swellings of the cheek • Bloating • Enuresis, dysuria • Oedema • Tinnitus, deafness
G.B.	• Hypochondrium • Flanks • Axilla • Supraclavicular fossa • Outer canthus of eye • Jaw • Head • Lower extremities	• Bitter taste in mouth • Blurred vision
LIV	Abdomen Back Vertex headache	Hernia Sensation of fullness in chest Enuresis, dysuria Dry throat Hiccups Mental confusion

2.7.4 Syndromes of the six meridian pairs

There are two kinds of 'meridian pairing':
Interiorly–exteriorly paired meridians, according to the Interior/Exterior (*Yin/Yang*) rule: LU/L.I., ST/SP, HE/S.I., BL/KID, P/T.B., LIV/G.B. (→ 4.2).
Corresponding meridians: according to the 'above and below' rule, corresponding meridians course along the upper and lower extremity respectively in anatomically corresponding areas. In TCM, this 'pairing' is considered so important that the 'partners' are even allocated the same name (→ 4.2).

TCM describes how the pathogenic factors penetrate the body from the Exterior, initially affecting the three *Yang* pairs, and subsequently the three *Yin* pairs. The deeper the pathogen penetrates into the body, the poorer the prognosis.

2.7.5 Syndromes of the eight extraordinary meridians

The eight extraordinary meridians (→ 4.5) are attributed the following functions:

- They support the connections between the 12 regular meridians.
- They regulate the *Qi* energy and function of the 12 regular meridians.
- They have a special connection to the Liver and Kidneys.
- They have a connection with the 'extraordinary' organs – the uterus, brain and marrow (of the bones and the spinal cord).

Syndromes that are associated with the extraordinary vessels often manifest with symptoms reflecting their pathway and function (→ Table 2.9).

Table 2.9 Symptoms of the extraordinary vessels

EXTRAORDINARY VESSEL	OPENING POINT	SYMPTOMS
Chong Mai	SP-4	• Abdominal pain and spasms • Menstrual disorders • Male/female infertility • Asthma
Yin Wei Mai	P-6	'Deep syndromes', e.g. chest, heart and epigastric pain
Ren Mai (conception vessel)	LU-7	• Epigastric and abdominal pain • Genital region: leukorrhoea, menstrual disorders, male/female infertility, spermatorrhoea • Enuresis, urinary retention • Hernia
Yin Qiao Mai	KID-6	• Abdominal/lumbar pain, hip pain; spasms • Impaired supination and internal rotation of the foot • Lethargy, epilepsy
Du Mai (governing vessel)	S.I.-3	• Impaired range of motion and pain of whole spine • Opisthotonos • Headache and epilepsy
Yang Qiao Mai	BL-62	• Back and knee pain • Spasms • Impaired pronation and external rotation of lower extremity • Insomnia • Epilepsy • Inflammation of inner canthus of eye
Dai Mai	G.B.-41	• Lumbar weakness • Weakness, atrophy and motor impairment of lower extremity • Bloating and sensation of fullness of abdomen and epigastrium • Leukorrhoea • Uterine prolapse
Yang Wei Mai	T.B.-5	'Superficial syndromes', e.g. chills and fever

2.7.6 Syndromes according to pathogenic factors

The five External pathogenic factors are:

- Wind
- Cold
- Summer-Heat
- Fire
- Dryness
- Dampness (Phlegm[1]).

Each syndrome manifests with characteristic symptoms that depend on the pathogenic factor involved.

> Significance of the pathogenic factors for acupuncture therapy:
> - Selection of the correct symptomatic points
> - Selection of the correct treatment method, for example moxibustion for Cold syndromes; draining, sedating for full-Heat syndromes,

Wind

| *Yang* pathogen | Corresponding meridian pair: LIV/G.B. |

Symptoms

- Sudden, severe disorders with changing location
- Affects the upper, superficial and lateral aspects of the body (LIV/G.B.).

Pathogenesis

- Moves the body like the wind moves the branches of a tree; affects particularly the upper part of the body
- Leads to disharmony within the body.

Therapy

- Acupuncture followed by moxibustion and cupping: S.I.-3, T.B.-5, G.B.-20, G.B.-31, G.B.-34, Du-16, Du-20
- Internal Wind: LIV-3, Du-20.

Internal Wind

- Originates in the Liver and has a rising tendency (it is *Yang*!)

[1] Phlegm is not an external pathogenic factor, but forms within the body. It resembles Dampness.

- Causes headaches, vertigo
- Muscle twitches, tremors, tics, spasms, sudden paralyses.

Cold

| *Yin* pathogen | Corresponding meridian pair: KID/BL |

Symptoms

- Aversion to cold, chills, being cold, cold extremities
- Copious clear discharge (urine, leukorrhoea)
- Watery diarrhoea with undigested foods
- **Tongue body:** pale
- **Tongue coating:** white
- **Pulse:** slow, deep, vibrating.

Internal cold

Corresponds to *Yang* Deficiency disorders; signs of weakness:

- **Tongue body:** pale with toothmarks
- **Tongue coating:** thin, white.

Pathogenesis

- Cold impairs the circulation of *Qi*, *Yang* and Blood (*Xue*) in the meridians and vessels.
- Qi stagnation leads to pain. Pain due to Cold (*Yin*) is severe with a fixed, deep, boring nature, better with warmth; stiff joints.

Combination

Cold may combine with Wind and Dampness.

Therapy

Moxibustion on relevant points.

Heat – Summer-Heat (Stomach Heat) and Fire (Liver Fire)

| *Yang* pathogen | Corresponding meridian pair: HE/S.I. |

Summer-Heat is a natural, seasonal pathogen. Fire represents an extreme manifestation of Heat; it can form at any time through the combination of several pathogens.

Symptoms

- Aversion to heat
- **Tongue body:** red
- **Tongue coating:** dry and yellow
- **Pulse:** rapid.

Pathogenesis

- Heat penetrates the body.
- Cold, Wind, stagnating *Qi* and/or stagnating Dampness lead to Internal Heat, Damp-Heat or Blood-Heat, injuring the *Yin* and Body Fluids.

Therapy

- Moxibustion is contraindicated.
- The first and, particularly, the second point proximal to the acras are so-called 'Heat points' (→ Table 2.7, Table 2.10).

Dryness

Yang pathogen	Corresponding meridian pair: LU–L.I.

Affects exclusively the Lungs; rare factor.

Symptoms

Everything is dry: cough, mouth, tongue, lips (cracked), nose (possible epistaxis), skin, constipation.

Pathogenesis

Heat, loss of Fluids (through bleeding, diarrhoea, vomiting) or injury of the *Yin* and Body Fluids.

Therapy

- Exclude dehydration/exsiccosis; fluid substitution
- Acupuncture: select points on the LU and L.I. meridians.

Dampness

Yin pathogen	Corresponding meridian pair: SP/ST

Symptoms

- Fullness in the chest and abdomen
- Dull, diffuse, fixed pain (e.g. headache)

- Foggy (not able to think clearly), heavy, numb
- Swellings of the extremities and joints; wound pain
- Diarrhoea.

Pathogenesis

- Generally, external Dampness will affect the Spleen, injuring the *Yang* and thus also the flow of *Qi*.
- The disturbed balance between SP, KID and LU leads to the impairment of transformation, transportation and purification.

Combination

- Dampness and Cold lead to stagnation.
- Dampness and Heat lead to severe acute disorders (dysentery) or chronic smouldering internal disorders.

Therapy

- Local moxibustion (make sure that there is no heat present!)
- Acupuncture: SP-9, Ren-9 (to drain Dampness); ST-36, SP-6, BL-20 to tonify *Qi* and the Spleen in order to improve the transformation and transportation of Dampness.

Endogenous Dampness

Symptoms

Always accompanied by signs of Energy Deficiency:
- Dampness
- Possibly turbidity; eczema with blisters
- **Tongue body:** damp, possibly puffy
- **Tongue coating:** thick, slippery
- **Pulse:** slippery.

Pathogenesis

Spleen *Qi/Yang* Deficiency.

Phlegm (not an External pathogen)

Yin pathogen	Corresponding meridian pair: SP/ST

Phlegm can manifest either as expectoration, lumps or stones (visible Phlegm), or as a mental/intellectual slowing down/blockage or disturbed speech (invisible Phlegm).

Symptoms

- Phlegm in the meridians and vessels: swellings (goitre, swollen lymph nodes)
- Numbness and heaviness of the limbs
- Heart: disturbed mind, psychosis
- Lung: cough with copious viscous phlegm
- Stomach: fullness, loss of appetite, possibly nausea, vomiting with a distending headache (as if wearing a headband)
- Spasms, possible unconsciousness, hemiplegia
- **Tongue coating:** thick, greasy, sticky
- **Pulse:** slippery.

Pathogenesis

Spleen *Qi/Yang* Deficiency:

- The Spleen can no longer transform and transport dampness.

- The Kidneys can no longer purify.
- The Lung can no longer descend turbid Fluids to the Kidneys.
- Phlegm forms and blocks the vessels; this leads to the stagnation of *Qi* and Blood (*Xue*).
- The Phlegm will injure further organs, which in turn will lead to the formation of more Phlegm.
- Phlegm may also form as result of *Yin* Deficiency, replacing the deficient *Yin*.

Therapy

As Dampness, but specifically ST-40, Ren-12.

2.7.7 Common TCM syndromes

As many authors frequently refer in their publications to TCM syndromes, the following table provides an overview of the syndromes, their signs and symptoms, and the resulting treatment principle (→ Table 2.10).

Table 2.10 Overview of the TCM syndromes and their treatment

SYNDROME OR AFFECTED MERIDIAN	TCM	TYPICAL SIGNS AND SYMPTOMS	EXAMPLES	TREATMENT PRINCIPLE
Qi deficiency	**Pulse:** without force **Tongue body:** pale, flabby, tooth marks **Complexion:** possibly pale	• Dyspnoea with exertion • Weak voice, dislike of speaking, lethargic, tired • Spontaneous sweating (*Qi* controls the pores!) • Worse with exertion	Lack of energy, poor stamina	• Tonify the *Qi*: ST-36, SP-6, Ren-4, Ren-6 • Tonify the SP, ST and (postnatal) Qi: SP-6, BL-20, Ren-12
Blood (*Xue*) deficiency HE, LIV	**Pulse:** thready, choppy **Tongue body:** pale **Complexion:** pale, lusterless	• Muddled • Weepy, lack of self-esteem • Paraesthesia • Visual disturbances, e.g. floaters • Weakness, dizziness, trembling • Dry skin and hair • Emaciation • Light periods	Anaemia, neurasthenia	• Tonify and nourish the Blood (*Xue*) • To tonify Blood: BL-17 • To produce Blood: SP-10, BL-17 • To tonify the SP and ST: ST-36, SP-6, SP-10, BL-17, BL-20
Yang deficiency KID, SP, HE	**Pulse:** slow, without force **Tongue coating:** white **Tongue body:** pale, moist, tooth marks **Complexion:** pale (differential diagnosis: *Yang* deficiency), bright pale (differential diagnosis: Blood (*Xue*) deficiency)	• Cold signs: aversion to cold, cold extremities • Sweating: spontaneous, during daytime, with exertion	Lack of energy accompanied by Cold signs and symptoms	• Tonify and warm the *Yang* and the foundation. The Kidneys are the source of the *Yang*! • Tonify the Kidney *Yang*: acupuncture and moxa on BL-23, Ren-4, Ren-6, Du-4

Table 2.10 Overview of the TCM syndromes and their treatment—cont'd

SYNDROME OR AFFECTED MERIDIAN	TCM	TYPICAL SIGNS AND SYMPTOMS	EXAMPLES	TREATMENT PRINCIPLE
Yin deficiency KID, HE, LIV, LU, ST	**Pulse:** rapid, thready, may be superficial **Tongue body:** red, thin **Tongue coating:** thin or no coating **Complexion:** malar flush	• Restless • Night sweating • Heat of the Five Hearts	Damage to parenchyma	• Nourish the Yin, strengthen the foundation, calm the mind • Moxa contraindicated! • Back-*Shu* point, *Yuan*-source point and may be Heat points of affected meridian (choose 1st or 2nd point proximal to tips of extremities) • Tonify the body and *Yin* in general: SP-6, BL-23, KID-3, KID-6, Ren-3
Jing deficiency KID	**Pulse:** weak in the *Chi* position **Tongue body, tongue coating:** depending on implicated pattern	Congenital: impaired Jing, developmental disabilities, deformities Acquired: Jing exhausted (always implies one or more deficiency syndromes: *Qi*, Blood (*Xue*), *Yin*, *Yang*)	developmental disabilities, deformities Senile dementia	• Tonify the marrow and bones: G.B.-39+, BL-11+ (osteoporosis), Du-20+, Du-13+ [Du-14 *Bi*] • Tonify the brain: BL-15

2.8 Diagnostic methods in TCM

2.8.1 The diagnostic process

TCM diagnostics and differential diagnosis rely on the sensory abilities of the therapist:

- Observation: vitality, complexion, demeanour, appearance of sensory organs, excretions and tongue diagnosis
- Listening: the sound of the voice, speech, breathing sounds, etc.
- Smelling: body odour, excretions
- Feeling/palpation: pulse, abdomen, meridians, acupuncture points
- Asking/medical history: temperature sensations, sweating, appetite and thirst, stool and urine, pain, sleep, menstruation.

> Other diagnostic methods requiring instrumentation or laboratory investigation are obviously not part of TCM, but should definitely be considered.

From the wealth of information gathered through the medical history and physical examination, the TCM therapist obtains an overall impression of the patient. This provides information about:

- the condition of the Blood (*Xue*) and *Qi* – the condition and functioning of the general life force, the attitude towards life, the state of health, and the body's defence system
- the state of the internal organs – if *Yin* and *Yang* are in balance and Blood (*Xue*) and *Qi* are flowing smoothly, the internal organs will also be in good health.

Tongue and pulse examination play a particularly important role in the diagnostic process and are therefore described in greater detail.

2.8.2 Tongue diagnosis

TCM considers the Heart to open into the tongue so that disorders of the Heart will frequently manifest in the tongue and, metaphorically, in the speech.

All of the internal organs are also linked to the tongue by the meridians and their collaterals. The tongue thus becomes the mirror of the state of the internal organs: the tongue, just like the ear, is a somatotopic representation, whereby changes in the interior of the body become visible.

Tongue diagnosis primarily allows the differentiation of syndromes and provides information about the course of the disease.

Tongue diagnosis according to the Eight Principles

- Exterior/Interior: Are there changes regarding the tongue body and the tongue coating?
- Heat/Cold: Is the tongue body red or pale? Is the tongue coating yellow or white?
- Excess/Deficiency: Are the tongue body and tongue coating thick or thin?

Differentiation according to location: which organ is affected? (→ Fig. 2.6)

- Tip of the tongue: Heart
- Edge of the tongue: Liver (on the left), Gall Bladder (on the right)
- Centre of the tongue: Stomach, Spleen
- Root of the tongue: Kidneys.

Toothmarks: a 'scalloped' tongue edge caused by indentations of the teeth is a typical symptom of Spleen *Qi* Deficiency, indicating neurasthenic syndromes, psychosomatic and/or gastrointestinal disorders, dyspepsia, chronic diarrhoea, general weakness during convalescence.

2.8.3 Pulse diagnosis

Pulse diagnosis represents an empirical method. Simple pulse diagnosis can easily be learnt with some practice (→ Table 2.11, Fig. 2.7).
Principle: according to TCM, the pulse is a manifestation of the circulation of *Qi* (Energy) and Blood (*Xue*). The Heart and Lung *Qi*, with the involvement of the Liver *Qi*, maintain the circulation of the Blood (*Xue*). The Spleen produces *Qi* (Energy) from food and 'essence' stored in the Kidneys. Thus, all *Zang* organs play a role in the

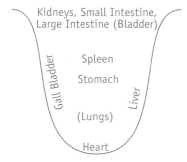

Fig. 2.6 Tongue diagnosis: division of the surface of the tongue body (from Focks & Hillenbrand 2003)

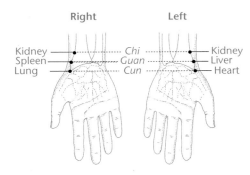

Fig. 2.7 Taking the pulse (from Focks & Hillenbrand 2003)

circulation of blood, so that the pulse is a sensitive indicator of any pathological changes within the body.
Technique: the pulse is felt by palpating the radial artery. From distal (slightly proximal to the wrist joint space, close to the styloid process of the radius) to proximal, place the index, middle and ring fingers on the artery. The palpation is carried out using three pressures: light, medium and firm.
Criteria
- Depth: superficial or deep
- Rate: slow or rapid
- Shape of the pulse wave: big or thready, long or short (longer or shorter than the three palpation sites)
- Flow: forceless or forceful, slippery or hesitant, soft or vibrating
- Rhythm: regular or irregular.

Interpretation according to TCM

- Differentiation of Exterior/Interior syndromes
- Determining the location of the disorder or the affected organ
- Differentiating Excess/Deficiency syndromes
- Differentiating *Yin/Yang* imbalance
- Determining the cause of the disorder and subjective symptoms
- Determining the course of the disorder and its stage: pulse diagnosis may provide information on whether acupuncture is still indicated for a patient or whether another, more effective, form of therapy, such as herbal therapy, should be applied.

2.9 General rules for point selection

A differential TCM diagnosis will result in a specific therapy, influencing point selection, needling depth and needle manipulation, as well as variations of the point prescription during individual treatments. Factors influencing point selection are:

The medical history based on TCM: questions regarding climatic pathogenic factors, symptoms based on *Yin/Yang* imbalances and syndromes.

Constitutional factors: consideration of the *Yin/Yang* type, congenital Energy, mental Energy, food Energy, defensive Energy.

Pulse and tongue diagnosis: see above.

> Western schools of acupuncture often use well-proven point prescriptions based on the Western diagnosis. For more severe or chronic disorders, a differential therapy with point prescriptions based on TCM criteria will often form the basis of the point selection.

2.9.1 TCM syndrome therapy

The syndrome directly guides to the treatment. In this respect, the following three criteria are of major importance for the acupuncture therapist.

Recognizing signs of Deficiency

In patients with an underlying Deficiency or deficiency of *Qi*, Blood (*Xue*), Body Fluids, etc., treatment should initially focus on tonifying. Any concurrent pain should be addressed with gentle reducing, sedating methods: weak patients should not be further weakened through aggressive draining and reducing techniques.

Recognizing discrete heat signs

The application of Heat or moxibustion is contraindicated with Heat. Discrete signs of Heat are:

- Weak, but rapid pulse
- Weak, but rapid body movements
- Red, but thin tongue body
- Little or no tongue coating
- Afternoon fever
- Hot palms or soles
- Restlessness.

Explanation: 'Heat' (a *Yang* pathogen) consumes Fluids (a *Yin* substance). If there is some form of pre-existing *Yin* Deficiency (loss of substance, damage to the parenchymatous tissue), this will result in the dominance of an already weakened *Yang* over an even weaker *Yin* (cooling aspect). In other words, a small Fire burns under a little Water. If, in this situation, additional Heat is applied to the Yang, for example by moxibustion, further consumption of *Yin* is unavoidable. In our example this means that stoking the Fire leads to further consumption of the small amount of Water.

Example: in pulmonary tuberculosis, the damage to the parenchymatous lung tissue (*Yin* Deficiency) leads to discrete Heat signs, requiring rest, cooling, tonifying, but not further Heat.

Recognizing when acupuncture is indicated

It is important to recognize cases in which acupuncture is the therapy of choice and those in which herbal therapy, Chinese or Western, should be given preference.

> Rule of thumb:
> - All patients with 'hyper' conditions (*Yang* Excess), acute disorders and pain conditions, and somatic disorders with a specific organ involvement (asthma, gastritis, duodenal/ventricular ulcer) are well suited to acupuncture therapy.
> - All patients with 'hypo' conditions (*Yin* Deficiency), general weakness (with reduced reactivity), hypofunctioning, neurasthenia or general morbidity without specific organ involvement need more than acupuncture.

2.9.2 The Vienna School after Bischko

The Vienna School combines therapeutic reflections based on TCM with experience in the treatment of Western patients. This has resulted in point combinations that can be applied for Western diagnoses familiar to therapists with a scientific background. This method can be learnt more easily and produces, in most cases, comparable results.

The 'Rule of Three' of the Vienna School presents a useful and practical way of approaching the diagnostic process:

Do the symptoms point to a particular meridian?

If yes, the syndrome is of an External nature (skin, musculoskeletal system).

Therapy: acupuncture. Select points on the affected meridian or on one of its 'partners' (→ 4.2, corresponding and paired meridians).

Do the symptoms point to an organ or a 'substance of life'?

If yes, the disorder is of an Internal nature. The next step is to differentiate a functional disorder with no substantial injury to the parenchymatous tissue (e.g. bloating, angina, bronchial asthma in children, etc.).
Therapy: Acupuncture and possibly Western medication. Point selection: substance-specific or organ-specific points, as well as points addressing the symptoms:

* *Fu* organs: front-*Mu* points as well as the lower *He*-sea points
* *Zang* organs: back-*Shu* points as well as *Yuan*-source points
* Functional disorder with parenchymatous tissue damage: pancreatic insufficiency following pancreatitis, tuberculosis (treated only in China with acupuncture, not in Western countries), etc. *Therapy:* primarily Western medication, acupuncture with mild stimulation as adjunctive therapy
* To improve the general condition: Ren-4, Ren-6, ST-36, SP-6
* Organ-specific points
* Substance-specific points: → Table 2.10.

What role is played by other modifying circumstances?

Sensitivity to wind and changes in the weather

Sensitivity to wind and changes in the weather is associated with the LIV/G.B. (→ Table 2.3).
Therapy: points that are indicated for 'wind':

* LIV meridian: LIV-3
* G.B. meridian: G.B.-20, G.B.-34, G.B.-31
* T.B. meridian: T.B.-5, T.B.-15
* Du (the *Du Mai* is most exposed to wind because it traverses the head): Du-20, Du-16; S.I.-3 – as opening point opens the *Du Mai* (needle either as first or last point)
* Points on other meridians with names referring to Wind: BL-12 (*Feng Men*/Wind Gate)

Heat symptoms

Fever, thirst, red tongue, tachycardia.

Therapy
* Heat points: first or second point proximal to the tips of the extremities
* Points that drain heat: L.I.-4, L.I.-11, Du-13
* No additional heat – no moxibustion!

Cold symptoms

Therapy: acupuncture and heat
* Tonify the Kidneys: KID-3, KID-6
* Moxibustion, warm drinks.

Dampness

As a trigger (symptoms worse with fog or damp weather) or as symptoms (myogelosis, fluid retention).

Therapy
* Tonify the Spleen: acupuncture and moxibustion on SP-6, SP-9
* For dampness: Ren-9.

Dryness

Therapy
* Tonify the Kidneys (association: Water): KID-3, KID-6 or KID-7, and BL-23
* 'Moisten' the Lungs: inhalation, herbal therapy, points on the Lung meridian, e.g. LU-5.

Phlegm

Therapy
* Tonify the Spleen: Ren-12, ST-40, SP-6
* Moxibustion – provided there are no Heat symptoms!

General condition/diet

* Good overall condition and good diet: localized musculoskeletal pain tends to be in the foreground
  Therapy: more acupuncture points depending on the location of the pain, stronger stimulation.
* Poor overall condition, poor diet
  Therapy: first of all strengthen the patient, only then apply treatment of local symptoms: Western medication and fewer acupuncture points, gentle stimulation.
* Strengthen the general/nutritional condition by tonifying the 'foundation': KID-3 or KID-7 and BL-23.
* Improve the appetite and assimilation of nutrition: ST-36, Ren-12, SP-6, BL-20.

Type and stage of the disorder

- Acute illness, severe symptoms: distal points with strong stimulation, possibly combined local points
- Chronic disorder, slow onset of symptoms: fewer points, less frequent treatments, mild stimulation.

Psyche

Therapy: emotionally harmonizing points:

- HE-3, HE-7 (the Heart governs the Spirit and the brain)
- BL-15
- ST-36.

Hormonal imbalance

Therapy

Points on the KID and BL meridians, e.g. KID-3, KID-11, BL-31, BL-32.

Allergies

Therapy

Metabolic points (selection according to location of the allergy): BL-54, BL-58, KID-2, KID-6, LIV-13, L.I.-2, L.I.-3, L.I.-4

- Corticotrophic points: BL-23, BL-47, Du-16.

3

Treatment methods and techniques

Boris Sommer

3.1 General

Preparation

A comfortable room temperature and a calm atmosphere will help the patient to relax and thereby enhance the therapeutic effect. Pillows and knee supports are also very helpful for the patient's comfort. It is self-evident that the patients should be provided with the necessary information regarding the treatment – this will ensure cooperation.

Positioning of the patient

Treatments are best given with the patient lying down, especially for the first appointment. This precludes a collapse and contributes to an effective relaxation.

Sometimes the patient may be needled in alternative positions:

- **Prone:** especially to treat points on the Bladder meridian or for moxibustion of points on the back
- **Seated:** good access to all points, but less relaxing and danger of collapse
- **Side-lying:** access to many points, but more difficult to locate points correctly on the abdomen and back; also less relaxing.

Points on the back can be needled at the beginning of the treatment, and the needles retained for a shorter period. Alternatively, they can be needled transversely (subcutaneously) so that the patient can lie cautiously on their back while the needles are retained.

Needles

Today, body acupuncture is generally performed with stainless steel needles that are 1–10 cm long and 0.15–0.3 mm thick. For auricular and facial acupuncture, needles with a length of 15–25 mm and a diameter of less than 0.2 mm are used. The internationally recognized standard acupuncture needle is 3 cm long with a diameter of 0.3 mm, making it suitable for all regions of the body. The handle should preferably be of coiled copper to facilitate stimulation techniques.

- **Disposable needles** are strongly recommended for safety reasons and for forensic considerations. They also help to allay patients' anxiety, for example regarding AIDS.
- **Three-edged needles** are used for bloodletting.
- **Intradermal needles** are only a few millimetres long and very fine. They are held in place with tape and can be retained for up to 1 week. They are used mainly in auricular acupuncture. Seeds such as rape seed (approximate size 1 × 1 mm) or magnetic pressballs, also held in place with tape, can be used instead.

Duration and course of treatment

Duration of treatment: an acupuncture treatment usually lasts for approximately 15–30 minutes. During this time, the needles may be stimulated 2–3 times.

Treatment frequency: treatments are generally administered once weekly, in acute cases more frequently, even daily.

Treatment course: depending on the case, a treatment course consists of 10–15 treatments. This may repeated as needed, usually after approximately 1 year, in chronic recurrent cases after only 3–6 months.

Unwanted side-effects of needling

Healing crisis: this is often caused by too strong a stimulus (too many needles, stimulation too vigorous), but can be considered as a positive sign, signalling the body's response to the treatment.

Painful insertions: can be avoided by improving the insertion technique (more rapid penetration of the skin) and caution when needling close to blood vessels and nerve or tendon sheaths.

Pain during needle retention: may occur due to wrong point location and movements by the patient. It can be avoided by advising the patient to avoid moving and by retracting or further inserting the needle (the latter if the needle is inserted in muscular tissue).

Bleeding upon removal of the needle: this is a desired effect in cases of Excess patterns. Sterile swabs should be kept ready.

Complications

Complications occur only rarely, the most common being infections, collapse or accidental injury.

The following measures should be taken to minimize the risk of infection:

- Use disposable needles.
- Clean any dirty skin areas.
- Disinfect the skin before deep needling or in patients with compromised immunity or diabetes mellitus.
- Use fewer points.
- When using intradermal needles, inform the patient about the risk of infection.

In case of a collapse ('needle fainting', *Yun-Cheng* phenomenon), take the following measures:

- Avoid a collapse by treating the patient lying down.
- If a collapse has already occurred, remove the needles; needle, or better massage, the following points: P-9, H-9 and Du-26 (at the upper third of the philtrum, needle in a superior direction).

Accidental injuries: serious complications, such as pneumothorax, which tend to be reported by the media, will not occur if acupuncture is applied by properly trained therapists.

3.2 *De Qi*

A sharp, epicritic pain may be experienced during insertion of the needle. After stimulation of the needle, this will be replaced by the *De Qi* sensation, caused by the protopathic sensitivity, also referred to as the propagated sensation along the channel (PSC). It feels as though 'something has arrived' and is often described as a dull, possibly warm, distending or paraesthetic feeling, which may occur at the point itself or along the course of the meridian. The feeling tends to propagate along the direction of the meridian in which the tip of the needle is pointing. Although an attempt should always be made to obtain the *De Qi* sensation, there are some points where it cannot be triggered. The differing degree of sensitivity between individual patients should always be taken into consideration: fragile patients require gentle needle insertions.

If, despite correct point location, no *De Qi* sensation can be obtained, the following techniques might be helpful:

- Lifting and thrusting the needle
- Twisting the needle
- A combination of lifting, thrusting and twisting
- Tapping and flying
- Scraping the handle of the needle
- Waving the needle
- 'Vibrating' the needle: the needle is grasped and vibrated with a small amplitude (rapid, small lifts and thrusts).

> Generally, a lack of *De Qi* sensation might indicate a lack of response due to *Qi* deficiency. Sometimes rest and a snack might help; sometimes the *Qi* has to be tonified with relevant herbs (example formula: *Si Jun Zi Tang*).

3.3 Acupuncture techniques

Insertion techniques

Insertion (→ Fig. 3.1)

With the left hand, palpate the acupuncture point and either stretch or pinch the skin so that a fold forms. Quickly insert the needle with the right hand, pushing it with twisting movements either to the required depth or until the *De Qi* sensation is obtained.

The 'very point technique' (after Gleditsch) finds the exact location of the point by letting the needle 'dance' on the surface of the skin. The needle is inserted where it glides most easily through the skin.

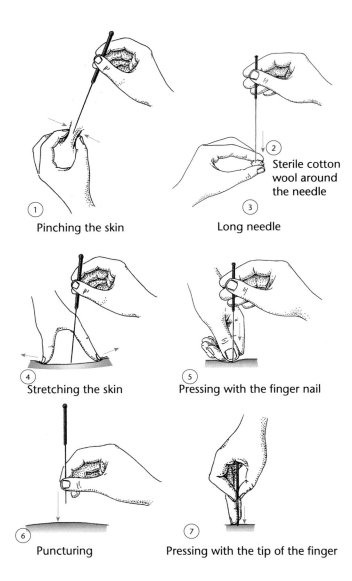

1 Pinching the skin

2 Long needle

3 Sterile cotton wool around the needle

4 Stretching the skin

5 Pressing with the finger nail

6 Puncturing

7 Pressing with the tip of the finger

Fig. 3.1 Insertion techniques (from Focks & Hillenbrand 2003)

Insertion depth

The insertion depth depends on the anatomical location: on the fingers needling will be very superficial, whereas on the bigger muscles (e.g. ST-36 on the tibialis anterior) insertions will be deeper. A thorough anatomical knowledge is an essential prerequisite for needling.

Direction of the insertion

The *De Qi* sensation should radiate towards the affected region; therefore, the tip of the needle should point in that direction.

Angle of insertion (→ Fig. 3.2)

The angle of needle insertion depends on the tissue under the point:

- Perpendicular insertion (90°): on muscles
- Oblique insertion (45°): on areas with less soft tissue, for example near joint spaces
- Transverse insertion (10°) for subcutaneous threading of several acupuncture points or in areas with sensitive anatomical structures such as intercostal spaces or on the cranium.

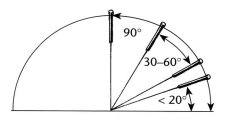

Angle of insertion: - Perpendicular (90°)
- Oblique (30–60°)
- Transverse/horizontal (< 20°)

Fig. 3.2 Angle of insertion (from Focks & Hillenbrand 2003)

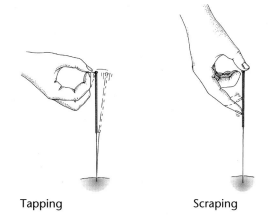

Tapping   Scraping

Needle removal

The needle should be removed with a gentle twisting movement. Removal of the needle can be used as a final stimulation.

Needle manipulation techniques (→ Fig. 3.3)

Sedating (*Xie*)

Indications: excess conditions (*Yang* syndromes), hyperfunctioning, acute disorders, acute pain, inflammatory disorders may be accompanied by fever (*caution:* only in patients with a robust constitution), hypertension, general irritability, tendency to muscle spasms. **Tongue:** rough, thick tongue coating (→ Table 3.1).
Technique: strong stimulation, slow thrust and rapid lift ('pulling something out'), stimulation for 10–30 minutes. No pressure should be put on the insertion site after needle removal: allow bleeding.
Electrostimulation: with high frequency.
Point selection: a sedating effect can also be achieved by using the sedation point on the relevant meridian and on the meridian corresponding to its 'son' (→ 4.2 Mother–Son rule).

Tonifying (*Bu*)

Indications: deficiency conditions, hypofunctioning, chronic or degenerative disorders, general weakness, tendency to night sweats, hypotension, apathy. **Tongue:** pale, thin tongue coating (→ Table 3.1).
Technique: gentle stimulus through cautious, quick insertion. Gentle stimulation with rapid thrust and slow

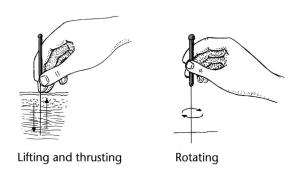

Lifting and thrusting   Rotating

Fig. 3.3 Stimulation technique (from Focks & Hillenbrand 2003)

lift ('pushing something in'), stimulation for 5–20 minutes. Put pressure on the insertion site after needle removal: avoid bleeding.
Electrostimulation: with low frequency.
Point selection: a tonifying effect can also be achieved by using the tonification point on the relevant meridian and on the meridian corresponding to its 'mother' (→ 4.2 Mother–Son rule); laser treatment (→ 3.7) is considered as tonifying.

3.4 Micromassage and tuina therapy

Micromassage

This technique stimulates acupuncture points through massage or pressure. It is also referred to as 'acupressure', a linguistically inconsistent term.

Table 3.1 Sedating, tonifying and even needling techniques

	TONIFYING METHOD	SEDATING METHOD	EVEN METHOD
Indication	• Weak patient • Chronic disorder • 'Deficiency' conditions	• Robust patient • Acute disorder • 'Excess' conditions	
Stimulus	Weak	Strong	Medium
De Qi	Obtain gently	Obtain strongly	Obtain fairly strongly
Manipulation	Short	Long	
Needle insertion	Quick	Slow	Fairly quickly
Needle removal	Slow	Quick	Medium
Stimulation	'Push' something into the body	'Pull' something out of the body	Even lifting and thrusting
Needle retention	5–20 min	10–30 min	15–20 min
Insertion site after needle removal	'Close' with a cotton bud and apply short micromassage	Do not 'close'	
Other methods	Moxa, laser	Electrostimulation	

Indications: general malaise, paediatric treatments, skin lesions due to too frequent acupuncture, self-treatment, either on a single point or in conjunction with other points.

Contraindications: local skin irritation and/or suspicion of malignant skin changes in the area to be treated.

Tuina (Chinese massage)

Tuina is a unique Chinese massage technique (*Tui*, to push; *Na*, to grasp) that can also be used in conjunction with acupuncture treatments.

Indications: as for acupuncture; in other words, functional and reversible disorders.

Contraindications: the same as for acupuncture – depression, neuroses, psychoses and other severe organ disorders.

3.5 Moxibustion

Moxibustion combines herbal therapy with the application of heat. Dried mugwort *(Artemesia vulgaris)* is burnt on acupuncture points, either on or above the skin. Moxa has the consistency of 'wool' (like fine tobacco). It is also available in the form of moxa cigars. Using small funnels, moxa wool can be shaped into cones.

Methods

- **Direct moxa:** moxa cones are placed directly on to the skin, burnt down by two-thirds, and then removed from the skin. In scarring moxa – used in China but contraindicated in the West – the cone is burnt down all the way, resulting in possible scarring.

- **Indirect moxibustion:** an insulating ginger slice is placed between the moxa cone and the skin. Another form of indirect moxibustion is the warming up of a particular area by using a moxa cigar. The moxa cigar is repeatedly brought close to the skin or to an inserted acupuncture needle, or a piece of moxa cigar (approximately 2.5 cm long) is applied to the handle of the needle.

Indications: Cold symptoms; for Full-Cold, for example during an acute infection with chills or severe musculoskeletal pain due to Cold, combine moxibustion with sedating needling techniques; in contrast, for Deficiency-Cold combine moxibustion with tonifying needling techniques.

Contraindications: Heat symptoms of an excess type; particular attention should be paid to deficient Heat symptoms (*Yin* deficiency), as applying more Heat will increase the *Yang* excess and further consume *Yin*. Example: Patients with tuberculosis (Lung and Kidney *Yin* deficiency) should avoid exposure to the sun, sauna and heat.

3.6 Electrostimulation

Electrostimulation is a method of applying electrical energy to inserted acupuncture needles. The commonly used devices employ frequencies of 1–200 Hz, with impulses emitted either continuously or intermittently. Special high-frequency equipment with an output of up to 2000 Hz is used for analgesic purposes; the strength of the electric current is 0–5 mA.

Indications: limp and spastic pareses, chronic pain in degenerative disorders, headaches, pain due to malignancy, postoperative pain syndromes, pain during labour.

Contraindications: pacemakers, arrhythmias, CNS disorders such as epilepsy and other spastic disorders, acute febrile diseases, pregnancy with the exception of labour pain and induction of labour.

3.7 Laser

The acronym 'laser' means 'Light Amplification for Stimulated Emission of Radiation' and refers to bundled, monochrome light of a defined wavelength. Lasers used in acupuncture are so-called 'soft lasers' of 2–30 mW, which are said to have a biostimulating effect. In contrast, lasers used in surgery have a strength of several watts and a coagulating effect on tissue. They are not used in laser acupuncture.

Red light lasers with a wavelength of 632 nm (helium–neon lasers) can be distinguished from infrared lasers, which have a wavelength of 780–1006 nm (diode lasers).

Advantages: pain-free, non-traumatic, aseptic and time saving, as only a short stimulation time is necessary.

Disadvantages: penetrates less deeply, not suitable for stronger stimulation. It may take longer to achieve the desired treatment success than with conventional acupuncture. Medical device regulations must be observed. High cost for equipment.

Methods

- **Laser on a particular point:** laser is used instead of needling as a form of 'gentle acupuncture'. Irradiation time: 10–30 seconds per point.

- **Laser treatment of a body area:** whole areas of the body are treated with laser.; particularly indicated for weeping dermatological disorders affecting larger skin areas.

Indications: in children (substitute for needling), in elderly and frail patients; dermatological disorders such as herpes simplex, herpes zoster; gingivitis, leg ulcers.

Contraindications: laser therapy is contraindicated on the head.

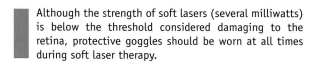 Although the strength of soft lasers (several milliwatts) is below the threshold considered damaging to the retina, protective goggles should be worn at all times during soft laser therapy.

3.8 PuTENS

Heydenreich's method of PuTENS refers to *pu*nctate *t*ranscutaneous *e*lectrical *n*erve *s*timulation, using a single point electrode. In contrast to classical transcutaneous electrical nerve stimulation (TENS), high-voltage impulses are used. PuTENS allows the precise location of points and is well suited to self-treatment.

Technical requirements

- Biphasic impulse with a maximum amplitude of 500 V through a 20-kOhm load

- Strength of the electric current: 0–10 mA

- Impulse duration: 85 ms, pulse power 0.86 mW through a 20-kOhm load

- Frequency: 2–200 Hz.

Technique: after choosing the correct frequency, the point stimulator is placed on the skin and the strength of the electric current adjusted until a slight tingling sensation can be felt by the patient. Stimulation once daily for 10–20 seconds.

Basic point combination: for general pain-relieving therapy the following points are recommended: LU-7, L.I.-4, ST-36, SP-6, HE-7, S.I.-3, BL-10, BL-62, KID-6 (3), PE-6, T.B.-5, G.B.-20, G.B.-41, LIV-3, *Yin Tang* accompanied by roller treatment with rollers of all reflex zones on the back, covering the back-*Shu* points on the Bladder meridian and the points on the *Du* Mai (governing vessel).

Indications: all indications that apply to acupuncture.

Contraindications: autoimmune disorders, therapy with immunosuppressive drugs, cytostatic medication, radiotherapy, pacemakers, arrhythmias, cardiovascular disorders, epilepsy, psychosis, shock, pregnancy (strictly contraindicated).

3.9 Injection acupuncture

Here, various substances are injected into acupuncture points.

Methods

- Aquapuncture: 0.1 mL pyrogen-free distilled water (aqua dest.) is injected into acupuncture points
- Herbal injections, for example with mistletoe preparations (e.g. Plenosol®)
- Injection of homeopathic agents
- Mesotherapy: various homeopathic and allopathic preparations as well as mixed preparations
- Drugs: local analgesics, for example 0.5% procaine.

Indications: pain syndromes; the same indications as for acupuncture.

Contraindications: allergies, pregnancy.

4

Summary of the 12 regular meridians and the 8 extraordinary meridians

G. Kubiena

4.1 The meridian system

The term 'meridian' is commonly used in the West for the Chinese term *Jing Luo'*, which describes a 'network of channels'. An anatomical structure for the meridians has not been established. They are interpreted as a system of reference lines for the location of acupuncture points. According to TCM, the meridians are the 'channels', in which *Qi* (pronounced 'chee'; energy, function) flows in a 24-hour rhythm. The numbering system used for the acupuncture points corresponds to the direction of flow of the *Qi*. Any disturbance of this flow will result in the manifestation of illness.

There are 12 primary meridians, which span the body bilaterally as vertical lines, as well as 8 extraordinary meridians (→ Table 4.1).

Table 4.1 Names of the meridians in English and Chinese (pinyin)

GERMAN		ENGLISH		CHINESE TERM	*PINYIN*
Lunge	Lu	Lung	LU	Great hand *Yin*	Shou Tai Yin Fei Jing
Dickdarm	Di	Large Intestine	L.I.	Bright hand *Yang*	Shou Yang Ming Da Chang Jing
Magen	Ma	Stomach	ST	Bright foot *Yang*	Zu Yang Ming Wei Jing
Milz	Mi	Spleen	SP	Great foot *Yin*	Zu Tai Yin Pi Jing
Herz	He	Heart	HE	Lesser hand *Yin*	Shou Shao Yin Xin Jing
Dünndarm	Dü	Small Intestine	S.I.	Great hand *Yang*	Shou Tai Yang Xiao Chang Jing
Blase	Bl	Bladder	BL	Great foot *Yang*	Zu Tai Yang Pang Guang Jing
Niere	Ni	Kidney	KID	Lesser foot *Yin*	Zu Shao Yin Shen Jing
Perikard	Pe	Pericardium	P	Terminal hand *Yin*	Shou Jue Yin Xin Bao Jing
Dreifacher Erwärmer, SanJiao	3E, SJ	Triple Burner	T.B.	Lesser hand *Yang*	Shou Shao Yang San Jiao Jing
Gallenblase	Gb	Gall Bladder	G.B.	Lesser foot *Yang*	Zu Shao Yang Dan Jing
Leber	Le	Liver	LIV	Terminal foot *Yin*	Zu Jue Yin Gan Jing
Lenkergefäß	Du, LG	Governing vessel	Du	*Du Mai*	Du Mai
Konzeptionsgefäß	Ren, KG	Conception vessel	Ren	*Ren Mai*	Ren Mai

In addition, there are several accompanying and connecting structures (including the primary meridians, a total of 72) that are located at different depths. These structures can be accessed through specific points and are indicated for various disorders (→ Table 4.2).

4.2 Relationships among the meridians

During the course of a day, the *Qi* will course in a bi-hourly rhythm through all 12 regular meridians. All regions of the body will be passed by the *Qi* three times daily, each circuit following the same sequence (→ Fig. 4.1, Table 4.3).

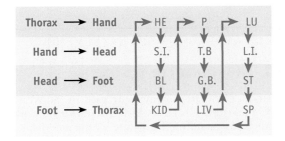

Fig. 4.1 The cyclical circulation of *Qi*

Table 4.2 The different types of channel in Chinese medicine

MERIDIAN	NUMBER	MAJOR POINTS	INDICATIONS
Cutaneous zones	12	Massage only	Massage, superficial disorders, sensitive patients
Luo Mai on the extremities[a]	12	*Luo*-connecting point	Spider veins (treat with plum blossom needle); disorders that progress from one meridian to its paired meridian; *Yin* meridians: sensory organs
Special *Luo* on the torso	4	Du-1, Ren-15, SP-21 and *Xu Li*[b] – the empty mile: Ren-12, Ren-17 (needle towards left, in the direction of the Heart	SP-21: affects all collaterals *Xu Li*: for the connection ST–HE, congenital allergies
Sinew meridians	12	*A-Shi* points (trigger points on the sinew meridians and ipsilateral *Jing*-well points	Acute invasion of pathogenic factors (e.g. acute cervical syndrome caused by draught)
Divergent meridians	12	Contralateral *Jing*-well points, *He*-sea points, Du-20	Psychosomatic disorders, unilateral disorders that occur each day at the same time and are associated with 'sensations' in the affected organ
Primary meridians	12	Meridian points	Meridian and organ disorders
Extraordinary meridians	8	Opening points	Deep-seated disorders, extraordinary meridian syndromes and 'diagonal' disorders (e.g. left shoulder/right knee)

[a]Besides the 72 'great' *Luo Mai* mentioned above, there exist a multitude of small *Luo*, so-called *Sun Luo* ('grandchild'), *Fu Luo* (superficial *Luo*) and *Xue Luo* (blood vessel network). For example, when spider veins become visible they are categorized as small *Luo Mai* and treated locally with a plum blossom needle. All of these small networks are connected directly to the great *Luo Mai* of the Spleen, SP-21, making it an important point for the treatment of generalized pain (new diseases are located in the meridians, old diseases in the collaterals!)
[b]This is not mentioned in all publications, but is a later addition

Organ–channel units

In TCM a functional unit is formed by two organs and their associated meridians. They have a common relationship to Internal and External factors, such as climatic and psychological aspects. In a functional unit, a solid organ (*Zang*) is always paired with a hollow organ (*Fu*) (→ 2.6, Table 2.3).

Corresponding meridians

However, it is not only the *Yin/Yang* pairing of meridians that is of importance. In addition, two meridians of the same polarity (*Yin/Yang*) form one of the 'six great meridians', sharing a common name (Fig. 4.2). Their pathways on the extremities are in anatomically

Interiorly–exteriorly paired meridians

The *Yin* and *Yang* meridians of the same functional unit are referred to as interiorly–exteriorly paired meridians. On the extremities, the *Yin* meridians course along the medial (inside) aspect and the *Yang* meridians along the lateral (outer) aspect. This is sometimes called the 'outer–inner rule'.

Lung (LU)	Large Intestine (L.I.)
Spleen (SP)	Stomach (ST)
Heart (HE)	Small Intestine (S.I.)
Kidney (KID)	Bladder (BL)
Pericardium (P)	Triple Burner (T.B.)
Liver (LIV)	Gall Bladder (G.B.)

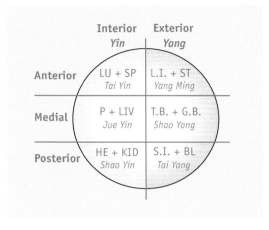

Fig. 4.2 Corresponding meridians

Table 4.3 Flow of *Qi* during the course of a day

CIRCUIT	FROM	TO	TIME (→ FIG. 2.3)	MERIDIAN SEQUENCE	ELEMENT
1st circuit	Thorax	Fingertips	3–5am	LU	Metal
	Fingertips	Head	5–7am	L.I.	
	Head	Tips of the toes	7–9am	ST	Earth
	Tips of the toes	Thorax	9–11am	SP	
2nd circuit	Thorax	Fingertips	11am–1pm	HE	Imperial Fire
	Fingertips	Head	1–3pm	S.I.	
	Head	Tips of the toes	3–5pm	BL	Water
	Tips of the toes	Thorax	5–7pm	KID	
3rd circuit	Thorax	Fingertips	7–9pm	PE	Ministerial Fire
	Fingertips	Head	9–11pm	T.B.	
	Head	Tips of the toes	11pm–1am	G.B.	Wood
	Tips of the toes	Thorax	1–3am	LIV	

Hand	Foot	Location		Meridian
Large Intestine (L.I.)	Stomach (ST)	Anterior	Outside	*Yang Ming*
Triple Burner (T.B.)	Gall Bladder (G.B.)	Medial	Outside	*Shao Yang*
Small Intestine (S.I.)	Bladder (BL)	Posterior	Outside	*Tai Yang*
Lung (LU)	Spleen (SP)	Anterior	Inside	*Tai Yin*
Pericardium (P)	Liver (LIV)	Medial	Inside	*Jue Yin*
Heart (HE)	Kidney (KID)	Posterior	Inside	*Shao Yin*

corresponding locations – hence the name 'corresponding meridians'. In China, their names are much more commonly used than in the West, where meridians are usually named after the organ to which they pertain. Thus, in China the Large Intestine meridian will be referred to as '*Hand Yang Ming*', the Stomach meridian as '*Foot Yang Ming*'.

Mother–Son rule

The Mother–Son rule is based on the generating sequence of the Five Phases: each element 'generates' the one succeeding it. Applying this principle to the meridians, the Mother–Son rule means that the meridians can be 'strengthened' or tonified in the following order: LIV/ G.B. (Wood) → HE/P/S.I./T.B. (Fire) → SP/ST (Earth) → LU/L.I. (Metal) → KID/BL (Water). The opposite direction has a 'weakening' or sedating effect. In other words, instead of tonifying the affected meridian directly, the Mother of the affected meridian can be tonified instead (or, for a sedating effect, the Son can be sedated instead) (→ 5.2.2; Fig. 2.2).

4.3 Meridian points

There is a total of 361 points located on the meridians, which can be seen as reflex zones of internal body structures. The 'points' (Chinese: *Xue*, a hole or point of access) are stimulated by the insertion of a needle or by other techniques, such as laser acupuncture (→ 3.7), injection acupuncture (→ 3.9) or micromassage (→ 3.4).

On each meridian there are therapeutically important points that belong to specific point categories. These are listed under the headings of the individual meridians (→ 5.2).

4.4 The 12 primary meridians and the 2 major extraordinary meridians

For each meridian, the following features are listed in the sections below:

- Chinese name
- Number of points
- Interiorly–exteriorly paired meridian and its corresponding meridian
- Main indications
- External and Internal pathway
- Specific points.

Main indications: each meridian is, of course, indicated for pain and other disorders along its pathway. The main indications of a meridian are based on TCM physiology and pathology of the corresponding organ. The major parameters for the more complex organs are thus shown in table format.

How to locate points

The individual body measurement 'cun' (which corresponds approximately to 1 inch or 1 thumbwidth) is used to determine the distance of an acupuncture point from anatomically defined reference points. However, 1 cun does not always equal 1 thumbwidth, it is also defined as a proportional measurement.

> Comparison of several Chinese and Western acupuncture charts can be a very confusing experience: there are no two identical versions, so do not get frustrated by minor variations.

Principally, there are three methods for locating points:

- Anatomical reference points, either fixed or movable
- Finger measurements (thumbwidth)
- Proportional cun measurements.

Anatomical reference points

Points are described in relation to anatomically defined reference points.

Fixed reference points include the nipples, umbilicus, head of the fibula, tip of the malleolus, etc. **Movable reference points** depend on a particular position of the body. For example, the external branch of the Bladder meridian is located 3 cun lateral to the posterior midline. Only in a relaxed position with the shoulders hanging down will this line correspond to the medial border of the scapula.

Finger cun measurements/thumbwidth (→ Figure)

One cun corresponds to the following:

- One thumbwidth, measured slightly distal to the interphalangeal joint
- The distance between the folds of the proximal and distal interphalangeal joints of the loosely flexed middle finger – this is a more exact measurement
- Commonly used is the 'four-finger method': the width of the four fingers (2nd to 5th fingers) at the level of the proximal interphalangeal joints corresponds to 3 cun, and two fingers correspond to 1.5 cun

> Always bear in mind that the 'cun' is an individual, patient-specific unit of measurement. In clinical practice, compare the width of your fingers with that of the patient and adjust your cun measurements accordingly.

Proportional cun (→ Figure)

It is always important to remember that, besides the finger cun, there are also proportional cun. Here a specific distance is divided into a specific number of proportional cun units, which do not always correspond to finger cun – one only has to think of the diverse shapes that stomachs might have. Thus, the distance from the pubic symphysis to the umbilicus is divided into 5 proportional cun, whereas the distance from the umbilicus to the xiphoid process is divided into 8 proportional cun. One unit of these distances corresponds

to 1 proportional cun. Kitzinger describes a useful measuring technique:

> An elastic band is marked at regular intervals. To locate points on the lower abdomen, the tape is stretched so that 5 units cover the distance between the pubic symphysis and the umbilicus. For points on the upper abdomen (between the umbilicus and the xiphoid process) it has to be stretched so that 8 units cover this distance.

Proportional cun are also used for locating points on the head, thorax and extremities:

- From the anterior to the posterior hairline: 12 cun
- From the midpoint between the eyebrows to the 7th cervical vertebra: 16 cun
- Between the nipples: 8 cun.

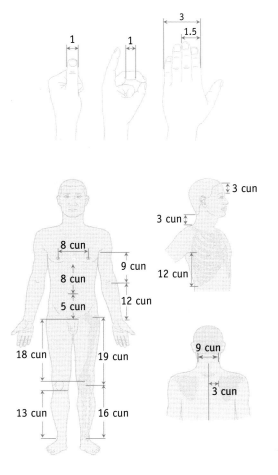

4.4.1 Lung meridian (LU)

Shou Tai Yin	Greater Yin of the hand	11 points

Partner

Interior–Exterior pairing according to the inside/outside rule (Yin/Yang)	Large Intestine meridian
Six great channel pairing according to the above/below rule (Yin/Yin) Together: Tai Yin	Spleen meridian

Main indications according to TCM organ physiology and pathology

Organ physiology	Pathology
Prime Minister in the 'body state' (Nei Jing)	Viscerovisceral reflex: isolated disorder hardly possible, mostly several organs will be affected
Governs the Qi and respiration, the 'foundation of Qi', descends the Qi	Dyspnoea
Regulates the Water passages	Oedema in the upper part of the body, face
Governs the surface: the skin and hair	Skin pathologies, susceptible to external pathogens
Opens into the nose	Impaired sense of smell, nasal flaring
Manifests in the voice	Hoarseness, low voice
Controls the defensive Qi (Wei Qi) and sweating	Sweating with exertion, lowered body defence, prone to infections and colds
Supports the Heart in circulating the Blood	Poor circulation, cold hands
The Lungs house the corporeal soul Po (autonomic nervous system)	Vegetative dystonia, pruritus
Based on its pathway and its pairing with the Large Intestine meridian	Headaches, sinusitis, common cold

External pathway

The Lung meridian begins on the thorax in the 2nd intercostal space (ICS) inferior to the clavicle ➔ anteromedial aspect of the arm ➔ ends on the thumb at the radial corner of the nail at LU-11 [after Bischko: at the ulnar corner of the nail].

Internal pathway and connections

Originates in the Middle Burner ➔ descends to the Large Intestine ➔ ascends to the cardia ➔ penetrates the diaphragm and reaches the Lung ➔ courses along the trachea to the larynx.

Specific points on the Lung meridian

Front-Mu point	LU-1
Back-Shu point	BL-13
Luo-connecting point	LU-7 to L.I.-4
Yuan-source point	LU-9
Opening point	LU-7 (for the Ren Mai)
Tonification point (+)	LU-9
Sedation point (–)	LU-5
Master points	LU-11 (disorders of the throat, Bischko) LU-7 (thorax) LU-9 (disorders of the vessels, arrhythmia)
Xi-cleft point	LU-6
Hui-meeting point	LU-9 (vascular disorders)
He-sea point	LU-5
Time of maximum activity	3–5 am

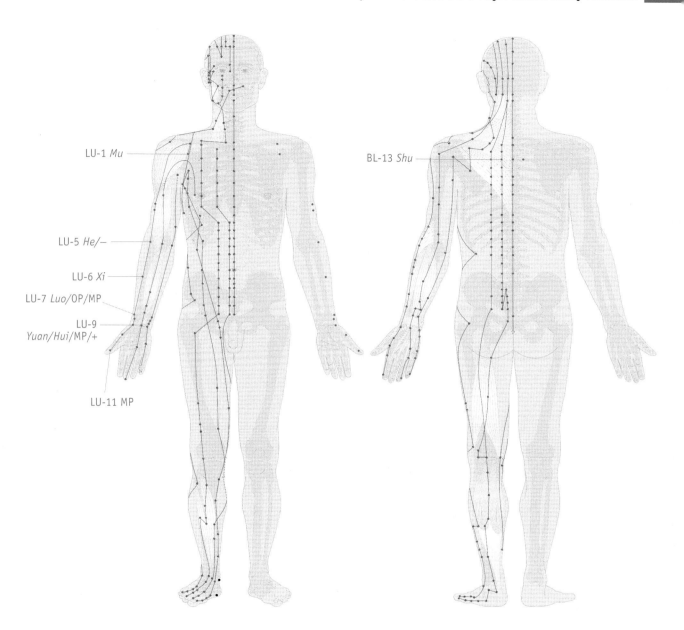

LU-1 *Mu*

BL-13 *Shu*

LU-5 *He/—*

LU-6 *Xi*

LU-7 *Luo*/OP/MP

LU-9
Yuan/Hui/MP/+

LU-11 MP

4.4.2 Large Intestine meridian (L.I.)

Shou Yang Ming	Bright Yang of the hand	20 points

Partner

Interior–Exterior pairing according to the inside/outside rule (Yin/Yang)	Lung meridian
Six great channel pairing according to the above/below rule (Yang/Yang) Together: Yang Ming	Stomach meridian

Main indications according to TCM organ physiology and pathology

Organ physiology	Pathology
Nei Jing: Palace of transmission	Constipation, diarrhoea
Governs the fluids	Absorption disorders (of water-soluble substances)
Based on its pathway and its pairing with the Lung meridian	Disorders of the wrist, elbow, shoulder, sinusitis, headaches (especially frontal), common cold

External pathway

The Large Intestine meridian begins on the index finger, at the radial corner of the nail ➔ lateral aspect of the arm ➔ as the most anterior Yang meridian passes the elbow at the radial end of the cubital crease ➔ anterior border of the deltoid muscle ➔ anterior aspect of the shoulder, ascends to the head ➔ terminates at L.I.-20 at the superior end of the nasiolabial groove.

According to TCM, the L.I. meridian crosses to the contralateral side of the body at the upper lip and ends contralaterally at L.I.-20.

Internal pathway and connections

Connects with the Lung ➔ penetrates the diaphragm ➔ Large Intestine ➔ from here, a branch descends to the lower He-sea point (ST-37).

Specific points on the Large Intestine meridian

Front-Mu point	ST-25
Back-Shu point	BL-25
Luo-connecting point	L.I.-6 to LU-9
Yuan-source point	L.I.-4
Tonification point (+)	L.I.-11
Sedation point (−)	L.I.-2
Metabolism points	L.I.-2,3,4 [Bischko]
Master points	L.I.-1 (toothache) L.I.-15 (any disorder of the upper extremity, shoulder) L.I.-11 (paresis of the upper extremity) L.I.-3 and L.I.-4 (acne)
Xi-cleft point	L.I.-7
He-sea point	L.I.-11
Lower He-sea point (Xia He)	ST-37
Time of maximum activity	5–7 am

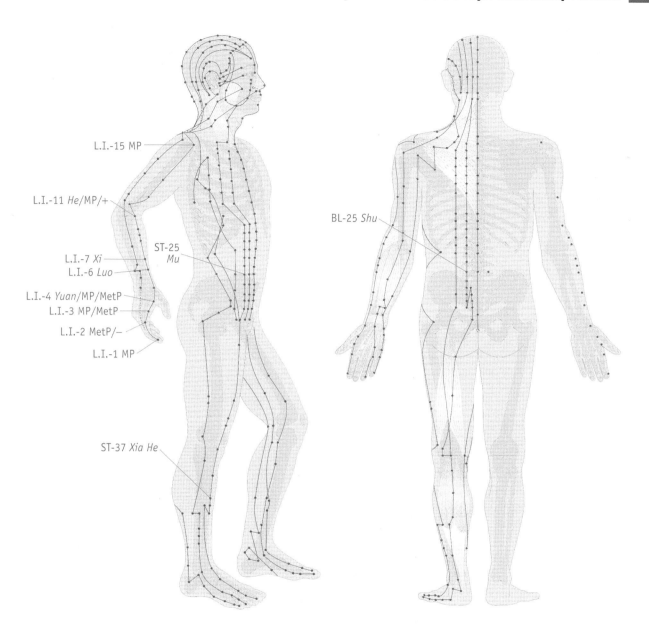

L.I.-15 MP

L.I.-11 *He*/MP/+

L.I.-7 *Xi*
L.I.-6 *Luo*

L.I.-4 *Yuan*/MP/MetP
L.I.-3 MP/MetP

L.I.-2 MetP/−

L.I.-1 MP

ST-25
Mu

ST-37 *Xia He*

BL-25 *Shu*

4.4.3 Stomach meridian (ST)

Zu Yang Ming	Bright Yang of the foot	45 points

Partner

Interior–Exterior pairing according to the inside/outside rule (Yin/Yang)	Spleen meridian
Six great channel pairing according to the above/below rule (Yang/Yang) Together: Yang Ming	Large Intestine meridian

Main indications according to TCM organ physiology and pathology

Organ physiology	Pathology
Works like a 'food processor' – controls fermentation and ripening of food, prepares ingested food for production of Qi and Blood by the Spleen	If the Stomach does not supply the Spleen with raw materials, this will result in Qi deficiency, Blood deficiency, muscular weakness, anorexia, wasting and death
Together with the Spleen controls the transport of the food essences to the whole body, especially to the extremities	Weakness of the extremities
Origin of the fluids derived from ingested food and drink	Disturbed fluid metabolism
Based on its pathway and its pairing with the Spleen meridian	Headaches (especially frontal), sinusitis, hoarseness, mastitis, lactation problems, intestinal disorders, disorders of the leg, knee, ankle and dorsum of the foot

External pathway

Forked origin on the head (in this section of the meridian differing numbering systems) ➔ both branches (one originating at the lower orbital margin, the other coursing from the lower jaw to the temporal region) merge at the mandibular angle (from ST-9 onwards unified numbering system) ➔ anterolateral aspect of the neck ➔ midpoint of clavicle ➔ descends along the midclavicular line to the 6th ICS ➔ from here descends closer to the midline (medial to the Spleen meridian) ➔ inguinal groove ➔ anterolateral aspect of the leg ➔ midpoint of transverse crease of the ankle joint (ST-41) ➔ highest point on the dorsum of the foot (ST-42) ➔ between the 2nd and 3rd metatarsal bones ➔ terminates at ST-45 on the 2nd toe, at the lateral corner of the nail.

Internal pathway and connections

Connects with the Stomach organ and Spleen meridian.

Specific points on the Stomach meridian

Front-Mu point	Ren-12
Back-Shu point	BL-21
Luo-connecting point	ST-40 to SP-3
Yuan-source point	ST-42
Tonification point (+)	ST-41
Sedation point (–)	ST-45
Master points	ST-36 [Bischko: 'Divine serenity, Great Healer of the feet and knee'; Meng: hormonal balance, hypertension, hypotension]
Xi-cleft point	ST-34
He-sea point	ST-36
Lower He-sea point (Xia He)	ST-37 (L.I.) ST-39 (S.I.)
Time of maximum activity	7–9 am

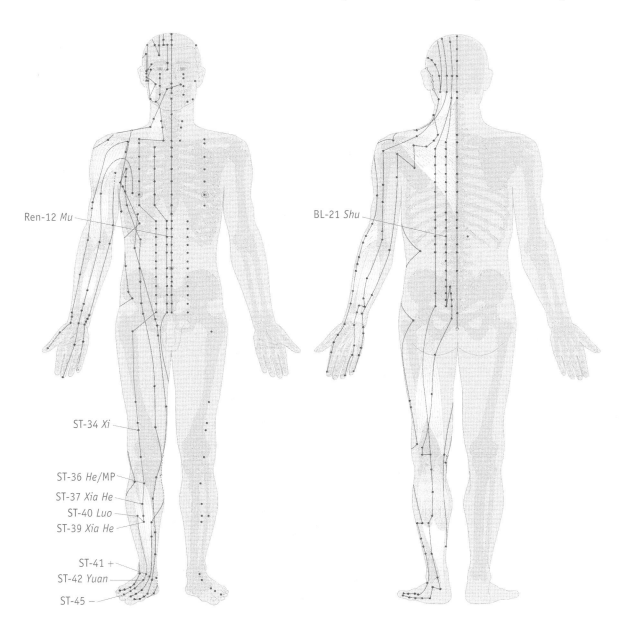

Ren-12 *Mu*

BL-21 *Shu*

ST-34 *Xi*

ST-36 *He*/MP
ST-37 *Xia He*
ST-40 *Luo*
ST-39 *Xia He*

ST-41 +
ST-42 *Yuan*

ST-45 −

4.4.4 Spleen meridian (SP)

Zu Tai Yin	Greater Yin of the foot	21 points

Partner

Interior–Exterior pairing according to the inside/outside rule (Yin/Yang)	Stomach meridian
Six great channel pairing according to the above/below rule (Yin/Yin) Together: Tai Yin	Lung meridian

Main indications according to TCM organ physiology and pathology

Organ physiology	Pathology
The Spleen is a synonym for digestion; it governs the transportation and transformation of the food and fluids	Trophic disorders, but also obesity, chronic diarrhoea and constipation, fluid retention, formation of Dampness and Phlegm
Provides the foundation for blood and flesh (muscles), holds the blood in the vessels	Anaemia, TCM: Blood deficiency, bleeding; lack of muscle tone
Governs the muscles, the flesh and limbs	Weakness of the muscles and limbs, heavy sensation in the limbs
Sends the pure Qi derived from food to the Lungs	If the transformation is impaired, Phlegm will form
Opens into the mouth, lips; controls taste	Lip pathologies, impaired sense of taste (sweet, sour, bitter, salty, pungent)
Controls the middle, holds the organs in place	Weak connective tissue, organ prolapses, ptosis
The Spleen houses the 'Yi', the soul of philosophers and bookkeepers (with an eye for detail but sometimes also pedantic)	Worrying, brooding, ruminating

External pathway

The Spleen meridian begins on the big toe, at the medial corner of the nail ➜ continues along the 1st metatarsal bone at the border of the red and white skin ➜ cuneiform I ➜ anterior to the medial malleolus ➜ to the posterior border of the tibia ➜ ascends the leg, inguinal groove, torso ➜ to the 2nd ICS ➜ descends again in a lateral direction ➜ terminates at SP-21, inferior to the axilla, in the 6th ICS.

Internal pathway and connections

Enters the abdomen superior to the inguinal groove ➜ ascends to the Spleen ➜ connects with the Stomach ➜ ascends, penetrating the diaphragm ➜ along the oesophagus to the root and underside of the tongue; a branch emerges at the Stomach, penetrates the diaphragm and reaches the Heart and the Heart meridian.

Specific points on the Spleen meridian

Front Mu-point	LIV-13
Back Shu-point	BL-20 (11th ICS)
Luo-connecting point	SP-4 to ST-42
Yuan-source point	SP-3
Opening point	SP-4 (for the Chong Mai)
Tonification point (+)	SP-2
Sedation point (–)	SP-5
Master points	SP-5 (weakness of connective tissue) SP-4 (any type of diarrhoea) SP-9 (female genitalia, urination)
Meeting points	SP-13 with the LIV, Yin Wei Mai SP-14, -15, -16 with the Yin Wei Mai
He-sea point	SP-9
Time of maximum activity	9–11 am

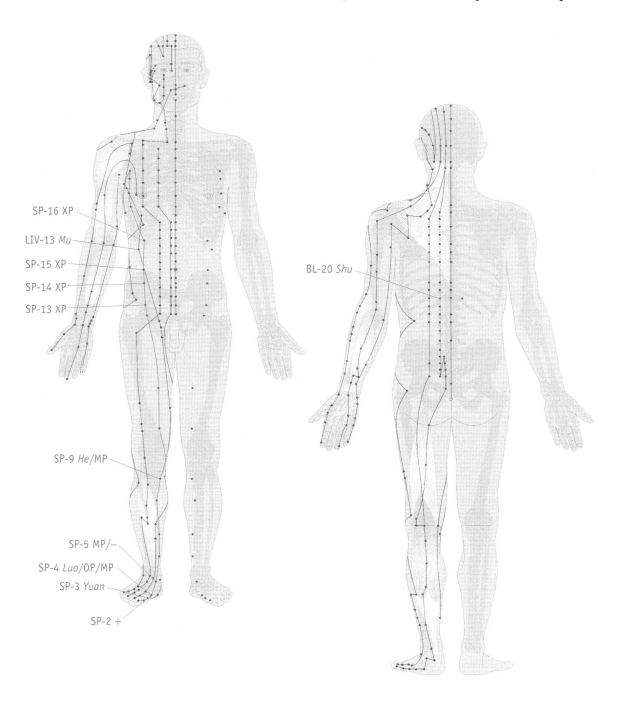

SP-16 XP

LIV-13 *Mu*

SP-15 XP

SP-14 XP

SP-13 XP

BL-20 *Shu*

SP-9 *He*/MP

SP-5 MP/−

SP-4 *Luo*/OP/MP

SP-3 *Yuan*

SP-2 +

4.4.5 Heart meridian (HE)

| Shou Shao Yin | Lesser Yin of the hand | 9 points |

Partner

Interior–Exterior pairing according to the inside/outside rule (Yin/Yang)	Small Intestine meridian
Six great channel pairing according to the above/below rule (Yin/Yin) Together: Shao Yin	Kidney meridian

Main indications according to TCM organ physiology and pathology

Organ physiology	Pathology
The Heart is the Emperor of the 'body state'	Isolated Heart symptoms are hardly possible; if the Emperor is diseased, the whole state (body) will be affected
Governs the Blood and the blood vessels	Circulatory disorders, palpitations
Opens into the tongue	Speech disorders
Manifests in the complexion	Pathological complexion (e.g. with a congenital heart defect)
Sweat is the fluid of the Heart	Uncontrolled sweating (due to psychological disorders)
The Heart houses the soul ('Shen')	Spirit disorders, psychoemotional disorders, nervousness, insomnia, poor memory

External pathway

Thorax (axilla) ➜ medioposterior aspect of the arm ➜ palmar aspect of the hand ➜ terminates at HE-9 on the little finger, at the radial corner of the nail.

Internal pathway and connections

Originates in the Heart ➜ traverses the Lung and continues to the axilla/HE-1 ➜ an internal branch ascends the oesophagus bilaterally and continues to the eyes ➜ descends, penetrates the diaphragm and reaches the Small Intestine.

Specific points on the Heart meridian

Front-Mu point	LIV-13
Back-Shu point	BL-15
Luo-connecting point	HE-5 to S.I.-4
Yuan-source point	HE-7
Tonification point (+)	HE-9
Sedation point (–)	HE-7
Master points	HE-3 (depression)
Xi-cleft point	HE-6
He-sea point	HE-3
Time of maximum activity	11 am–1 pm

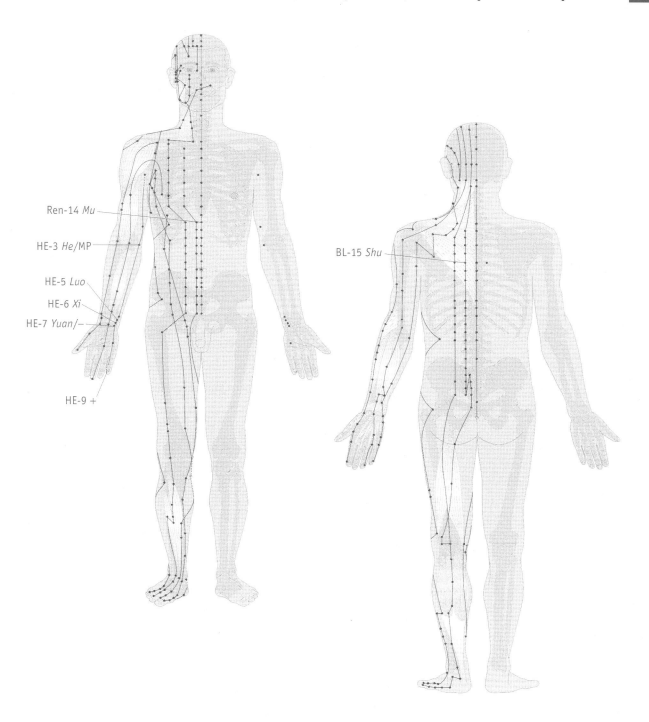

Ren-14 *Mu*

HE-3 *He*/MP

HE-5 *Luo*

HE-6 *Xi*

HE-7 *Yuan*/−

HE-9 +

BL-15 *Shu*

4.4.6 Small Intestine meridian (S.I.)

Shou Tai Yang	Greater *Yang* of the hand	19 points

Partner

Interior–exterior pairing according to the inside/outside rule (*Yin/Yang*)	Heart meridian
Six great channel pairing according to the above/below rule (*Yang/Yang*) Together: Tai Yang	Bladder meridian

Main indications according to TCM organ physiology and pathology

Organ physiology	Pathology
The Small Intestine is a hollow organ (*Fu*)	Element: Fire – susceptible to both Excess and Deficiency Cold; either can result in *Qi* stagnation and therefore pain
It is the 'official' responsible for separating the clear from the turbid: absorbs the 'dirty water' that is transformed to urine by the Kidneys and transported to the Bladder	Cloudy urine, urinary disorders
Interiorly–exteriorly paired with the Heart	Heart–Fire transmitted to the Small Intestine, causing cystitis and haematuria
Based on the meridian pathway	Pain in the wrist, elbow, shoulder, scapula, cervical syndrome, trismus, disorders of the ear such as otitis, tinnitus, deafness, eye disorders such as conjunctivitis

External pathway

The Small Intestine meridian originates on the little finger, at the ulnar corner of the nail ➜ ascends the outside of the arm ➜ passes the postero-ulnar aspect of the olecranon ➜ passes the posterior aspect of the axillary fold ➜ posterior border of the scapular spine ➜ deviates inferiorly and medially to the centre of the infraspinous fossa ➜ passes the lateral aspect of the neck, where S.I.-15 is located close to T.B.-16 and G.B.-21 on the trapezius [according to Bi identical] ➜ terminates anterior to the earlobe at S.I.-19.

Internal pathway and connections

Connects with Du-14 [Bischko: Du-13]; continues via the supraclavicular fossa to the Heart ➜ penetrates the diaphragm and enters the Stomach and Small Intestine ➜ from here, a branch descends to ST-39, the Lower *He*-sea point of the meridian; from the supraclavicular fossa (ST-12) a branch ascends to the cheek ➜ divides into two branches, one continuing to the outer canthus of the eye and the inner ear, the other to the medial canthus of the eye (BL-1).

Specific points on the Small Intestine meridian

Front-*Mu* point	Ren-4
Back-*Shu* point	BL-27
Luo-connecting point	S.I.-7 to HE-7
Yuan-source point	S.I.-4
Opening point	S.I.-3 (for the *Du Mai*)
Tonification point (+)	S.I.-3
Sedation point (−)	S.I.-8
Master points	S.I.-3 (spasms, mucous membranes)
He-sea point	S.I.-8
Lower *He*-sea point (*Xia He*)	ST-39
Time of maximum activity	1–3 pm

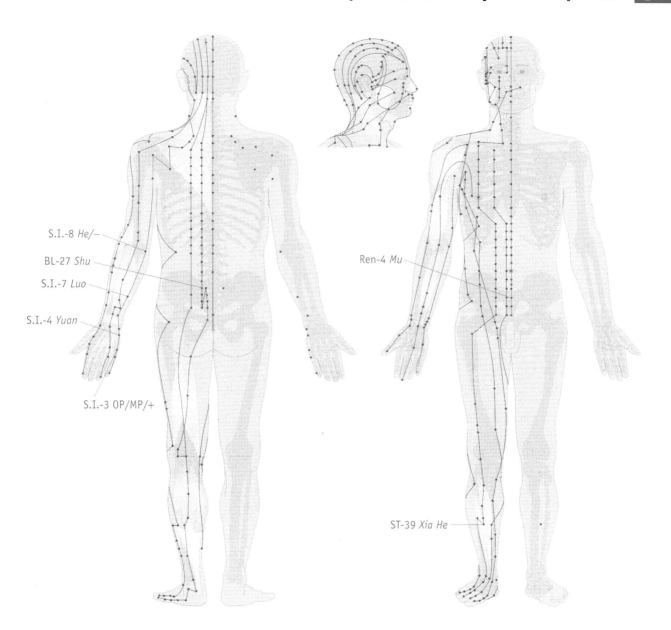

S.I.-8 *He/–*

BL-27 *Shu*

S.I.-7 *Luo*

S.I.-4 *Yuan*

S.I.-3 OP/MP/+

Ren-4 *Mu*

ST-39 *Xia He*

4.4.7 Bladder meridian (BL)

Zu Tai Yang	Greater *Yang* of the foot	67 points

Partner

Interior–Exterior pairing according to the inside/outside rule (*Yin/Yang*)	Kidney meridian
Six great channel pairing according to the above/below rule (*Yang/Yang*) Together: *Tai Yang*	Small Intestine meridian

Main indications according to TCM organ physiology and pathology

Organ physiology	Pathology
The Bladder provides contact with the outside world	Susceptible to external pathogenic factors
With the support of the Kidney *Yang* transforms water, which has been separated by the intestines, into urine	Kidney *Yang* deficiency: copious clear urine, enuresis
Qi holds urine in the Bladder and activates urination	Incontinence, urinary retention
Based on the meridian pathway	Headaches, cervical syndrome, back pain, lumbago
Based on the back-*Shu* points	Disorders of the internal organs

External pathway

Head (inner canthus of the eye, traverses the head paramedially towards the posterior) ➔ occiput ➔ descends the back paramedially ➔ posterior aspect of the leg ➔ terminates on the little toe, at BL-67, at the lateral border of the nail.

Internal pathway and connections

Five branches, some with superficial, some with internal pathways; connects with the vertex, brain and shoulder.

Specific points on the Bladder meridian

Front-*Mu* point	Ren-3
Back-*Shu* point	BL-28
Luo-connecting point	BL-58
Yuan-source point	BL-64
Opening point	BL-62 (for the *Yang Qiao Mai*)
Tonification point (+)	BL-67
Sedation point (–)	BL-65
Master points	BL-21 (Stomach) BL-31 (menopause) BL-40 (skin disorders) BL-43 (haematopoiesis) BL-60 (any kind of pain) BL-62 with KID-6 (insomnia)
Metabolic points	BL-58, BL-40 [Bischko: BL-54]
He-sea point	BL-40 [Bischko: BL-54]
Lower *He*-sea point (*Xia He*)	BL-39 [Bischko: BL-53] – Triple Burner
Time of maximum activity	3–5 pm

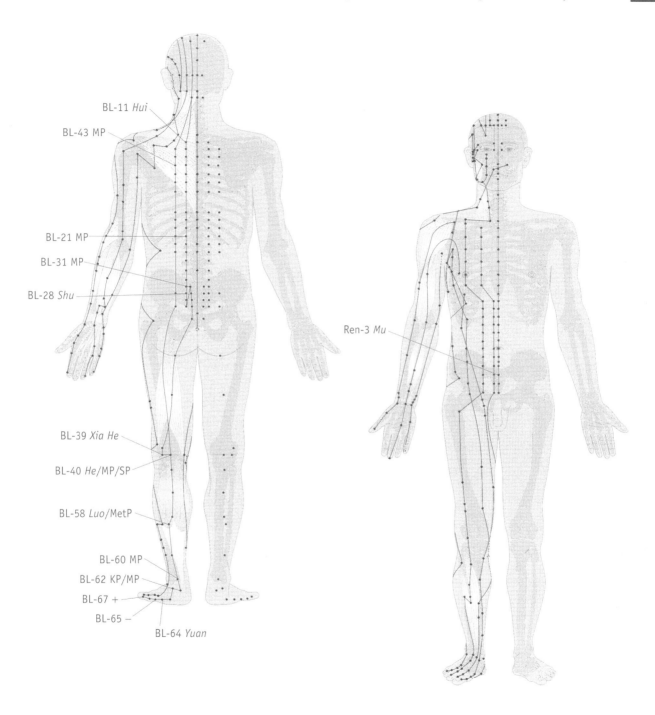

BL-11 *Hui*

BL-43 MP

BL-21 MP

BL-31 MP

BL-28 *Shu*

Ren-3 *Mu*

BL-39 *Xia He*

BL-40 *He*/MP/SP

BL-58 *Luo*/MetP

BL-60 MP

BL-62 KP/MP

BL-67 +

BL-65 −

BL-64 *Yuan*

4.4.8 Kidney meridian (KID)

| *Zu Shao Yin* | Lesser *Yin* of the foot | 27 points |

Partner

| Interior–Exterior pairing according to the inside/outside rule (*Yin/Yang*) | Bladder meridian |
| Six great channel pairing according to the above/below rule (*Yin/Yin*) Together: *Shao Yin* | Heart meridian |

Main indications according to TCM organ physiology and pathology

Organ physiology	Pathology
The lower back is the abode of the Kidneys	Chronic lumbago, especially with weakness of the lumbar spine and knees (Kidney *Qi/Yin/Yang/Jing* deficiency)
The Kidneys are the abode of Water and Fire (Water Kidney, Fire Kidney)	Fluid metabolism disorders as well as hormonal imbalances
Stores the essence (*Jing*): endocrine system	Infertility, congenital disorders, premature greying
Governs and fills the bones – influences the marrow and the brain	Osteoporosis, premature physeal closure, open fontanelles, leukaemia, anaemia, Alzheimer's disease
Manifests in the teeth (Essence/*Jing*)	Tooth anomalies, poor teeth
Governs the water metabolism	Oedema, diarrhoea, constipation, polyuria/oliguria, urinary difficulties
'Grasps' the *Qi* descended from the Lungs (breathing)	Dyspnoea, asthma, especially following steroid therapy
Opens into the ears and the 'two *Yin*' (anus and urethra)	Tinnitus, deafness, incontinence
Manifests in the hair	Premature greying and/or balding
Nourishes Liver *Yin*	Kidney *Yin* deficiency is often the root of a hyperactive Liver *Yang*

| The Kidneys are the origin of all the body's *Yin* and *Yang* | The Kidneys are always the root of general *Yin/Yang* deficiency; any organ deficiency can also affect the Kidneys |
| Based on the meridian pathway, particularly the internal pathway | Disorders of the lower abdomen as well as disorders of the pharynx and root of the tongue |

External pathway

Originates on the sole of the foot between the pads of the foot → circles the medial malleolus → ascends the medial aspect of the leg (most posterior *Yin* meridian) → ascends the abdomen and thorax, meridian closest to the *Ren Mai* → terminates at the sternoclavicular joint at KID-27.

Internal pathway and connections

To Du-1 → from there, the internal pathway ascends to the Kidneys, Liver, diaphragm, root of the tongue, Pericardium, thorax.

Specific points on the Kidney meridian

Front-*Mu* point	G.B.-25
Back-*Shu* point	BL-23
Luo-connecting point	KID-4 to BL-64
Yuan-source point	KID-3
Opening point	KID-6 (for the *Yin Qiao Mai*)
Tonification point (+)	KID-7
Sedation point (–)	KID-1
Metabolic points	KID-2, KID-6
Master points	KID-6 with BL-62 (insomnia)
Xi-cleft point	KID-5 (Kidney), KID-8 (*Yin Qiao Mai*), KID-9 (*Yin Wei Mai*)
He-sea point	KID-10
Time of maximum activity	5–7 pm

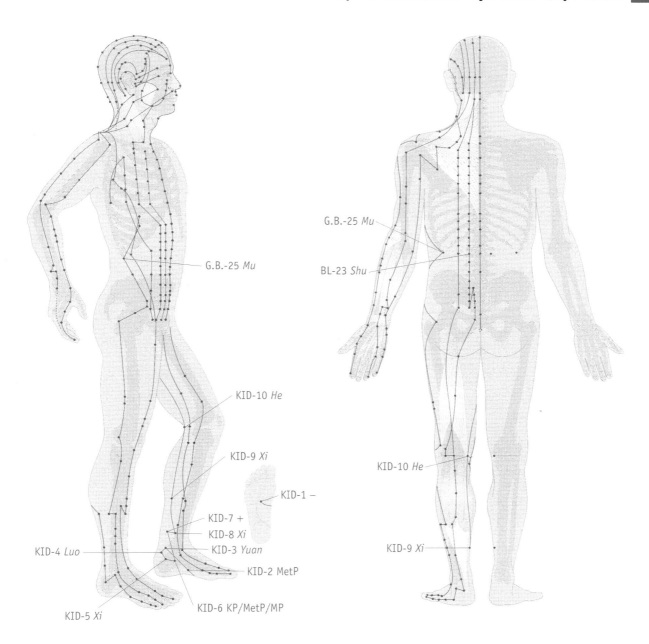

G.B.-25 *Mu*

G.B.-25 *Mu*

BL-23 *Shu*

KID-10 *He*

KID-9 *Xi*

KID-1 –

KID-7 +
KID-8 *Xi*
KID-3 *Yuan*

KID-4 *Luo*

KID-2 MetP

KID-10 *He*

KID-9 *Xi*

KID-5 *Xi*

KID-6 KP/MetP/MP

4.4.9 Pericardium meridian (P)

Shou Jue Yin	Reverting Yin of the hand	9 points

Partner

Interior–Exterior pairing according to the inside/out-side rule (Yin/Yang)	Triple Burner meridian
Six great channel pairing according to the above/below rule (Yin/Yin) Together: Jue Yin	Liver meridian

Main indications according to TCM organ physiology and pathology

Organ physiology	Pathology
'Heart protector' – essentially represents the heart as an organ in the Western sense	Cardiovascular disorders, hypertension, hypotension, 'rising' sensation on the anterior aspect of the body: nausea, vomiting, flushes
The Heart according to TCM	See Heart meridian
Protects the Heart from external pathogenic factors	Pericardium patterns are used to describe conditions characterized by coma and delirium caused by Heat (fever) and/or Phlegm
Transports the Yang/Yin Qi to the Yin organs; activates, controls and supplies the Yin meridians with energy	Collapse (P-9)

External pathway

Originates in the thorax (in the 4th ICS, 1 cun lateral to the nipple) → continues lateral to the HE meridian → anteromedial aspect of the arm → terminates at P-9 on the middle finger.

Internal pathway and connections

Originates in the centre of the chest → connects with the Pericardium → descends, penetrating the diaphragm → connects with all Three Burners (respiration, digestion and urogenital/endocrine system).

Specific points on the Pericardium meridian

Front-Mu point	Ren-17
Back-Shu point	BL-14
Luo-connecting point	P-6 to T.B.-4
Yuan-source point	P-7
Opening point	P-6 (for the Yin Wei Mai)
Tonification point (+)	P-9
Sedation point (−)	P-7
Master point	P-6 (nausea)
Xi-cleft point	P-4
He-sea point	P-3
Time of maximum activity	7–9 pm

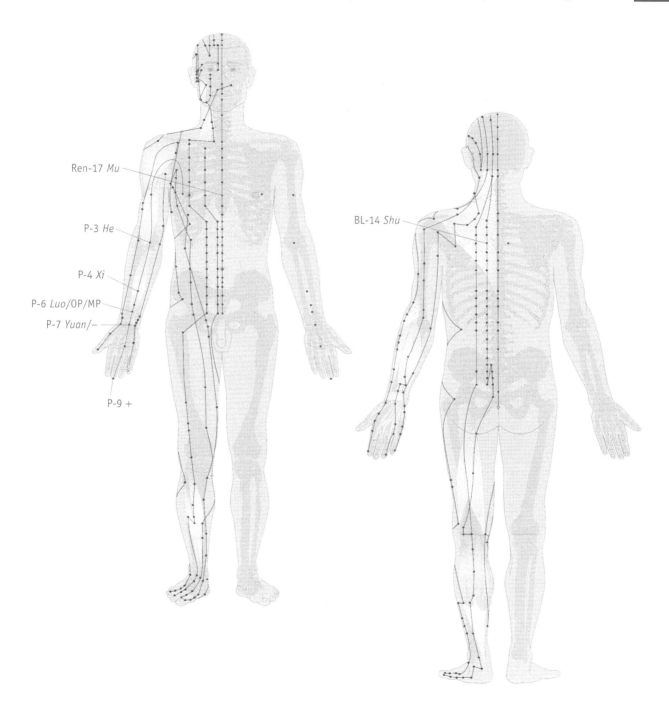

Ren-17 *Mu*

P-3 *He*

P-4 *Xi*

P-6 *Luo/OP/MP*

P-7 *Yuan/−*

P-9 +

BL-14 *Shu*

4.4.10 Triple Burner meridian (T.B.)

Shou Shao Yang	Lesser *Yang* of the hand	23 points

Partner

Interior–Exterior pairing according to the inside/outside rule (*Yin/Yang*)	Pericardium meridian
Six great channel pairing according to the above/below rule (*Yang/Yang*) Together: *Shao Yang*	Gall Bladder meridian

Main indications according to TCM organ physiology and pathology

Organ physiology	Pathology
The name refers to the three 'storeys' of the body and their organs: **Upper Burner:** Heart and Lung **Middle Burner:** Spleen, Stomach **Lower Burner:** Liver, Kidneys	Allows differentiation of Damp–Heat according to the 'three storeys': **Upper Burner:** e.g. chronic sinusitis **Middle Burner:** e.g. chronic pancreatitis, hepatitis **Lower Burner:** e.g. chronic prostatitis
Has a connection with the Water passages: governs Water metabolism by securing the free flow of fluids	The lower *He*-sea point BL-39 is effective for urinary retention
Controls the production of defensive *Qi* (*Wei Qi*), transports the Essence (*Jing*) or original *Qi* from the Kidneys to all other organs via the *Yuan*-source points of their pertaining meridians	Colds, aversion to wind and susceptibility to changes in weather; T.B.-5 can expel all pathogenic factors
Based on its pathway	Temporal headaches, migraines; eye disorders such as conjunctivitis; ear disorders such as otitis, tinnitus, deafness; facial paralysis; pain on the posterior aspect of the shoulder, flank pain, intercostal neuralgia

External pathway

Originates on the ring finger, at the ulnar border of the nail ➔ traverses the hand between the 4th and 5th metacarpal bones ➔ ascends the outside of the arm, between the L.I. and S.I. meridians ➔ passes the tip of the olecranon ➔ reaches the shoulder ➔ anterior border of the mastoid ➔ curves around the ear ➔ continues anteriorly to the supratragic incisure between the ear and the G.B. meridian ➔ terminates at T.B.-23 at the lateral end of the eyebrow.

Internal pathway and connections

Reaches Du-12 and Du-14 [Bi: Du-13], also reaches G.B.-21; continues to the mediastinum ➔ Ren-17, penetrates the diaphragm ➔ connects with all three Burners ➔ a branch descends to its Lower *He*-sea point BL-39 ➔ [Bi: BL-53].

Specific points on the Triple Burner meridian

Front-*Mu* point	Ren-5
Back-*Shu* point	BL-22
Luo-connecting point	T.B.-5 to P-7
Group *Luo*-connecting point (**Luo**)	T.B.-8: for the three *Yang* meridians of the arm (S.I., T.B., L.I.)
Yuan-source point	T.B.-4
Opening point	T.B.-5 (for the *Yang Wei Mai*)
Tonification point (+)	T.B.-3
Sedation point (–)	T.B.-10
Master point	T.B.-4 (vasomotor headache) T.B.-5 (rheumatism) T.B.-15 (susceptibility to weather changes, upper extremities)
Xi-cleft point	T.B.-7
He-sea point	T.B.-10
Lower *He*-sea point (*Xia He*)	BL-39 [Bischko: BL-53]
Time of maximum activity	9–11 pm

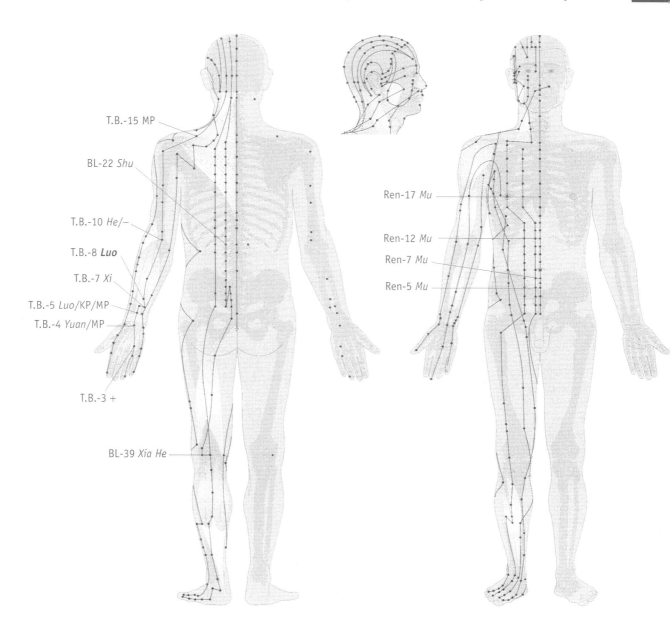

T.B.-15 MP

BL-22 *Shu*

T.B.-10 *He/–*

T.B.-8 **Luo**

T.B.-7 *Xi*

T.B.-5 *Luo/KP/MP*

T.B.-4 *Yuan/MP*

T.B.-3 +

BL-39 *Xia He*

Ren-17 *Mu*

Ren-12 *Mu*

Ren-7 *Mu*

Ren-5 *Mu*

4.4.11 Gall Bladder meridian (G.B.)

Zu Shao Yang	Lesser *Yang* of the foot	44 points

Partner

Interior–exterior pairing according to the inside/outside rule (*Yin/Yang*)	Liver meridian
Six great channel pairing according to the above/below rule (*Yang/Yang*) Together: *Shao Yang*	Triple Burner meridian

Main indications according to TCM organ physiology and pathology

Organ physiology	Pathology
Upright 'official' in charge of judgement and decision-making (right/wrong) (*Nei Jing*)	**Deficiency:** difficulty making decisions **Excess:** aggressive personality
Stores and excretes bile	Bile flow disorders
The G.B. meridian activates the *Yang* aspect of the Liver functions	Liver disorders, joint disorders, disorders of movement
The Gall Bladder is both a *Fu* and also an extraordinary *Fu* – '*Fu* of inner purity'; it is the only *Yang* organ not transforming a dirty substance	Disorders of the *Fu* and extraordinary *Fu*
Based on its pathway	Eye disorders such as conjunctivitis, glaucoma (in emergencies needle G.B.20); ear disorders such as deafness, tinnitus; dizziness; headaches, migraines affecting the temporal region and the eyes, especially around the eyebrows; cervical syndrome, flank pain, lumbago, disorders of the big joints, particularly the hip joint

External pathway

Originates at the lateral orbital margin → zigzags on the lateral aspect of the head → anterior to the ear (intertragic incisure) → continues to the temples →zigzags around the ear to the mastoid (G.B.-12) → returns to the forehead (G.B.-14) → courses back to the mastoid (G.B.-20) → continues between the BL and T.B. meridians to the occiput → passes the highest point of the shoulder → intersection of three *Yang* meridians (G.B.-21, T.B.-16 and S.I.-15) → continues to the anterior → crosses the L.I. meridian at the upper border of the trapezius → traverses the clavicle lateral to the ST meridian and continues to the axilla → courses anteriorly to the mamillary line (G.B.-24, 7th ICS) → then posteriorly to the free end of the 12th rib (G.B.-25) → again courses towards the anterior, continues in an inferior direction → passes the iliac crest and continues to the anterior superior iliac spine → again runs towards the posterior, passes the greater trochanter of the femur posteriorly → descends the lateral aspect of the leg to the anterior border of the head of the fibula → traverses the dorsum of the foot between the 4th and 5th metatarsal bones → terminates at G.B.-44 on the 4th toe, at the lateral corner of the nail.

Internal pathway and connections

Enters the interior of the body at the supraclavicular fossa → penetrates the diaphragm → connects with the Gall Bladder, Liver, genital region and inner ear.

Specific points on the Gall Bladder meridian

Front-*Mu* point	G.B.-24
Back-*Shu* point	BL-19
Luo-connecting point	G.B.-37 to LIV-3
Group *Luo*-connecting point (***Luo***)	G.B.-39 (BL, ST and G.B. meridians)
Yuan-source point	G.B.-40
Opening point	G.B.-41 (for the *Dai Mai*)
Tonification point (+)	G.B.-43
Sedation point (−)	G.B.-38
Master point	G.B.-34 (musculature) G.B.-41 (big joints) G.B.-30 (sciatica, pareses of the legs)
Xi-cleft point	G.B.-36
Hui-meeting point	G.B.-39: marrow (bones, spinal cord, brain)
He-sea point	G.B.-34
Time of maximum activity	11 pm–1 am

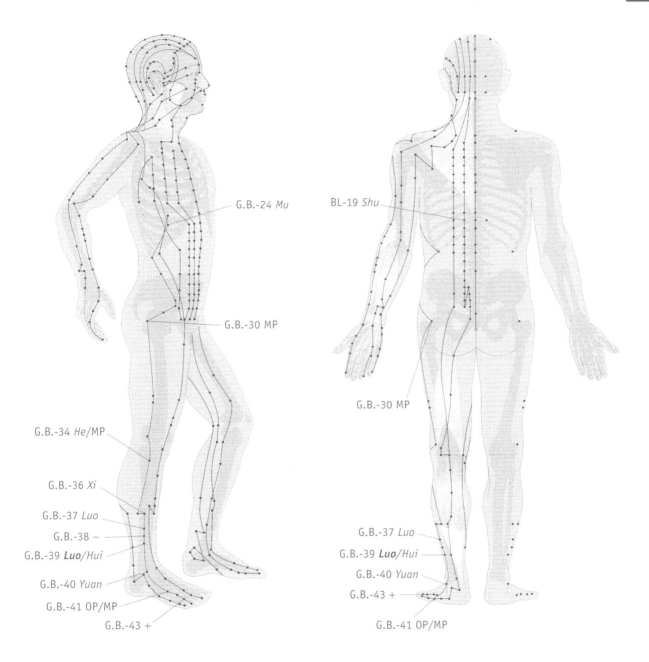

G.B.-24 *Mu*

BL-19 *Shu*

G.B.-30 MP

G.B.-30 MP

G.B.-34 *He*/MP

G.B.-36 *Xi*

G.B.-37 *Luo*

G.B.-38 –

G.B.-39 **Luo**/*Hui*

G.B.-40 *Yuan*

G.B.-41 OP/MP

G.B.-43 +

G.B.-37 *Luo*

G.B.-39 **Luo**/*Hui*

G.B.-40 *Yuan*

G.B.-43 +

G.B.-41 OP/MP

4.4.12 Liver meridian (LIV)

| Zu Jue Yin | Reverting Yin of the foot | 14 points |

Partner

Interior–Exterior pairing according to the inside/outside rule (Yin/Yang)	Gall Bladder meridian
Six great channel pairing according to the above/below rule (Yin/Yin) Together: Jue Yin	Pericardium meridian

Main indications according to TCM organ physiology and pathology

Organ physiology	Pathology
'General': responsible for planning, strategies and action	Lack of planning
Stores the Blood – during rest, the Blood returns to the Liver	Symptoms worse with rest, e.g. palpitations
Regulates the Qi flow; responsible for the smooth flow of Qi, bile and emotions	Qi stagnation equals pain, e.g. dysmenorrhoea, abdominal cramps
Controls activity, suppleness of the muscles, tendons and ligaments	Pathologies affecting movement
Influences the digestive function of the Stomach and Spleen	Digestive disorders due to emotions
Opens into the eyes	Eye symptoms
Manifests in the nails	Poor nails
Based on its pathway, particularly its internal pathway (circles the genitalia, sends inner branches to the eyes and Du-20)	Disorders of the external genitalia, vertex headaches, eye disorders

External pathway

Originates on the big toe, at the lateral corner of the nail ➔ passes the medial malleolus, ascends the medial aspect of the leg ➔ on the lower part of the foreleg anteriorly, from its medial section between the KID and SP meridians ➔ ascends the abdomen lateral to the ST meridian ➔ crosses the SP meridian twice ➔ terminates at LIV-14 on the thorax, in the 6th ICS, on the midclavicular line.

Internal pathway and connections

Reaches the diaphragm, Stomach, thoracic cavity, Lungs, retrobulbar space, Du-20.

Specific points on the Liver meridian

Front-Mu point	LIV-14
Back-Shu point	BL-18
Luo-connecting point	LIV-5 to G.B.-40
Yuan-source point	LIV-3
Tonification point (+)	LIV-8
Sedation point (–)	LIV-2
Metabolic point	LIV-13
Master point	LIV-14 (nausea)
Xi-cleft point	LIV-6
He-sea point	LIV-8
Hui-meeting point	LIV-13: for the viscera (Zang) (associated with the Yin meridians: LU, SP, HE, KID, P, LIV)
Time of maximum activity	1–3 am

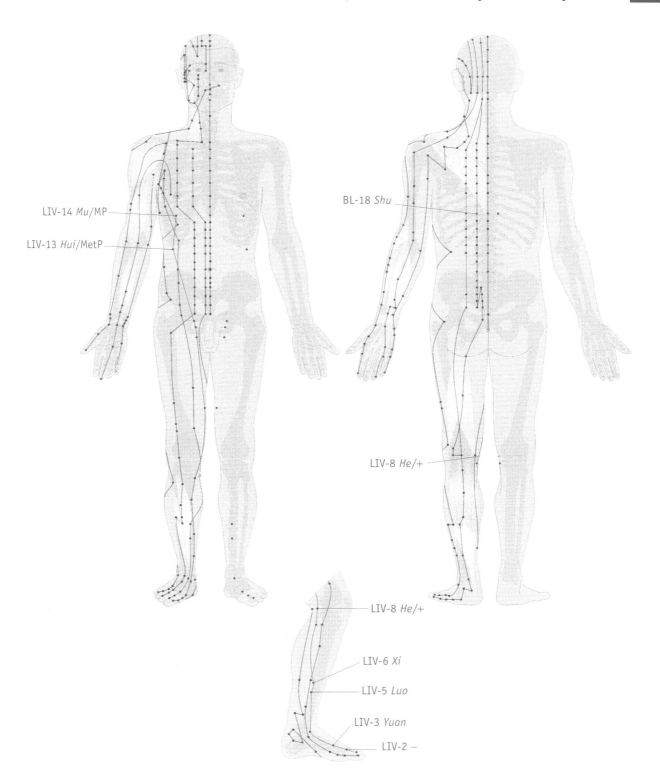

LIV-14 *Mu*/MP

LIV-13 *Hui*/MetP

BL-18 *Shu*

LIV-8 *He*/+

LIV-8 *He*/+

LIV-6 *Xi*

LIV-5 *Luo*

LIV-3 *Yuan*

LIV-2 −

4.5 The 8 extraordinary meridians

The extraordinary meridians are not associated with any particular organ. They are not special meridians as such, but represent the deepest and most primordial meridian structures, which can be compared to energy reservoirs. With the exception of the *Du Mai* and the *Ren Mai*, they do not have their own points, but utilize points on the regular meridians, thus establishing a connection among them.

Unlike in the regular meridians, there is no constant flow of energy in the extraordinary meridians; instead they are activated by needling their opening points. To achieve this, the more important of the two opening points is needled first, then the second most important point is needled, preferably followed by further points on the now 'open' extraordinary meridians.

For maximum effect, they are used in pairs with either two *Yin* or two *Yang* dominated opening points/vessels forming a pair (→ 5.2.2).

4.5.1 Chong Mai

Penetrating vessel	Opening point:	13 points
Distributor of energy	SP-4	
Wide road of consolation		
Sea of the 12 meridians		
Sea of Blood		
Sea of organs		

Points

Ren-1	KID-11 to KID-21	ST-30

Partner

Yin Wei Mai

Function

- Reservoir for Essence (*Jing*), Blood (*Xue*) and *Qi* for all 12 meridians
- Has a connection to all 12 regular meridians, especially to the two sources of Essence (*Jing*): Kidney and Stomach.

Indications

- Digestive disorders: bloating, borborygmus, belching; heart disorders; blood and venous disorders
- Common indication with its partner, the *Yin Wei Mai* (→ 4.5.2).

External pathway

Ren-1 → ST-30 → KID-11 to KID-21.

Internal pathway

Originates in the *Dan Tian* → descends to Ren-1 → courses along the spine → continues to ascend; from KID-21 (terminal point of the external pathway) internally ascends the neck and circles the mouth.

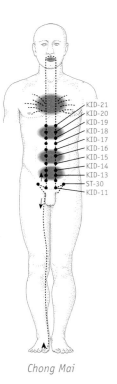

KID-21
KID-20
KID-19
KID-18
KID-17
KID-16
KID-15
KID-14
KID-13
ST-30
KID-11

Chong Mai

4.5.2 *Yin Wei Mai*

Yin linking vessel   Opening point: P-6   7 points
Keeper of the *Yin*

Points

KID-9   SP-13   SP-15   SP-16   LIV-14   Ren-22   Ren-23

Partner

Chong Mai

Function

* Connects the three *Yin* meridians and holds them together
* Governs the interior of the body.

Indications

* Key symptom: heart pain
* Pain in the thorax, stomach and abdomen
* Nausea, vomiting, diarrhoea
* General weakness
* Prolapse of the rectum
* Goitre
* Hypertension.

Pathway

Ascends from KID-9 along the medial aspect of the lower leg and the thigh ➜ ascends in a broad band anterolaterally ➜ SP-13 ➜ SP-15 ➜ SP-16 ➜ LIV-14 ➜ Ren-22 ➜ terminates at Ren-23.

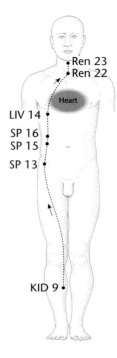

Yin Wei Mai

4.5.3 Ren Mai – conception vessel (Ren)

Sea of *Yin*	Opening point: LU-7	24 points

Function

- Governs the *Qi* and Blood (*Xue*) of all *Yin* meridians.

Indications

- The indications reflect its pathway; they are also influenced by the front-*Mu* points of the Three Burners, which are located on the *Ren Mai*.
- Respiration
- Abdominal: digestion, diarrhoea
- Urogenital region: as the Sea of *Yin*, the *Ren Mai* is attributed the function of a compensatory reservoir for the *Qi* (energy) of the *Yin* meridians.

External pathway

Originates at the perineum, just anterior to the anus ➜ ascends the anterior midline, traversing the abdomen, chest and neck ➜ terminates at Ren-24 in the centre of the mentolabial groove.

Internal pathway and connections

Originates in the lower abdomen ➜ ascends the torso externally as well as internally ➜ circles the lips ➜ traverses the cheek to ST-1 on the infraorbital foramen; one branch enters the spine at Du-1 and ascends the spinal cord. At Ren-15, all collaterals disperse over the whole abdomen in an inferior direction.

Specific points on the *Ren Mai*

Back-*Shu* point	BL-24 for Ren-6, BL-26 for Ren-4
Opening point	LU-7
Hui-meeting point	Ren-12 for the *Fu* organs; Ren-17 for the *Qi*, respiratory tract

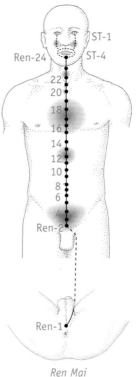

Ren Mai

4.5.4 *Yin Qiao Mai*

Yin motility vessel   Opening point: KID-6   5 points

Points

KID-2   KID-6   KID-8   ST-12   BL-1

Partner

Ren Mai

Function

- Promotes the smooth flow of *Qi* along the medial aspect of the leg, thereby supporting harmonious movement
- Auxiliary meridian of the *Ren Mai*
- Internal rotation of the leg
- Closing the eyelid, sleep.

Indications

Menstrual disorders, gynaecological disorders, abdominal pain/colic; lower extremity: medial contracture, lateral weakness; if deficient, difficulty closing the eyes, insomnia; if in excess, difficulty opening the eyes, somnolence.

Pathway

From KID-2 ➔ KID-6 ➔ KID-8 ➔ leg ➔ torso ➔ ST-12 ➔ ST-9 ➔ BL-1 (meeting point with the *Yin Qiao Mai*).

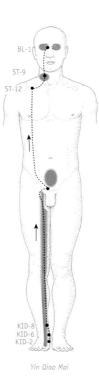

Yin Qiao Mai

4.5.5 Du Mai – governing vessel (Du)

Sea of *Yang*	Opening point: S.I.-3	28 points

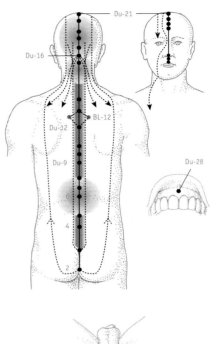

Function

- Governs and supervises all *Yang* and the *Yang* meridians, which meet at Du-14.

Indications

Disorders due to Wind and Cold, fever, spinal pain, psychoemotional disorders.

External pathway

Emerges between the anus and the tip of the coccyx → ascends along the posterior midline → passing the spinous processes, it reaches the external occipital protuberance → follows the midline of the sagittal sinus → traverses the head to its anterior aspect → descends the forehead, nose and upper lip → terminates at Du-28 inside the mouth at the superior frenulum.

Internal pathway and connections

Originates in the lower abdomen (as with the *Ren Mai* and *Chong Mai*, the uterus and penis respectively are considered as its origin) → emerges at the perineum; ascends within the spine to the occiput (Du-16) → there enters the brain → ascends to the vertex → reaches the nose via the forehead.

The *Du Mai* connects with the BL meridian in the scapular region (BL-12). On the thorax, branches emerge segmentally from the spine. From Du-1, a branch ascends the anterior midline parallel to the *Ren Mai* and *Chong Mai*.

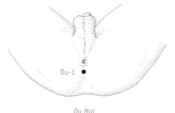

Du Mai

Specific points on the *Ren Mai*

Back-*Shu* point	BL-16
Opening point	S.I.-3
Master point	Du-4 (sexuality point), Du-14 (exhaustion), Du-19 (mental exhaustion, lack of concentration)
Time of maximum activity	None

4.5.6 *Yang Qiao Mai*

Yang motility vessel   Opening point: BL-62   13 points

Points

BL59 to	G.B.-	G.B.-	S.I.-	L.I.-	L.I.-	ST-4	ST-3	BL-1	Du-16
BL-62	20	29	10	15	16				

Partner

Du Mai

Function

- Promotes the smooth flow of *Qi* along the lateral aspect of the leg, thereby supporting harmonious movement
- Auxiliary meridian of the *Du Mai*
- External rotation of the leg
- Opening the eyelid.

Indications

- Epilepsy, headaches
- Redness of the inner canthus of the eye
- Vertigo, mental restlessness, insomnia
- Lower extremity: lateral contracture, medial weakness; highly acute arthritis, severe lumbago
- If deficient, difficulty opening the eyes – somnolence; if in excess, difficulty closing the eyes – insomnia.

Pathway

Predominantly uses points on the BL and G.B. meridians: BL-62 ➔ BL-61 ➔ BL-59 ➔ G.B.-29 ➔ S.I.-10 ➔ L.I.-15 ➔ L.I.-16 ➔ ST-4 ➔ ST-3 ➔ ST-1 ➔ BL-1 ➔ G.B.-20.

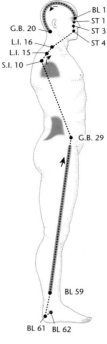

Yang Qiao Mai

4.5.7 Dai Mai

Girdling vessel	Opening point: G.B.-41	4 points

Points

LIV-13	G.B.-26	G.B.-27	G.B.-28

Partner

Yang Wei Mai

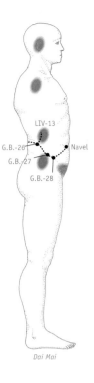

Dai Mai

Function

- Holds together all extraordinary and regular meridians at the waist
- Provides balance between Above and Below.

Indications

- Musculoskeletal system: disorders of the big joints, highly acute lumbago, weakness of the lower extremities
- Pelvic spasms, uterine prolapse, leukorrhoea, abdominal distension, sagging waist
- Headaches and abdominal stagnation (in women).

Pathway

Encircles the middle of the body like a corset ➜ iliac crest, connects all meridians on the torso.

4.5.8 *Yang Wei Mai*

Keeper of the *Yang*   Opening point: T.B.-5   15 points

Points

G.B.-13 to   G.B.-35   S.I.-10   BL-63   T.B.-15   Du-15   Du-16
G.B.-21

Partner

Dai Mai

Function

• Controls the Exterior (surface of the body)

• Connects the *Yang* meridians and holds them together.

Indications

• Acute infection with fever and chills

• Subacute or chronic arthritis, cervical syndrome

• Torticollis, shoulder pain

• Disorders affecting the small joints

• Dermatological disorders with hot sensations – acne, boils

• Headaches, migraines, vertigo.

Pathway

Wide pathway, ascending the dorsolateral aspect of the body → BL-63 → G.B.-35 → S.I.-10 (meeting point with the *Yang Qiao Mai*) → T.B.-15 → G.B.-21 → G.B.-13 → G.B.-14 → G.B.-15 → G.B.-16 → G.B.-17 → G.B.-18 → G.B.-19 → G.B.-20 → Du-16 → Du-15.

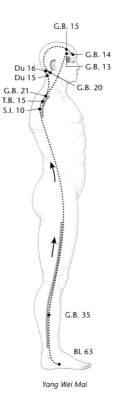

Yang Wei Mai

4.5.9 The extraordinary meridians: overview
(→ Table 2.9)

Extraordinary meridian	Pathway	Partner	Opening point	Common indications
Yin Wei Mai Yin-regulating meridian	Ascends in a broad band antero-laterally ➔ leg ➔ torso; points on the LIV, KID, SP meridians, Ren Mai	**Chong Mai**	P-6	• Disorders of the thorax and the Heart, Stomach[a] • Congenital organ insufficiency (Jing disorders), hypothyroidism (Ren-22 or Ren-23)[b]
Chong Mai Distributor of Energy, Sea of the 12 meridians, Sea of Blood, and the organs	External branch: Ren-1, KID-11 to KID-21 Internal branch: along the spine!	**Yin Wei Mai**	SP-4	
Ren Mai Conception vessel, Sea of Yin meridians	Ascends the anterior midline: perineum ➔ chin An internal branch ascends the spine, parallel to the Du Mai and Chong Mai	**Yin Qiao Mai**	LU-7	• Disorders of the neck, thorax, Lungs[a] • Yin disorders, in women combined with fluid disorders[b]
Yin Qiao Mai Yin motility vessel	A narrow strip on the front of the body, from leg ➔ torso Points: (KID-2), KID-6, KID-8, BL-1 (meeting point with the Yin Qiao Mai)	**Ren Mai**	KID-6	
Du Mai Governing vessel, Sea of Yang meridians	On the posterior midline: perineum ➔ philtrum	**Yang Qiao Mai**	S.I.-3	• Disorders of the occiput, shoulders, back, inner canthus of the eye[a] • Especially in men: spasms, contractures, joint disorders, disorders of the central nervous system[b]
Yang Qiao Mai Yang motility vessel	On the posterior aspect of the body, narrow ➔ parallel to the Du Mai Points: especially on the BL and G.B. meridians	**Du Mai**	BL-62	
Yang Wei Mai Yang-regulating meridian	On the posterolateral aspect of the flanks, wide pathway ascending the dorsolateral aspect of the body ➔ temple Points: especially on the BL, G.B., T.B. meridians and the Du Mai	**Dai Mai**	T.B.-5	• Disorders in the retroauricular region, cheek and outer canthus of the eye[a] • Migraines plus menstrual disorders, joint disorders[b]
Dai Mai Girdling vessel	Like a corset around the middle of the body ➔ iliac crest ➔ connects all meridians at the level of the waist Points: LIV-13, G.B.-26 to G.B.-28	**Yang Wei Mai**	G.B.-41	

[a]Cheng Xinnong 1987
[b]Low 1983

5

Acupuncture points

G. Kubiena

5.1 Meridian points

A total of 361 acupuncture points ($\to$ 5.2.6), which can be considered as reflex zones or projection zones of internal structures, are located on the meridians. In acupressure, the 'points' (Chinese: openings, areas of access) are stimulated through massage, whereas in acupuncture, stimulation is achieved by the insertion of needles ($\to$ 3.3 for methods and techniques).

As well as the meridian points, there is a multitude of extra points originating from different sources. In addition, there are so-called 'extra-meridian', 'new points' or 'auxiliary points'. Section 5.3 uses the nomenclature that has recently achieved legal status in China, as well as the synonymous point names (extra points $\to$ 5.3).

All acupuncture points have a **local effect**, for example on the knee, and a **regional effect**, for example on the leg. The latter is determined by the meridian pathway. When selecting a point for its regional effect, not only the individual meridian, but also the corresponding meridian (six channel pairing), should be taken into consideration. Many points have additional, more universal, actions; for example, they might affect general or fluid metabolism, or they might have a calming effect. Among the meridian points there are several groups of specific point categories that are selected for use with special techniques or point combinations.

5.2 Specific point categories

On each meridian, important points with specific therapeutic indications can be found. The names of these groups of points often describe their specific characteristics, for example sedating/tonifying points or whether a point is indicated for acute or more chronic conditions.

5.2.1 Specific points on the torso – segmentally active points

Back-*Shu* points

These points are generally located at the same level as the organ after which they are named. The textural quality of the point – convex, concave, or sensitive on pressure – indicates either excess or deficiency, but in any case a disharmony of the associated organ. Treatment should be tailored accordingly.

Location: on the back, on the inner branch of the Bladder meridian.

Indications: Primarily for disorders of the *Yin* organs (*Zang*), often used in combination with the relevant *Yuan*-source points.

Front-*Mu* points

Like the back-*Shu* points, these indicate disharmonies of the internal organs.

Location: on the anterior aspect of the torso (exception: G.B.-25 for the Kidneys). They are located in either of the following three locations:

1. On the corresponding meridian:

Lung	Gall Bladder	Liver
LU-1	G.B.-24	LIV-14

2. On the *Ren Mai*:

Stomach	Heart	Small Intestine
Ren-12	Ren-14	Ren-4
Bladder	**Pericardium**	**Triple Burner**
Ren-3	Ren-17	Ren-5

3. On another meridian:

Large Intestine	Spleen	Kidneys
ST-25	LIV-13	G.B.-25

Indications: Primarily for treatment of the *Yang* organs (*Fu*), often in combination with the corresponding lower *He*-sea point (→ 5.2.2). Front-*Mu* points are commonly used together with the associated back-*Shu* point to ensure an organ is reached.

Yuan-source points (top row, blue) and back-*Shu* points (bottom row, black)

Lung	Large Intestine	Stomach	Spleen	Heart	Small Intestine	Bladder	Kidney	Pericardium	Triple Burner	Gall Bladder	Liver	Ren Mai
BL-13	BL-25	BL-21	BL-20	BL-15	BL-27	BL-28	BL-23	BL-14	BL-22	BL-19	BL-18	BL-24 (Ren-6)
LU-9	L.I.-4	ST-42	SP-3	HE-7	S.I.-4	BL-64	KID-3	P-7	T.B.-4	G.B.-40	LIV-3	BL-26 (Ren-4)

Front-*Mu* points, back-*Shu* points (blue); 3rd row: *He*-sea points and lower *He*-sea points (in brackets)

Lung	Large Intestine	Stomach	Spleen	Heart	Small Intestine	Bladder	Kidney	Pericardium	Triple Burner	Gall Bladder	Liver
LU-1	ST-25	Ren-12	LIV-13	Ren-14	Ren-4	Ren-3	G.B.-25	Ren-17, (P-1, KID-11)	Ren-5,7,12,17	G.B.-24	LIV-14
BL-13	BL-25	BL-21	BL-20	BL-15	BL-27	BL-28	BL-23	BL-14	BL-22	BL-19	BL-18
	(ST-37)	ST-36			(ST-39)	BL-40			(BL-39)	G.B.-34	

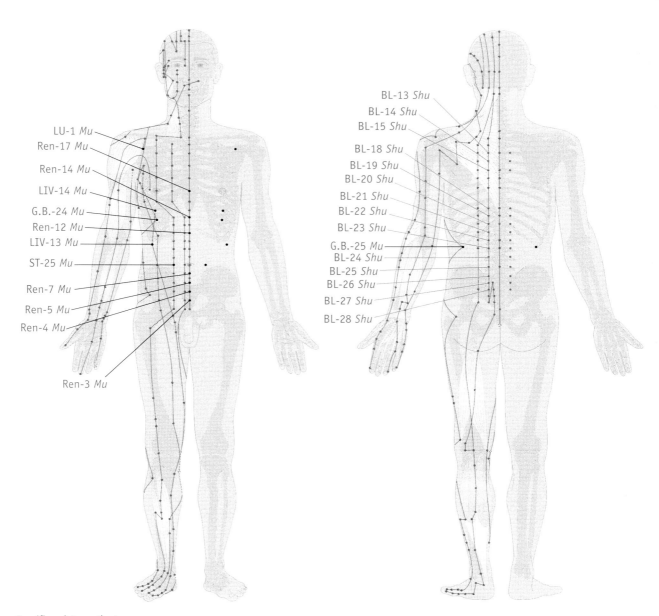

LU-1 *Mu*
Ren-17 *Mu*
Ren-14 *Mu*
LIV-14 *Mu*
G.B.-24 *Mu*
Ren-12 *Mu*
LIV-13 *Mu*
ST-25 *Mu*
Ren-7 *Mu*
Ren-5 *Mu*
Ren-4 *Mu*
Ren-3 *Mu*

BL-13 *Shu*
BL-14 *Shu*
BL-15 *Shu*
BL-18 *Shu*
BL-19 *Shu*
BL-20 *Shu*
BL-21 *Shu*
BL-22 *Shu*
BL-23 *Shu*
G.B.-25 *Mu*
BL-24 *Shu*
BL-25 *Shu*
BL-26 *Shu*
BL-27 *Shu*
BL-28 *Shu*

Specific points on the torso

5.2.2 Specific points on the extremities

Yuan-source points

Each of the 12 regular meridians has a Yuan-source point. The name refers to the source Qi (Yuan Qi), which originates in the Essence (Jing). If a Yuan-source point is found to be swollen, depressed or sensitive to pressure, this indicates a disharmony of the relevant organ.

Location: on the Yin meridians the Yuan-source point is identical with the Shu-stream point. It is therefore always the 3rd point proximal to the tips of the extremities (e.g. HE-7). This rule does not apply to the Yang meridians, where the Yuan-source points are the 4th point proximal to the tips of the extremities (exception: G.B.-40).

Indications: predominantly for disorders affecting the Yin organs; often used in combination with the relevant back-Shu point.

Yuan-source points

Lung	Large Intestine	Stomach	Spleen	Heart	Small Intestine	Bladder	Kidney	Pericardium	Triple Burner	Gall Bladder	Liver
LU-9	L.I.-4	ST-42	SP-3	HE-7	S.I.-4	BL-64	KID-3	P-7	T.B.-4	G.B.-40	LIV-3
BL-13	BL-25	BL-21	BL-20	BL-15	BL-27	BL-28	BL-23	BL-14	BL-22	BL-19	BL-18

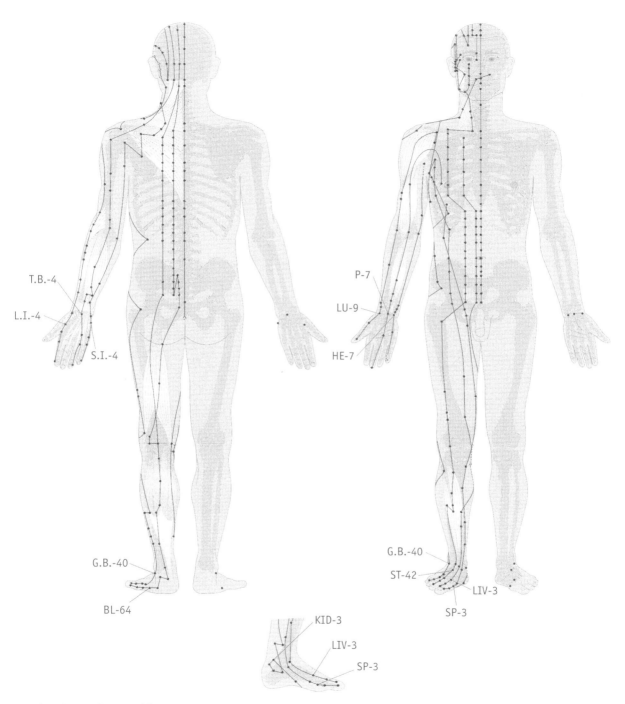

T.B.-4

L.I.-4

S.I.-4

P-7

LU-9

HE-7

G.B.-40

BL-64

G.B.-40

ST-42

LIV-3

SP-3

KID-3

LIV-3

SP-3

Specific points on the extremities

Luo-connecting points

Each regular meridian has a *Luo*-connecting point. Those on *Yin* meridians have a special relationship, via the divergent channels, to the sensory organ associated with the relevant meridian. *Luo*-connecting points can also be found on two of the extraordinary meridians, the *Du Mai* (Du-1) and the *Ren Mai* (Ren-15).

In addition there are the great *Luo*-connecting points of the Spleen (SP-21) and, less frequently mentioned, the Stomach (Ren-12, Ren-17 needled towards the left ST-18).

Location: proximal to the *Yuan*-source points.

Indications: disorders of the sensory organs, disorders progressing from one *Yin/Yang* partner to the other, for example onset of a common cold with sneezing/coughing (Lung), followed by diarrhoea (Large Intestine). In this case, the selected points would be the *Yuan*-source point of the initially affected meridian (here, LU-9) combined with the *Luo*-connecting point of the secondarily affected organ (here, L.I.-6).

Group *Luo*-connecting points

Group *Luo*-connecting points create a connection between all meridians of one polarity (*Yin* or *Yang*) on a specific extremity. They are selected when the whole group of meridians is affected.

Location: → Figure.

Luo-connecting points of the 12 regular meridians, the *Du Mai* and *Ren Mai*

Lung	Large Intestine	Stomach	Spleen	Heart	Small Intestine	Bladder	Kidney	Pericardium	Triple Burner	Gall Bladder	Liver	Du Mai	Ren Mai
LU-7	L.I.-6	ST-40	SP-4	HE-5	S.I.-7	BL-58	KID-4	P-6	T.B.-5	G.B.-37	LIV-5	Du-1	Ren-15

The four group *Luo*-connecting points

Upper extremity		Lower extremity	
3 *Yin* meridians	3 *Yang* meridians	3 *Yin* meridians	3 *Yang* meridians
P-5	T.B.-8	SP-6	G.B.-39

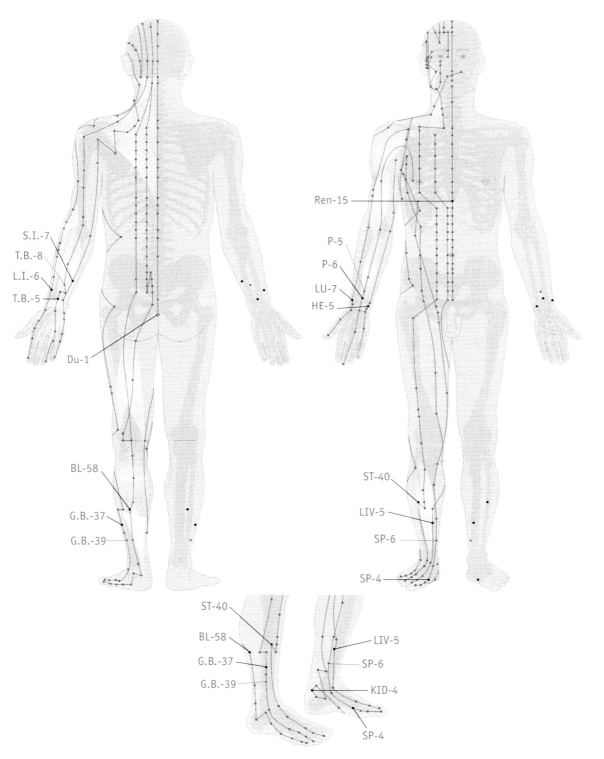

S.I.-7
T.B.-8
L.I.-6
T.B.-5
Du-1

Ren-15
P-5
P-6
LU-7
HE-5

BL-58
G.B.-37
G.B.-39

ST-40
LIV-5
SP-6
SP-4

ST-40
BL-58
G.B.-37
G.B.-39

LIV-5
SP-6
KID-4
SP-4

Group *Luo*-connecting points

The 5 *Shu*-transporting points (5 antique points)

Each regular meridian has 5 points located on the extremities that are assigned to the five elements. The names of these points symbolize the concept that energy increases as it moves from distal to proximal, similar to a smaller stream of water that grows to form a river. At the elbows and knees respectively, the 'rivers' flow (*He* = confluence) into the sea – the energy enters the deeper levels of the body. The sequence of the elements begins distally with Wood (*Yin* meridians) or Metal (*Yang* meridians).

The tonification point corresponds to the element of the 'Mother', whereas the sedation point corresponds to that of the 'Child' of the relevant meridian.

Location: The 1st, 2nd and 3rd meridian points proximal to the tips of the extremities correspond to the 1st to the 3rd *Shu*-transporting points. The 5th point is always located near the knee or the elbow. The 4th *Shu*-transporting point is not necessarily the 4th point on the meridian, but will be located somewhere between the 3rd and 5th points.

Indications:

- All *Jing*-well points: epigastric fullness, irritability, restlessness, insomnia
- All *Ying*-spring points: febrile diseases, heat symptoms
- All *Shu*-stream points: joint disorders, especially if caused by dampness
- All *Jing*-river points: cough due to cold or heat, respiratory disorders, asthma
- All *He*-sea points: counterflow *Qi*, disorders of the *Zang-Fu* organs.

Needling

Shu-transporting points play an important role in chronopuncture (treatment according to the time of day). The most simple method uses the concept of the organ clock and can be easily applied in clinical practice. The *Shu*-transporting point with the correct indication is needled at the time of maximum activity of its meridian (organ clock → 2.3).

Example: for joint disorders, the *Shu*-stream point is selected. If treatment takes place at 8am (time of maximum activity of the Stomach), ST-43 is needled. However, if the patient comes at 2pm, S.I.-3 (time of maximum activity of the Small Intestine) is needled instead.

Tonification points

The tonification points are recruited from the *Shu*-transporting points. Each meridian is associated with a particular element, as are the *Shu*-transporting points. The tonification point is the *Shu*-transporting point, which is associated with the Mother element of the meridian.

1. Meridian points: *Jing*-well points (tonification points [blue], sedation points [black], both in bold)

LU-11	L.I.-1	**ST-45**	SP-1	HE-9	S.I.-1	BL-67	**KID-1**	P-9	T.B.-1	G.B.-44	LIV-1

2. Meridian points: *Ying*-spring points

LU-10	**L.I.-2**	ST-44	SP-2	HE-8	S.I.-2	BL-66	KID-2	P-8	T.B.-2	G.B.-43	**LIV-2**

3. Meridian points: *Shu*-stream points

LU-9	L.I.-3	ST-43	SP-3	**HE-7**	S.I.-3	**BL-65**	KID-3	**P-7**	T.B.-3	G.B.-41	LIV-3

4. Meridian points: *Jing*-river points

LU-8	L.I.-5	ST-41	**SP-5**	HE-4	S.I.-5	BL-60	KID-7	P-5	T.B.-6	**G.B.-38**	LIV-4

5. Meridian points: *He*-sea points

LU-5	L.I.-11	ST-36	SP-9	HE-3	**S.I.-8**	BL-40	KID-10	P-3	**T.B.-10**	G.B.-34	LIV-8

Tonification points (+)

LU-9	L.I.-11	ST-41	SP-2	HE-9	S.I.-3	BL-67	KID-7	P-9	T.B.-3	G.B.-43	LIV-8

Sedation points (−)

LU-5	L.I.-2	ST-45	SP-5	HE-7	S.I.-8	BL-65	KID-1	P-7	T.B.-10	G.B.-38	LIV-2

Sedation points

The same principle applies as for tonification points, except that the sedation point is the point that corresponds to the Child element of the meridian.

Indications: tonification or sedation, particularly in conjunction with chronopuncture.

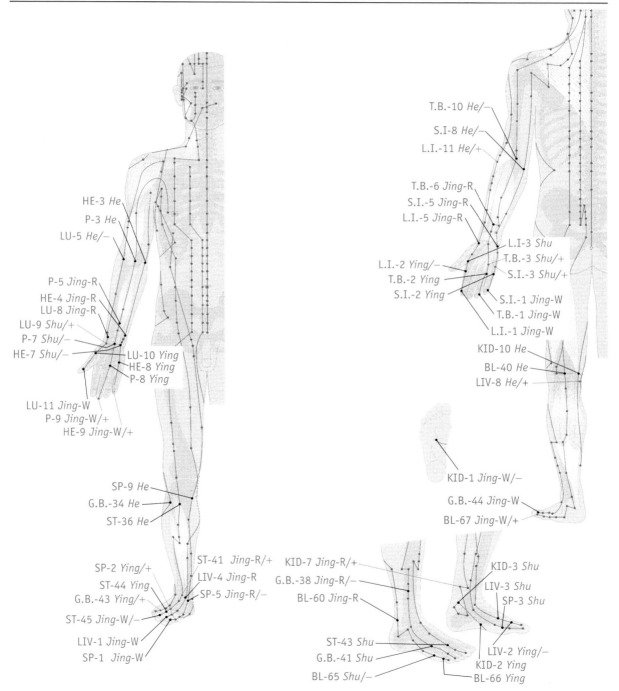

T.B.-10 *He/−*
S.I.-8 *He/−*
L.I.-11 *He/+*

T.B.-6 *Jing-R*
S.I.-5 *Jing-R*
L.I.-5 *Jing-R*

L.I.-3 *Shu*
T.B.-3 *Shu/+*
S.I.-3 *Shu/+*

L.I.-2 *Ying/−*
T.B.-2 *Ying*
S.I.-2 *Ying*

S.I.-1 *Jing-W*
T.B.-1 *Jing-W*
L.I.-1 *Jing-W*

KID-10 *He*
BL-40 *He*
LIV-8 *He/+*

HE-3 *He*
P-3 *He*
LU-5 *He/−*

P-5 *Jing-R*
HE-4 *Jing-R*
LU-8 *Jing-R*
LU-9 *Shu/+*
P-7 *Shu/−*
HE-7 *Shu/−*

LU-10 *Ying*
HE-8 *Ying*
P-8 *Ying*

LU-11 *Jing-W*
P-9 *Jing-W/+*
HE-9 *Jing-W/+*

KID-1 *Jing-W/−*

G.B.-44 *Jing-W*
BL-67 *Jing-W/+*

SP-9 *He*
G.B.-34 *He*
ST-36 *He*

KID-7 *Jing-R/+*
G.B.-38 *Jing-R/−*
BL-60 *Jing-R*

KID-3 *Shu*
LIV-3 *Shu*
SP-3 *Shu*

ST-41 *Jing-R/+*
SP-2 *Ying/+*
LIV-4 *Jing-R*
ST-44 *Ying*
SP-5 *Jing-R/−*
G.B.-43 *Ying/+*
ST-45 *Jing-W/−*
LIV-1 *Jing-W*
SP-1 *Jing-W*

ST-43 *Shu*
G.B.-41 *Shu*
BL-65 *Shu/−*

LIV-2 *Ying/−*
KID-2 *Ying*
BL-66 *Ying*

The 5 *Shu*-tansporting points

Lower He-sea points (Xia He)

In addition to their regular *He*-sea point near the elbow, the three *Yang* meridians of the upper extremity have a lower *He*-sea point below the knee. Although not considered a *Shu*-transporting point, it has a strong action on its associated *Fu* (hollow organ).
Indications: disorders of the *Fu* organs, often combined with the corresponding front-*Mu* point.

The 8 opening points

The 8 opening points (synonym: cardinal points) 'switch on' the extraordinary meridians.
Indications: → Table 4.2.

Xi-cleft points

Xi-cleft points can be found on all 12 regular meridians as well as on four of the extraordinary meridians.
Indications: acute pain conditions or therapy-resistant disorders.

5.2.3 The 8 Hui-meeting points

The *Hui*-meeting points influence organ systems and tissues.
Location: → Figure.
Indications: Disorders affecting the relevant organ system or tissue.

Lower *He*-sea points (*Xia He*)

Large Intestine	Small Intestine	Triple Burner
ST-37	ST-39	BL-39

The 8 opening points (OP)

Chong Mai	Du Mai	Yang Qiao Mai	Yin Qiao Mai	Yin Wei Mai	Yang Wei Mai	Dai Mai	Ren Mai
SP-4	S.I.-3	BL-62	KID-6	P-6	T.B.-5	G.B.-41	LU-7

Xi-cleft points

Lung	Large Intestine	Stomach	Spleen	Heart	Small Intestine	Bladder	Kidney	Pericardium	Triple Burner	Gall Bladder	Liver	Yang Qiao Mai	Yin Qiao Mai	Yang Wei Mai	Yin Wei Mai
LU-6	L.I.-7	ST-34	SP-8	HE-6	S.I.-6	BL-63	KID-5	P-4	T.B.-7	G.B.-36	LIV-6	BL-59	KID-8	G.B.-35	KID-9

The 8 *Hui*-meeting points

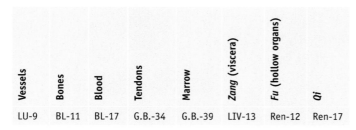

Vessels	Bones	Blood	Tendons	Marrow	Zang (viscera)	Fu (hollow organs)	Qi
LU-9	BL-11	BL-17	G.B.-34	G.B.-39	LIV-13	Ren-12	Ren-17

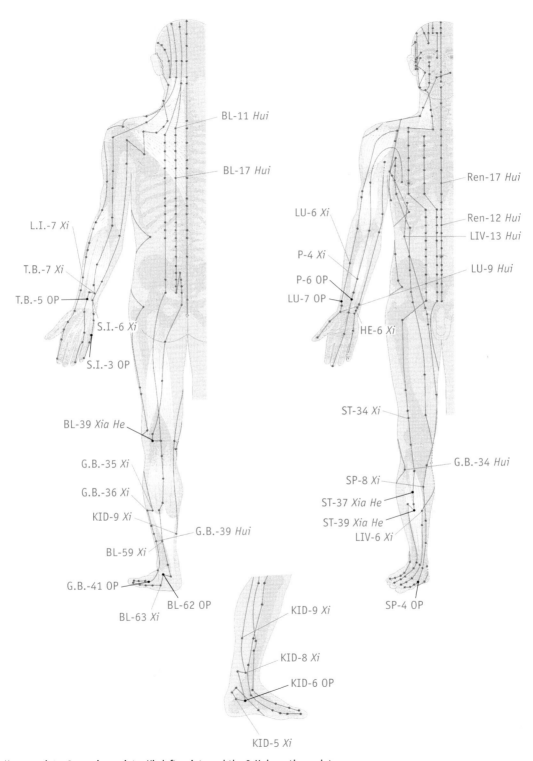

BL-11 *Hui*

BL-17 *Hui*

Ren-17 *Hui*

LU-6 *Xi*

Ren-12 *Hui*

LIV-13 *Hui*

L.I.-7 *Xi*

P-4 *Xi*

LU-9 *Hui*

T.B.-7 *Xi*

P-6 OP

LU-7 OP

T.B.-5 OP

S.I.-6 *Xi*

HE-6 *Xi*

S.I.-3 OP

ST-34 *Xi*

BL-39 *Xia He*

G.B.-34 *Hui*

G.B.-35 *Xi*

SP-8 *Xi*

G.B.-36 *Xi*

ST-37 *Xia He*

KID-9 *Xi*

ST-39 *Xia He*

G.B.-39 *Hui*

LIV-6 *Xi*

BL-59 *Xi*

G.B.-41 OP

BL-62 OP

BL-63 *Xi*

SP-4 OP

KID-9 *Xi*

KID-8 *Xi*

KID-6 OP

KID-5 *Xi*

Lower *He*-sea points, 8 opening points, *Xi*-cleft points and the 8 *Hui*-meeting points

5.2.4 Points according to TCM indications

The six command points

For specific regions of the body/indications.

Chinese master points

These include the 8 *Hui*-meeting points and the opening points, as well as the group *Luo*-connecting points.

5.2.5 Point categories according to European patterns

European master points

This is a European compilation of empirically effective points for specific Western indications (Zeitler 1983).

Metabolic points (after Bischko)

According to Bischko, these points have a particular effect on metabolism. The point selection is determined by the location of the disorder and the specific organ indication.

Metabolic points after Bischko (MetP)

L.I.-2	BL-54	KID-2	LIV-13
L.I.-3	BL-58	KID-6	
L.I.-4			

The 6 command points (CP)

Abdomen	Back (upper and lower)	Head, neck	Face, mouth	Thorax, ribcage	Restoring consciousness
ST-36	BL-40	LU-7	L.I.-4	P-6	Du-26

European master points (euMP); indications in alphabetical order

Indications	Point	Indications	Point
Acne	L.I.-3	Menopause	BL-31
Arm, abduction	L.I.-14	Metabolism point, analgesic point for upper half of body	L.I.-4
Arm, extension	S.I.-9		
Arm, particularly pareses	L.I.-15	Metabolism, activation of	LIV-13
Arm, worse with change in weather	T.B.-15	Musculature	G.B.-34
Arteries, veins	ST-32	Nausea	P-6
Autonomic nervous system, disorders in right-handed persons	Left KID-27	Obstructions, swellings	LU-7
		Pain along Bladder meridian	BL-60
Cardiovascular system, analgesic point for upper half of body	P-6	Pareses of upper extremity	L.I.-15
		Pareses of lower extremities, sciatica (especially lateral), reactive with bone disorders (together with BL-11)	G.B.-30
Claudication, intermittent	BL-58		
Collapse, epileptic seizures	Du-26		
Concentration (difficulty); (Du-20 – in centre of point combination *Si Shen Cong*/Four Alert Spirit)	Du-20	Sexuality, mental and physical exhaustion	Du-4
		Skin disorders affecting the face	LU-5
Connective tissue	SP-5	Sleep, Opening point of the *Yin Qiao Mai*	KID-6
Cough (dry)	Ren-22	Spasmolysis, has effect on mucous membranes (opening point of the *Du Mai*)	S.I.-3
Depression	HE-3		
Diaphragm (breathing)	BL-17	Spasms	LIV-2
Diarrhoea	SP-4	Spasms and colics affecting the epigastrium	Ren-13
Digestion, tonification of the sexual system	ST-30	Spasms, balances the emotions (together with L.I.-4)	LIV-3
Ear: Gate of the ear	T.B.-21		
Exhaustion, impotence, dizziness	Ren-6	Stammering, drooling	Ren-24
Gall Bladder disorders, reactive test point in Gall Bladder disorders	G.B.-14	Stomach (back-*Shu* point)	BL-21
		Stomach and epigastric disorders	Ren-12
Hypertension, hormones	ST-36	Thorax	Ren-17
Hypertension, intercostal neuralgia	P-7	Throat (sore)	LU-11
Insomnia (basic point)	BL-62	Toothache	L.I.-1
Joints (big), opening point of the *Dai Mai*	G.B.-41	Trismus	S.I.-18
Joints (small), opening point of the *Yang Wei Mai*	T.B.-5	Vascular headache, pain following removal of cast	T.B.-4
Knee and foot, analgesic point for lower half of body (together with SP-6); balances the emotions	ST-36		
		Vital energy, sedation: regulates the energy of the nervous system, balances the emotions	Ren-15
Marrow	G.B.-39		

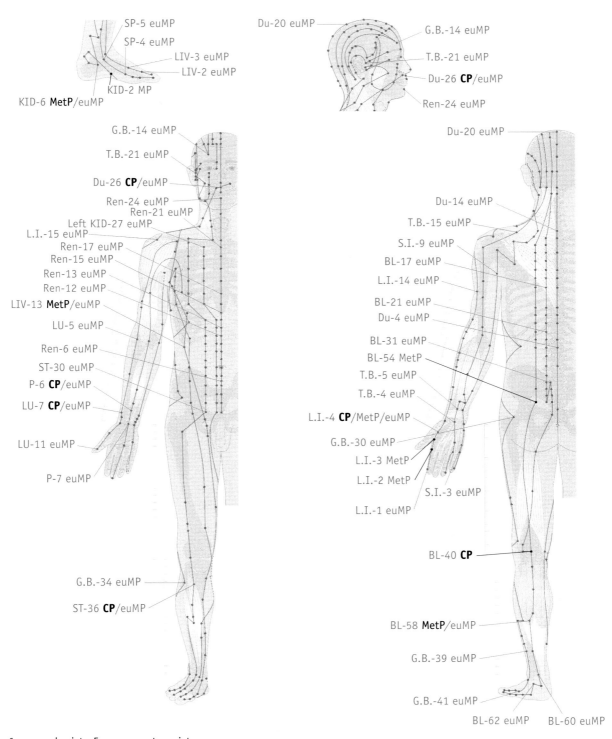

SP-5 euMP
SP-4 euMP
LIV-3 euMP
LIV-2 euMP
KID-2 MP
KID-6 **MetP**/euMP

Du-20 euMP
G.B.-14 euMP
T.B.-21 euMP
Du-26 **CP**/euMP
Ren-24 euMP

G.B.-14 euMP
T.B.-21 euMP
Du-26 **CP**/euMP
Ren-24 euMP
Ren-21 euMP
Left KID-27 euMP
L.I.-15 euMP
Ren-17 euMP
Ren-15 euMP
Ren-13 euMP
Ren-12 euMP
LIV-13 **MetP**/euMP
LU-5 euMP
Ren-6 euMP
ST-30 euMP
P-6 **CP**/euMP
LU-7 **CP**/euMP
LU-11 euMP
P-7 euMP

Du-20 euMP
Du-14 euMP
T.B.-15 euMP
S.I.-9 euMP
BL-17 euMP
L.I.-14 euMP
BL-21 euMP
Du-4 euMP
BL-31 euMP
BL-54 MetP
T.B.-5 euMP
T.B.-4 euMP
L.I.-4 **CP**/MetP/euMP
G.B.-30 euMP
L.I.-3 MetP
L.I.-2 MetP
S.I.-3 euMP
L.I.-1 euMP

BL-40 **CP**

G.B.-34 euMP
ST-36 **CP**/euMP

BL-58 **MetP**/euMP
G.B.-39 euMP
G.B.-41 euMP
BL-62 euMP   BL-60 euMP

6 command points, European master points

5.2.6 Table of the specific meridian points according to their location on the meridians

	Lung	Large Intestine	Stomach	Spleen	Heart	Small Intestine	Bladder	Kidney	Pericardium	Triple Burner	Gall Bladder	Liver	Ren Mai	Du Mai
Back-*Shu* points	1						13–28							
Front-*Mu* points	9		25					11			24, 25	13, 14	3–5, 7, 12, 14, 17	
Yuan-source points	7	4	42	3	7	4	64	3	7	4	40	3		
Luo-connecting points		6	40	4	5	7	58	4	6	5	37	5		
Group *Luo*-connecting points				6					5	8	39			
Jing-well points	11	1	45	1	9	1	67	1	9	1	44	1		
Ying-spring points	10	2	44	2	8	2	66	2	8	2	43	2		
Shu-stream points	9	3	43	3	7	3	65	3	7	3	41	3		
Jing-river points	8	5	41	5	4	5	60	7	5	6	40	4		
He-sea points	5	11	36	9	3	8	40	10	3	10	34	8		
Tonification points	9	11	41	2	9	3	67	7	9	3	43	8		
Sedation points	5	2	45	5	7	8	65	1	7	10	38	2		
Lower *He*-sea points (*Xia He*)			36, 37, 39				39, 40				34			
Opening points	7			4		3	62	6	6	5	41			
Xi-cleft points	6	7	34	8	6	6	63	5	4	7	36	6		
8 *Hui*-meeting points	9						11, 17				34, 39	13	12, 17	

	Lung	Large Intestine	Stomach	Spleen	Heart	Small Intestine	Bladder	Kidney	Pericardium	Triple Burner	Gall Bladder	Liver	*Ren Mai*	*Du Mai*
6 command points	7	4	36				40		6					26
European master points	5, 7,11	1, 4, 14, 15	30, 36	4, 5		3, 6	17, 21, 31, 58, 60, 62	6, 27	6, 7	4, 5	14, 30, 34, 39, 41	2, 3, 13	6, 12, 13, 15, 17, 22, 24	4, 14, 20, 26
Metabolic points		2, 3, 4					54, 58	2, 6				13		

5.3 Extra points

As well as the 361 meridian points, there are also the so-called 'extra points'. An attempt to unravel their nomenclature has now led to the creation of a new system, which was confirmed by law in China in 1991, listing 48 extra points. In the meantime, several authors have introduced other terms for these points, such as '**non-meridian points**' (Punkte außerhalb der Meridiane: König and Wancura), '**points curieux**' (Petricek and Zeitler) and '**new points**' (Neu-Punkte: König and Wancura, Schnorrenberger). The location of these points partially overlaps with the now commonly used nomenclature of extra points. In cases where the old nomenclature is still used frequently, this is also listed in the table of extra points (→ Figure).

Head and neck

Point abbreviation	Pinyin	Translation	Location
Ex-HN-1	*Si Shen Cong*	Four Alert Spirit	1 cun lateral, anterior and posterior to Du-20
Ex-HN-2	*Dang Yang*	Towards the Sun	On the forehead, on the pupil line, 1 cun superior to the anterior hairline
Ex-HN-3	*Yin Tang*	Seal Hall [Bi: *'Point de Merveille'* – miracle point][b]	At the midpoint between the eyebrows
Ex-HN-4	*Yu Yao*	Fish waist	At the midpoint of the eyebrows
Ex-HN-5	*Tai Yang*	Sun (supreme *Yang*)	On the temple, in a depression approx. 1 cun lateral to the midpoint of a line connecting the lateral extremity of the eyebrow and the outer canthus of the eye
Ex-HN-6	*Er Jian*	Tip of the ear	At the highest point of the apex of the ear ('allergy point')
Ex-HN-7	*Qiu Hou*	Behind the eyeball	On the lower margin of the orbit, at the junction of the lateral quarter and medial three-quarters
Ex-HN-8	*Shang Ying Xiang*	Upper *Ying Xiang*[c]	At the superior end of the nasiolabial groove
Ex-HN-9[a]	*Nei Ying Xiang*	Inner *Ying Xiang*[c]	In the nasal cavity, at the junction of the bone and cartilage
Ex-HN-10[a]	*Ju Quan*	Gathering spring	In the centre of the tongue body
Ex-HN-11[a]	*Hai Quan*	Sea spring	In the centre of the frenulum of the tongue
Ex-HN-12[a]	*Jin Jin*	Golden liquid	On the underside of the tongue, on the great lingual vein to the left of the frenulum
Ex-HN-13	*Yu Ye*	Jade fluid	On the underside of the tongue, on the great lingual vein to the right of the frenulum
Ex-HN-14	*Yi Ming*	Shielding brightness	1 cun posterior to T.B.-17 (at the anterior border of the mastoid). Same location as G.B.-12
Ex-HN-15	*(Jing) Bai Lao*	Hundred taxations	2 cun superior to the lower border of the spinous process of C7 and 1 cun lateral to the midline

[a]Not shown in figure
[b]After Bischko: 'miracle point' due to its rapid action for blocked nose and headaches
[c]*Ying Xiang* = L.I.-20

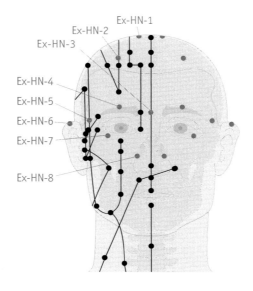

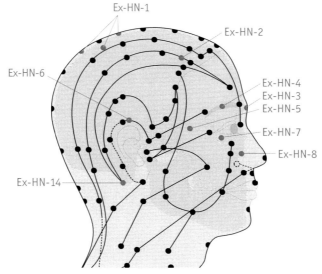

Abdomen

Name	Pinyin	Translation	Location
Ex-CA-1	*Zi Gong*	Palace of the Child, uterus	On the abdomen, 1 cun superior to the upper border of the pubic symphysis (level of Ren-3) and 3 cun lateral to the midline

Back

Name	Pinyin	Translation	Location
Ex-B-1	*Ding Chuan*	Calm dyspnoea	0.5 cun lateral to the spinous process of C7
Ex-B-2	*Hua Tuo Jia Ji*	*Hua Tuo*'s paravertebral points	17 point pairs, 0.5 cun lateral to the lower borders of the spinous processes of T1 to L5; medial to the inner Bladder line
Ex-B-3	*Wei Wan Xia Shu*	Stomach controller lower *Shu*	1.5 cun lateral to the lower border of the spinous process of T8
Ex-B-4	*Pi Gen*	Tumour root	3.5 cun lateral to the lower border of the spinous process of L1
Ex-B-5	*Xia Ji Shu*	*Shu* point for lower back	On midline, below the spinous process of L3
Ex-B-6	*Yao Yi*	Lower back wellbeing	3 cun lateral to the midline, at the level of lower border of the spinous process of L4
Ex-B-7	*Yao Yan*	Lumbar eyes	In the depression that appears when bending over, 3.5 cun lateral to the midline, at the level of the lower border of the spinous process of L4
Ex-B-8	*Shi Qi Zhui*	Below the 17th vertebra	On the midline, below the spinous process of L5
Ex-B-9	*Yao Qi*	Miraculous lumbar point	In a depression 2 cun superior to the tip of the coccyx

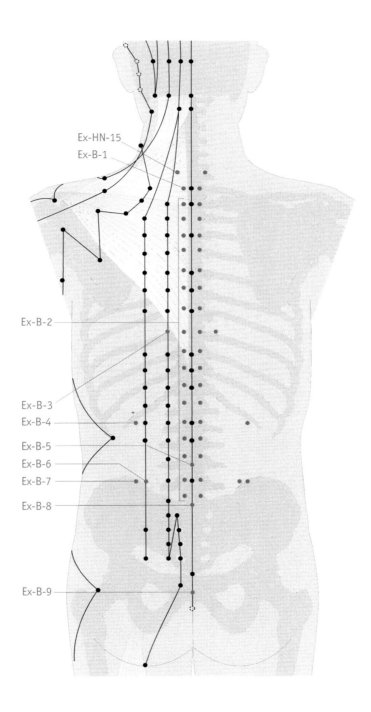

Ex-HN-15

Ex-B-1

Ex-B-2

Ex-B-3

Ex-B-4

Ex-B-5

Ex-B-6

Ex-B-7

Ex-B-8

Ex-B-9

Upper extremity

Name	Pinyin	Translation	Location
Ex-UE-1	Zhou Jian	Elbow tip	On the ulnar aspect of the tip of the olecranon (on the T.B. meridian)
Ex-UE-2	Er Bai	Two whites	A pair of points 4 cun proximal to the wrist crease, on either side of the tendon of the flexor carpi radialis muscle (one point is located on the P meridian)
Ex-UE-3	Zhong Yuan	Middle spring	On the dorsal aspect of the wrist joint, in the depression between the 'anatomical snuffbox' and the centre of the joint space
Ex-UE-4	Zhong Kui	Middle eminence	On the dorsal aspect of the middle finger, in the centre of the proximal interphalangeal joint
Ex-UE-5	Da Gu Kong	Greater bone opening	On the dorsal aspect of the thumb, in the centre of the interphalangeal joint
Ex-UE-6	Xiao Gu Kong	Lesser bone opening	On the dorsal aspect of the hand, in the centre of the proximal interphalangeal joint of the little finger
Ex-UE-7	Yao Tong Xue/Yao Tong Dian	Lumbar pain point	Two points on the dorsal aspect of the hand, between the 2nd/3rd and 4th/5th metacarpal bones, midway between the wrist crease and the metacarpophalangeal joints
Ex-UE-8	Wai Lao Gong/Luo Zhen	Outer Palace of Toil	On the dorsal aspect of the hand, between the 2nd and 3rd metacarpal bones, 0.5 cun proximal to the metacarpophalangeal joints
Ex-UE-9	Ba Xie	Eight pathogens	When a loose fist is made, 4 points on the dorsum of each hand, slightly proximal to the margins of the webs between the heads of the 1st to 5th metacarpal bones
Ex-UE-10	Si Feng	Four seams	On the palmar aspect of the 2nd to 5th fingers, at the midpoint of the transverse creases of the proximal interphalangeal joints
Ex-UE-11	Shi Xuan	Ten diffusions	At the tips of the 10 fingers, approx. 0.1 cun from the free margin of the nail

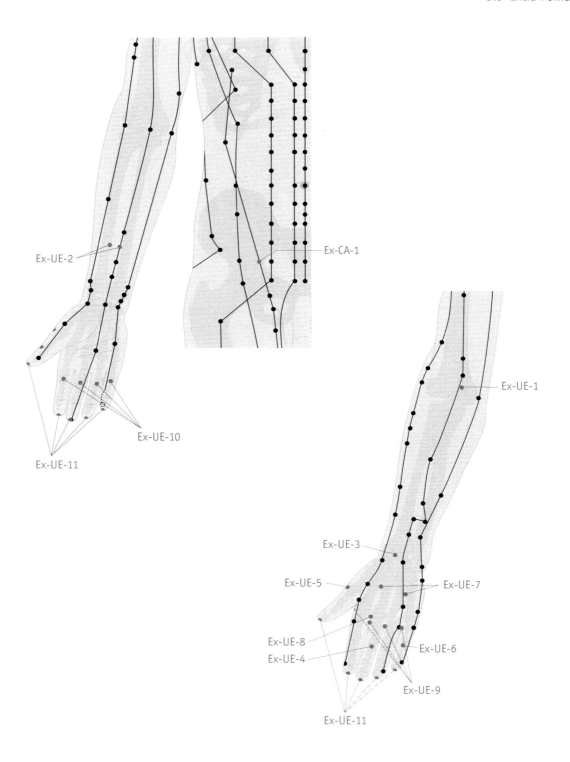

Ex-UE-2

Ex-CA-1

Ex-UE-10

Ex-UE-11

Ex-UE-1

Ex-UE-3

Ex-UE-5

Ex-UE-7

Ex-UE-8

Ex-UE-4

Ex-UE-6

Ex-UE-9

Ex-UE-11

Lower extremity

Name	Pinyin	Translation	Location
Ex-LE-1	*Kuan Gu*	Patella bone	A pair of points 1.5 cun lateral and medial to ST-34 (ST-34: with the knee flexed 2 cun superior to the upper lateral border of the patella)
Ex-LE-2	*He Ding*	Crane's summit	At the midpont of the upper border of the patella
Ex-LE-3	*Bai Chong Wo*	Hundred insect burrow	1 cun superior to SP-10 (SP-10: with the knee flexed 2 cun superior to the upper medial border of the patella, in a depression on the quadriceps femoris)
Ex-LE-4	*Nei Xi Yan*	Inner eye of the knee	With the knee flexed in a depression medial to the patellar ligament (also inner eye of the knee after Bachmann)
Ex-LE-5	*Xi Yan*	Eyes of the knee	With the knee flexed, the inner eye of the knee is medial to the tendon, the outer eye of the knee lateral to the tendon; the latter is identical with ST-35
Ex-LE-6	*Dan Nang Xue*	Gall Bladder point	On the G.B. meridian, 1–2 cun inferior to G.B.-34 (G.B.-34: on anterior border of the head of the fibula)
Ex-LE-7	*Lan Wei Xue*	Appendix point	2 cun inferior to ST-36, on the ST meridian (ST-36: 0.5 cun lateral to anterior crest of the tibia, 1.5 cun inferior to the lower border of the head of the fibula)
Ex-LE-8	*Nei Huai Jian*	Tip of medial malleolus	On the prominence of the medial malleolus
Ex-LE-9	*Wai Huai Jian*	Tip of lateral malleolus	On the prominence of the lateral malleolus
Ex-LE-10	*Ba Feng*	Eight Winds	4 points on the dorsum of the foot, 0.5 cun proximal to the interdigital folds
Ex-LE-11	*Du Yin*	Solitary *Yin*	On the sole of the foot, in the centre of the distal interphalangeal joint of the 2nd toe
Ex-LE-12	*Qi Duan*	*Qi* extremity	On the tips of the 10 toes, approx. 0.1 cun from the free border of the nail; a total of 10 points

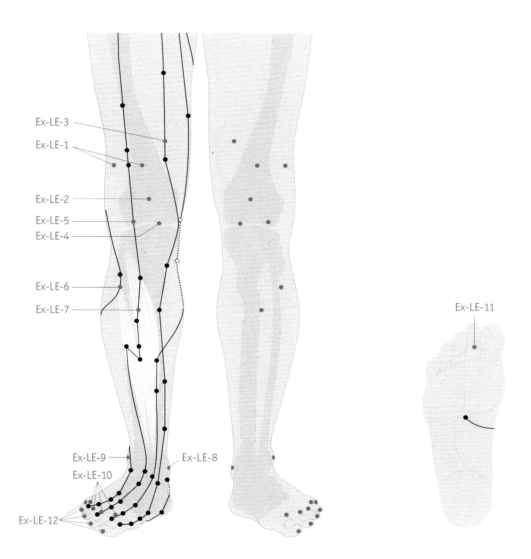

Ex-LE-3

Ex-LE-1

Ex-LE-2

Ex-LE-5
Ex-LE-4

Ex-LE-6

Ex-LE-7

Ex-LE-11

Ex-LE-9
Ex-LE-8
Ex-LE-10

Ex-LE-12

5.4 Auricular points

Adrenal glands (13)
Analgesia (teeth) (7)
Ankle (48)
Anti-aggression (PT1)
Anti-depression (PT3)
Apex of ear (78)
Asthma (31)
Autonomic nervous system (51)
Bladder (92)
Blood pressure regulating point (59)
Blood pressure lowering groove (105)
Brain (hypophysis) (28)
Breast (44)
Carpal bones (67)
Cervical spine (37)
Colon (91)
Elbow (66)
Endocrine system (22)
Fear/jealousy (PT2)

Heel (47)
Heart (21)
Heart (100)
Hip (57)
Hunger (18)
Kidney (95)
Knee (49)
Larynx and pharynx (15)
Liver (97)
Liver I (76)
Liver II (77)
Lumbar pain (54)
Lumbar spine (40)
Lungs (101)
Mandible (6)
Maxilla (5)
Mouth (84)
Ovaries (23)
Pancreas/Gall Bladder (96)

Pituitary gland (26a)
Posterior aspect of head/pillow (29)
Sacrum/coccyx (38)
Shoulder (65)
Shoulder joint (64)
Spirit Gate (*Shen Men*) (55)
Spleen (98)
Stomach (87)
Subcortex (grey matter) (34)
Thoracic spine (39)
Toes (46)
Tonsils I (73)
Tonsils II (74)
Tonsils III (75)
Trachea (103)
Urticaria zone (71)
Uterus (58)

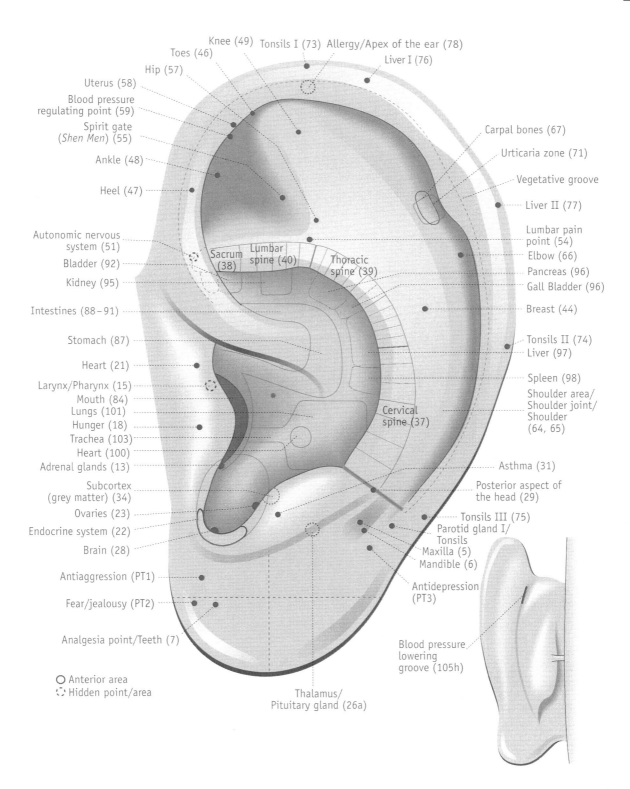

Knee (49) Tonsils I (73) Allergy/Apex of the ear (78)
Toes (46) Liver I (76)
Hip (57)
Uterus (58)
Blood pressure regulating point (59)
Spirit gate (Shen Men) (55)
Ankle (48)
Heel (47)
Autonomic nervous system (51)
Bladder (92)
Kidney (95)
Intestines (88–91)
Stomach (87)
Heart (21)
Larynx/Pharynx (15)
Mouth (84)
Lungs (101)
Hunger (18)
Trachea (103)
Heart (100)
Adrenal glands (13)
Subcortex (grey matter) (34)
Ovaries (23)
Endocrine system (22)
Brain (28)
Antiaggression (PT1)
Fear/jealousy (PT2)
Analgesia point/Teeth (7)

Sacrum (38)
Lumbar spine (40)
Thoracic spine (39)
Cervical spine (37)

Carpal bones (67)
Urticaria zone (71)
Vegetative groove
Liver II (77)
Lumbar pain point (54)
Elbow (66)
Pancreas (96)
Gall Bladder (96)
Breast (44)
Tonsils II (74)
Liver (97)
Spleen (98)
Shoulder area/ Shoulder joint/ Shoulder (64, 65)
Asthma (31)
Posterior aspect of the head (29)
Tonsils III (75)
Parotid gland I/ Tonsils
Maxilla (5)
Mandible (6)
Antidepression (PT3)
Blood pressure lowering groove (105h)

○ Anterior area
⚬ Hidden point/area

Thalamus/ Pituitary gland (26a)

95

5.5 Important points in hand acupuncture

1	*Yao Tui Dian*	Lumbar and leg point	2 points on the dorsum of the hand, between the 2nd/3rd and 4th/5th metacarpal bones, in the depressions just distal to the bases of the metacarpals	Acute lower back pain
2	*Huai Dian*	Ankle point	On the radial aspect of the metacarpophalangeal joint of the thumb, at the junction of the red and white skin (LU)	Any pain or disorder of the ankle
3	*Xiong Dian*	Chest point	On the radial aspect of the thumb joint (LU)	Intercostal neuralgia, any pain of the thoracic region, e.g. herpes zoster, contusion; vomiting, diarrhoea, epilepsy
4	*Yan Dian*	Eye point	On the ulnar aspect of the thumb joint, at the junction of the red and white skin (between LU and L.I.)	Any inflammatory eye disorder: conjunctivitis, hordeolum, keratitis; acute glaucoma attack
5	*Jian Dian*	Shoulder point	On the metacarpophalangeal joint of the index finger, at the junction of the red and white skin, between L.I.-2 and L.I.-3	Any shoulder pain, especially if due to Cold; humeroscapular periarthritis
6	*Qian Tou Dian*	Forehead point	On the radial aspect of the proximal interphalangeal joint of the index finger, at the junction of the red and white skin	Frontal headaches, stomach cramps, acute gastroenteritis, toe and knee pain
7	*Tou Ding Dian*	Vertex point	On the radial aspect of the proximal interphalangeal joint of the middle finger, at the junction of the red and white skin (P)	Neuralgic vertex headaches
8	*Pian Tou Dian*	Hemicrania point	On the ulnar aspect of the proximal interphalangeal joint of the ring finger, at the junction of the red and white skin (T.B.)	Temporal headaches, migraines, flank pain, biliary colic
9	*Hui Yin Dian*	Perineum	On the radial aspect of the proximal interphalangeal joint of the little finger, at the junction of the red and white skin (HE)	Pain in the perineum, e.g. due to fissures, haemorrhoids, boils
10	*Hou Tou Dian*	Back of the head point	On the ulnar aspect of the proximal interphalangeal joint of the little finger, at the junction of the red and white skin (S.I.)	Occipital headaches, occipital neuralgia, acute tonsillitis, cheek/arm pain; belching
11	*Ji Zhu Dian*	Spine point	Between S.I.-2 and S.I.-3, directly above the metacarpophalangeal joint of the little finger (S.I.)	Disorders of the spine, e.g. following distortion or surgery; lumbago, coccygodynia; tinnitus, blocked nose
12	*Zuo Gu Shen Jing Dian*	Sciatic nerve point	On the dorsum of the hand, between the metacarpophalangeal joints of the 4th and 5th finger, but closer to the 4th	Sciatica, pain in the gluteal region and hip joint
13	*Xan Hou Dian*	Pharynx, larynx and neck point	On the dorsum of the hand, between the metacarpophalangeal joints of the 3rd and 4th finger, but closer to the 3rd (between P and T.B.)	Acute tonsillitis, pharyngitis, laryngitis, trigeminal neuralgia, tooth pain
14	*Jing Xiang Dian*	Neck and throat point	On the dorsum of the hand, between the metacarpophalangeal joints of the 2nd and 3rd finger, but closer to the 2nd (between P and L.I.)	Cervical syndrome, distortion of the cervical spine

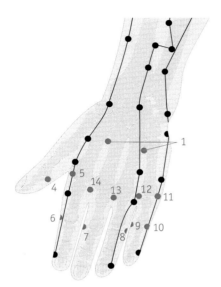

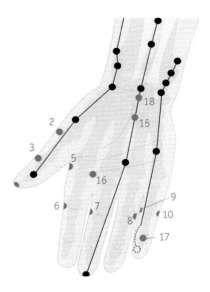

15	*Wei Chang Dian*	Gastrointestinal point	On the palm, on the midpoint between P-7 and P-8 (P)	Acute or chronic gastroenteritis, duodenal/ventricular ulcers, dyspepsia, ascarides in the biliary tract
16	*Ke Chuan Dian*	Cough and asthma point	On the palm, on the ulnar aspect of the metacarpophalangeal joint of the 2nd finger	Bronchitis, bronchial asthma, (neuralgic) headaches
17	*Ye Niao Dian*	Nocturia point	On the palmar aspect of the little finger, on the midpoint of crease of the distal interpahlangeal joint (HE)	Nocturia, frequent micturition
18	*Zu Gen Dian*	Heel point	On the palm, midway between Hand-15 and P-7 (on the life line, midway between Hand-15 and P-7)	Heel pain

5.6 Meridian points

Point	Pinyin	Translation	Location	Action
Lung meridian				
LU-1	*Zhong Fu*	Middle Palace	Find LU-2 first, LU-1 is located directly below in the 1st intercostal space (ICS). Caution: pneumothorax!	• Front-*Mu* point of the Lung • Meeting point with the Spleen meridian
LU-2	*Yun Men*	Cloud Gate	On the lower border of the clavicle, 6 cun lateral to the anterior midline. Caution: pneumothorax!	
LU-3	*Tian Fu*	Palace of Heaven	On the lateral border of the biceps, 3 cun inferior to the axillary fold. Zeitler: when the biceps is pressed against the nose, it will rest on LU-3	
LU-4	*Xia Bai*	Clasping the white	On the lateral border of the biceps, 4 cun inferior to the axillary fold	
LU-5	*Chi Ze*	Cubit marsh	On the cubital crease, radial to the tendon of the biceps	• Sedation point • *He*-sea point
LU-6	*Kong Zui*	Maximum opening	7 cun superior to the wrist crease, on a line connecting LU-5 (on the cubital crease, radial to the tendon of the biceps) and LU-9 (on the wrist crease, radial to the radial artery)	*Xi*-cleft point
LU-7	*Lie Que*	Broken sequence	1.5 cun proximal to the wrist crease, radial to the radial artery	• *Luo*-connecting point • Opening point of the *Ren Mai* • European master point stagnation
LU-8	*Jing Qu*	Channel gutter	Radial to the radial artery, 1 cun proximal to the wrist crease	*Jing*-river point
LU-9	*Tai Yuan*	Supreme abyss	On the wrist crease, radial to the radial artery	• *Shu*-stream point • *Yuan*-source point • *Hui*-meeting point of the vessels • Master point: blood vessels • Tonification point
LU-10	*Yu Ji*	Fish border	At the midpont of the 1st metacarapal bone, at the junction of the red and white skin	*Ying*-spring point
LU-11	*Shao Shang*	Lesser *Shang*	On the thumb, next to the radial corner of the nail [Bi: ulnar]	• *Jing*-well point • Master point for throat disorders

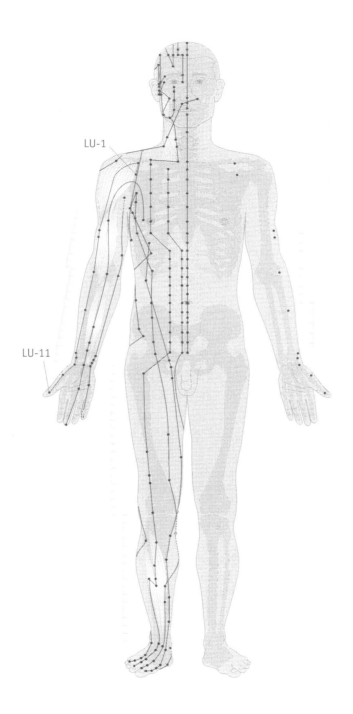

LU-1

LU-11

Point	Pinyin	Translation	Location	Action
Large Intestine meridian				
L.I.-1	*Shang Yang*	*Shang Yang*	On the index finger, next to the radial corner of the nail	• *Jing*-well point • European master point for toothache
L.I.-2	*Er Jian*	Second space	With the hand in a fist that curls around the thumb, in the depression distal to the metacarpophalangeal joint, at the junction of the red and white skin	• *Ying*-spring point • Sedation point • Metabolic point
L.I.-3	*San Jian*	Third space	With the hand in a fist that curls around the thumb, in the depression distal to the metacarpophalangeal joint, at the junction of the red and white skin	• *Shu*-stream point • Metabolic point • European master point for acne
L.I.-4	*He Gu*	Joining valley	On the dorsum of the hand, at the highest point of the muscle bulge between the 1st and 2nd metacarpal bones	• *Yuan*-source point • Standard fever protocol: L.I.-4, L.I.-11, Du-14 • Connection to the *Luo*-connecting point of the Lung (LU-7)
L.I.-5	*Yang Xi*	Yang-stream	On the radial aspect of the wrist crease, in a depression between the tendons of the extensor pollicis brevis and extensor carpi radialis longus. Tip for locating the wrist crease: hold the patient's wrist between two fingers and ask him or her to flex the wrist. S.I.-5 is on its ulnar aspect, L.I.-5 on its radial aspect	*Jing*-river point
L.I.-6	*Pian Li*	Veering passage	On the radial aspect of the forearm, on the lateral border of the radius, 3 cun proximal to the wrist crease. Tip: cross the thumbs so that the webs between the thumb and index finger touch; with the index finger reach over the dorsum of the hand so that the tip of the middle finger rests on LU-7 (radial pulse), the tip of the index finger on L.I.-6	*Luo*-connecting point (to LU-9)
L.I.-7	*Wen Liu*	Warm flow	On a line connecting L.I.-5 and L.I.-11, 5 cun proximal to the wrist crease (or L.I.-5)	*Xi*-cleft point
L.I.-8	*Xia Lian*	Lower angle	On a line connecting L.I.-5 and L.I.-11, 4 cun distal to L.I.-11	
L.I.-9	*Shang Lian*	Upper angle	2 cun distal to L.I.-11, on the lateral border of the muscle belly of the extensor digitorum communis	

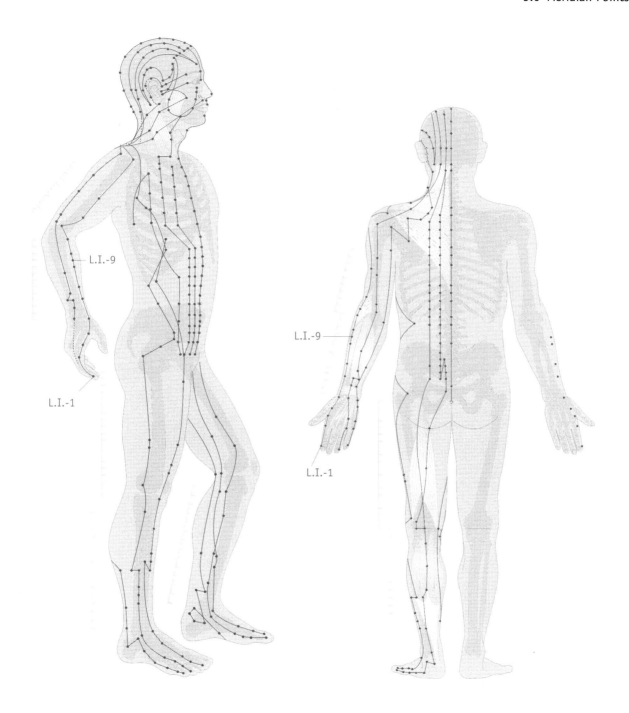

L.I.-9

L.I.-1

L.I.-9

L.I.-1

Point	Pinyin	Translation	Location	Action
Large Intestine meridian				
L.I.-10	*Shou San Li*	Arm three miles	On the radial aspect of the forearm, 3 cun distal to L.I.-11, on the belly of the extensor muscles	
L.I.-11	*Qu Chi*	Pool at the crook	With the arm fully flexed at the radial end of the cubital crease	• *He*-sea point • Tonification point
L.I.-12	*Zhou Liao*	Elbow crevice	With the elbow flexed 1 cun superior to L.I.-11, 2 cun superior to the lateral epicondyle, on the border of the brachioradialis	
L.I.-13	*Shou Wu Li*	Arm five miles	3 cun superior to L.I.-11, on the line connecting L.I.-11 (at the lateral end of the cubital crease) and L.I.-15 (in the depression anterior to the acromioclavicular joint)	
L.I.-14	*Bi Nao*	Upper arm	On the lateral aspect of the upper arm, slightly superior and anterior to the insertion of the deltoid	Meeting point with the ST, L.I. meridians and the *Yang Qiao Mai*
L.I.-15	*Jian Yu*	Shoulder bone	With the arm abducted, in the anterior of the two depressions inferior to the acromioclavicular joint, between the anterior and medial third of the deltoid (T.B.-14 is located in the posterior depression)	• European master point: paresis of the upper extremity • Meeting point with the *Yang Qiao Mai*
L.I.-16	*Ju Gu*	Great bone	With the arm abducted in a depression between the acromial end of the clavicle and the scapular spine	Meeting point with the *Yang Qiao Mai*
L.I.-17	*Tian Ding*	Heaven's tripod	On the posterior border of the sternocleidomastoid, 3 cun lateral to the anterior midline, at the level of the lower border of the laryngeal prominence. ST-10 is located on the anterior border of the muscle (level with the midpoint of the thyroid cartilage)	
L.I.-18	*Fu Tu*	Support the prominence	At the level of the laryngeal prominence, between the sternal and clavicular heads of the sternocleidomastoid; ST-9 is located at the same level on the anterior border of the muscle	
L.I.-19	*Kou He Liao*	Mouth grain crevice	Below the lower margin of the nostril. According to Chinese texts the L.I. meridian crosses to the contralateral side at Du-26 – L.I.-19 and L.I.-20 are therefore located on the other side of the body	
L.I.-20	*Ying Xiang*	Welcome fragrance	In the nasiolabial groove, at the level of the midpoint of the lateral border of the ala nasi	Meeting point with the ST meridian

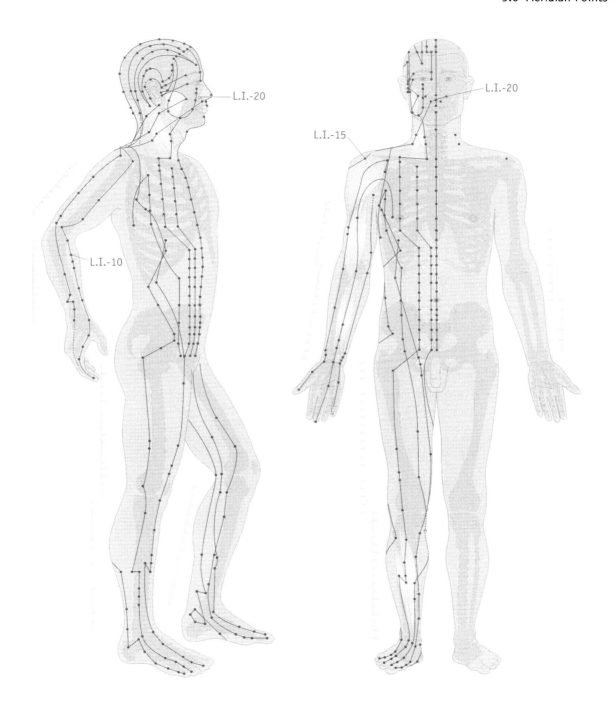

L.I.-20

L.I.-20

L.I.-15

L.I.-10

Point	Pinyin	Translation	Location	Action
Stomach meridian				
ST-1	*Cheng Qi*	Container of tears	On the pupil line, on the lower border of the orbital ridge	Meeting point with the *Ren Mai, Yang Qiao Mai*
ST-2	*Si Bai*	Four whites	On the pupil line, in the depression on the infraorbital foramen	
ST-3	*Ju Liao*	Great crevice	At the intersection of the pupil line and a horizontal line level with the lower border of the ala nasi	Meeting point with the *Yang Qiao Mai*
ST-4	*Di Cang*	Earth granary	1 cun lateral to the corner of the mouth, needle towards the mandibular angle	
ST-5	*Da Ying*	Great welcome	On the anterior border of the mandibular insertion of the masseter – ask the patient to blow their cheeks; the point is where the facial artery can be felt	
ST-6	*Jia Che*	Jaw bone	1 cun anterior and superior to the mandibular angle	
ST-7	*Xia Guan*	Below the joint	At the midpoint of the lower border of the zygomatic arch	
ST-8	*Tou Wei*	Head's binding	At the corner of the forehead, 3 cun superior and 1 cun posterior to the frontozygomatic suture	• Meeting point with the G.B. channel • For dizziness due to Phlegm
ST-9	*Ren Ying*	Man's welcome	On the anterior border of the sternocleidomastoid muscle, at the level of the laryngeal prominence	
ST-10	*Shui Tu*	Water prominence	At the level of the midpoint of the thyroid cartilage, on the anterior border of the sternocleidomastoid; 'Singer's point'	
ST-11	*Qi She*	Abode of *Qi*	On the upper border of the clavicle, at the junction of the shaft and the head, between the clavicular and sternal insertions of the sternocleidomastoid	
ST-12	*Que Pen*	Empty basin	In the centre of the supraclavicular fossa, on the mamillary line	
ST-13	*Qi Hu*	*Qi* door	On the lower border of the clavicle, on the mamillary line, below ST-12	
ST-14	*Ku Fang*	Storehouse	On the mamillary line, in the 1st ICS, at the level of Ren-20	
ST-15	*Wu Yi*	Room screen	On the mamillary line, in the 2nd ICS, at the level of Ren-19	
ST-16	*Ying Chuang*	Breast window	On the mamillary line, in the 3rd ICS, at the level of Ren-18	
ST-17	*Ru Zhong*	Middle of the breast	On the mamillary line, in the 4th ICS, in the centre of the nipple, at the level of Ren-17	

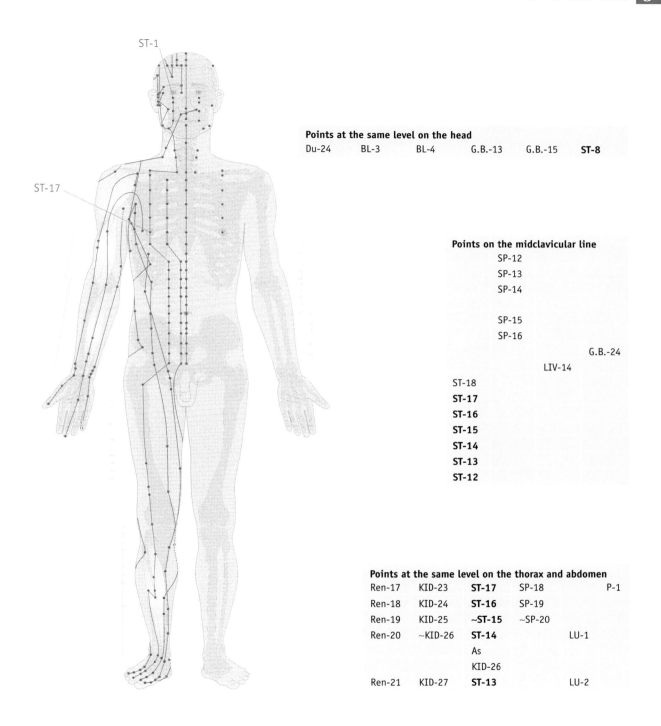

Points at the same level on the head

Du-24	BL-3	BL-4	G.B.-13	G.B.-15	**ST-8**

Points on the midclavicular line

SP-12		
SP-13		
SP-14		
SP-15		
SP-16		
		G.B.-24
	LIV-14	
ST-18		
ST-17		
ST-16		
ST-15		
ST-14		
ST-13		
ST-12		

Points at the same level on the thorax and abdomen

Ren-17	KID-23	**ST-17**	SP-18		P-1
Ren-18	KID-24	**ST-16**	SP-19		
Ren-19	KID-25	**~ST-15**	~SP-20		
Ren-20	~KID-26	**ST-14**		LU-1	
		As			
		KID-26			
Ren-21	KID-27	**ST-13**		LU-2	

105

Point	Pinyin	Translation	Location	Action
Stomach meridian				
ST-18	*Ru Gen*	Root of the breast	On the mamillary line, in the 5th ICS, at the level of Ren-16	
ST-19	*Bu Rong*	Not contained	2 cun lateral to the anterior midline, in the 7th ICS, 6 cun superior to the umbilicus, level with Ren-14	
ST-20	*Cheng Men*	Supporting fullness	2 cun lateral to the anterior midline, 5 cun superior to the umbilicus, level with Ren-13	
ST-21	*Liang Men*	Beam gate (cardia)	2 cun lateral to the midline, level with Ren-12, at the midpoint of the distance between the umbilicus and the xiphoid process	
ST-22	*Guan Men*	Pass gate	2 cun lateral to the midline, level with Ren-11, 3 cun superior to the umbilicus	
ST-23	*Tai Yi*	Supreme unity	2 cun lateral to the midline, level with Ren-10, 2 cun superior to the umbilicus	
ST-24	*Huo Rou Men*	Slippery flesh gate	2 cun lateral to the midline, level with Ren-9, 1 cun superior to the umbilicus	
ST-25	*Tian Shu*	Heaven's pivot	2 cun lateral to the centre of the umbilicus (Ren-8) [Bi: at the midpoint of a line connecting the umbilicus and upper iliac crest]	Front-*Mu* point of the Large Intestine
ST-26	*Wai Ling*	Outer mound	2 cun lateral to the midline, level with Ren-7, 1 cun inferior to the umbilicus [Bi: at the midpoint of a line connecting the umbilicus and anterior superior iliac spine]	
ST-27	*Da Ju*	The great	2 cun lateral to the midline and 2 cun inferior to the umbilicus, level with Ren-5 and KID-14	
ST-28	*Shui Dao*	Water passage	2 cun lateral to the midline and 3 cun inferior to the umbilicus, level with Ren-4	
ST-29	*Gui Lai*	Return	2 cun lateral to the midline and 4 cun inferior to the umbilicus, level with Ren-3 and KID-12	
ST-30	*Qi Chong*	Rushing *Qi*	On the upper border of the pubic symphysis, 2 cun lateral to the midline, level with Ren-2 and KID-11	
ST-31	*Bi Guan*	Thigh gate	At the level of the perineum, on a line connecting the anterior superior iliac spine and the lateral upper border of the patella	
ST-32	*Fu Tu*	Crouching rabbit	6 cun superior to the patella, on the rectus femoris muscle	Meeting point of the arteries and veins

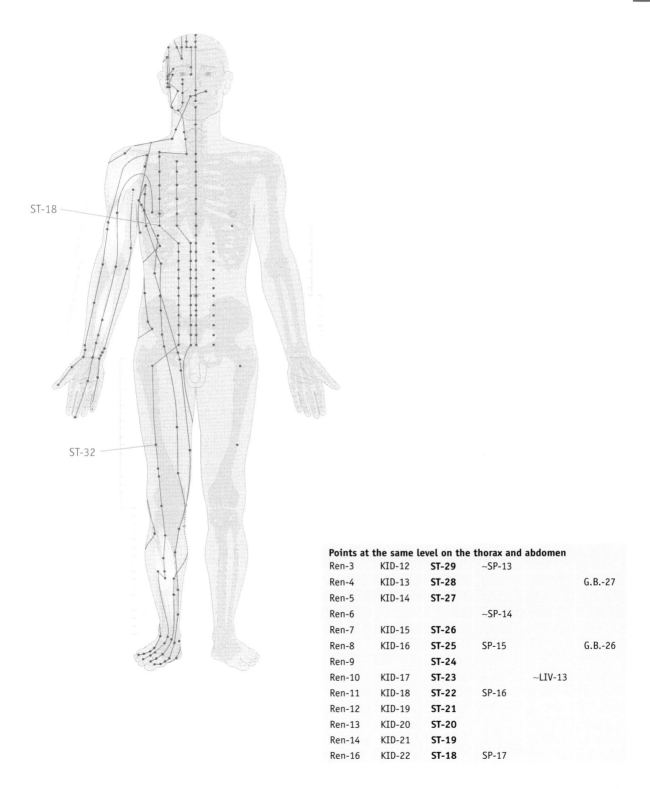

ST-18

ST-32

Points at the same level on the thorax and abdomen

Ren-3	KID-12	**ST-29**	~SP-13		
Ren-4	KID-13	**ST-28**			G.B.-27
Ren-5	KID-14	**ST-27**			
Ren-6			~SP-14		
Ren-7	KID-15	**ST-26**			
Ren-8	KID-16	**ST-25**	SP-15		G.B.-26
Ren-9		**ST-24**			
Ren-10	KID-17	**ST-23**		~LIV-13	
Ren-11	KID-18	**ST-22**	SP-16		
Ren-12	KID-19	**ST-21**			
Ren-13	KID-20	**ST-20**			
Ren-14	KID-21	**ST-19**			
Ren-16	KID-22	**ST-18**	SP-17		

Point	Pinyin	Translation	Location	Action
Stomach meridian				
ST-33	*Yin Shi*	*Yin* market	With the knee flexed, 3 cun superior to the lateral upper border of the patella (in the depression when kneeling)	
ST-34	*Liang Qiu*	Ridge mound	With the knee flexed, in the depression 2 cun superior to the lateral upper border of the patella	*Xi*-cleft point
ST-35	*Du Bi*	Calf's nose	With the knee flexed, in a depression at the lower border of the patella, lateral to the patellar ligament	Part of the extra point 'eyes of the knee'
ST-36	*Zu San Li*	Leg three miles	1 cun lateral to the anterior crest of the tibia, 1.5 cun inferior to the lower border of the head of the fibula (G.B.-34)	• *He*-sea point • European master point: hormones, blood pressure
ST-37	*Shang Ju Xu*	Upper great void	1 cun lateral to the anterior crest of the tibia, 4 cun inferior to the lower border of the head of the fibula or 3 cun inferior to ST-36	Lower *He*-sea point of the Large Intestine
ST-38	*Tiao Kou*	Lines opening	1 cun lateral to the anterior crest of the tibia, 7 cun inferior to lower border of the head of the fibula. At the midpoint of the distance between the highest prominence of the medial malleolus and the knee joint space	For acute shoulder pain
ST-39	*Xia Ju Xu*	Lower great void	1 cun inferior to ST-38	Lower *He*-sea point of the Small Intestine
ST-40	*Feng Long*	Abundant bulge	At the midpoint of the distance between the highest prominence of the medial malleolus and the knee joint space, 2 cun lateral to the anterior crest of the tibia	• *Luo*-connecting point (to SP-3) • Major point for transforming Phlegm • Nickname: 'Bisolvon of acupuncture'
ST-41	*Jie Xi*	Stream divide	At the midpoint of the anterior aspect of the ankle, between the tendons of the extensor hallucis longus and extensor digitorum longus	• Tonification point • *Jing*-river point
ST-42	*Chong Yang*	Rushing *Yang*	On the highest point of the dorsum of the foot, where the dorsalis pedis artery can be palpated	*Yuan*-source point
ST-43	*Xian Gu*	Sunken valley	In the depression distal to the junction of the 2nd and 3rd metatarsal bones	*Shu*-stream point
ST-44	*Nei Ting*	Inner court	On the interdigital fold between the 2nd and 3rd toes, near the metatarsophalangeal joint of the 2nd toe	*Ying*-spring point
ST-45	*Li Dui*	Literally: long passage/strict exchange[a]/ epithet: cruel payment	On the 2nd toe, near the lateral corner of the nail	• *Jing*-well point • Sedation point

[a]Deadman 1998 (p. 172)

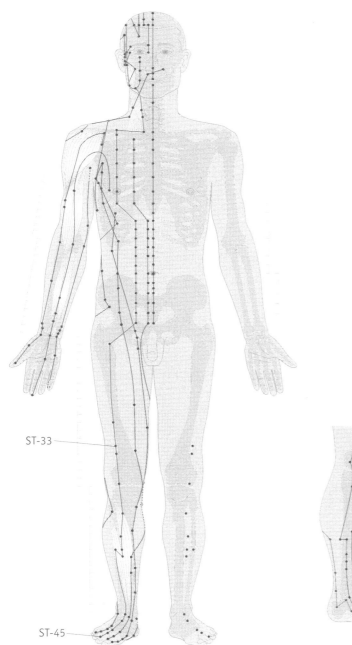

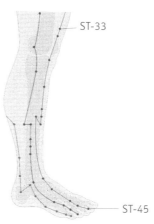

ST-33

ST-45

ST-33

ST-45

Points at the same level on the leg

	G.B.-40	BL-60
	G.B.-39	BL-59
ST-39	G.B.36, G.B.-35	BL-58
ST-38, ST-40		
		BL-39, BL-40

Point	Pinyin	Translation	Location	Action
Spleen meridian				
SP-1	*Yin Bai*	Hidden white	On the big toe, next to the medial corner of the nail	*Jing*-well point
SP-2	*Da Du*	Great metropolis	In the depression over the metatarsophalangeal joint of the big toe, at the junction of the red and white skin	• *Ying*-spring point • Tonification point
SP-3	*Tai Bai*	Supreme white	Just proximal to the metatarsophalangeal joint of the big toe, over the tendon of the abductor hallucis longus	• *Shu*-stream point • *Yuan* source point
SP-4	*Gong Sun*	Grandfather grandson	In the depression at the junction of the base and the shaft of the 1st metatarsal bone, at the junction of the red and white skin	• *Luo*-connecting point • Opening point of the *Chong Mai* • European master point for diarrhoea
SP-5	*Shang Qiu*	Shang mound[a]	With the foot in dorsiflexion in the depression between the tendons of the tibialis anterior and medial malleolus, on the navicular bone	• *Jing*-river point • Sedation point • European master point: connective tissue
SP-6	*San Yin Jiao*	Three *Yin* intersection	3 cun superior to the highest prominence of the medial malleolus, on the posterior border of the tibia	• Group *Luo*-connecting point of the 3 leg *Yin* meridians • Meeting point of the SP, KID, LIV meridians
SP-7	*Lou Gu*	Dripping valley	6 cun superior to the greatest circumference of the medial malleolus (SP-6)	
SP-8	*Di Ji*	Earth pivot	On the posterior border of the tibia, 3 cun inferior to SP-9 (at the same level as G.B.-34, but medial)	*Xi*-cleft point
SP-9	*Yin Ling Quan*	*Yin* mound spring	With the knee flexed, in the depression inferior to the medial condyle of the tibia, at the same level as G.B.-34	*He*-sea point
SP-10	*Xue Hai*	Sea of Blood	With the knee flexed, 2 cun superior to the upper patellar border, medial to the vastus medialis	
SP-11	*Ji Men*	Winnowing gate	With the knee flexed on the medial aspect of the thigh, 8 cun superior to the medial section of the upper patellar border, in the middle of the thigh, in a depression between the sartorius and vastus medialis, close to the femoral artery	

[a]'*Shang*' is the sound associated with the Metal element; SP-5 is the Metal point

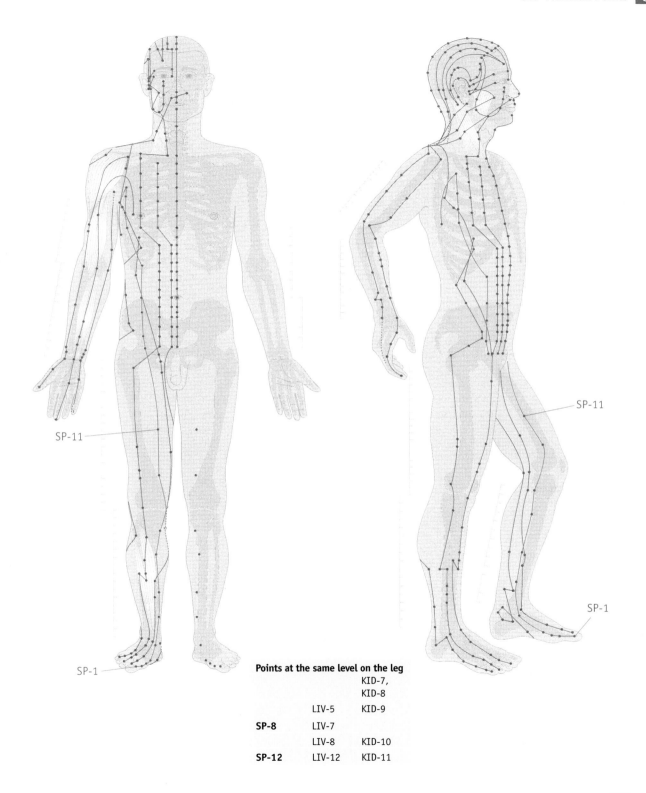

SP-11

SP-11

SP-1

SP-1

Points at the same level on the leg

		KID-7,
		KID-8
	LIV-5	KID-9
SP-8	LIV-7	
	LIV-8	KID-10
SP-12	LIV-12	KID-11

Point	Pinyin	Translation	Location	Action
Spleen meridian				
SP-12	*Chong Men*	Rushing gate	3.5 cun lateral to the centre of the pubic symphysis, at the same level as Ren-2, in the inguinal groove, lateral to the femoral artery	
SP-13	*Fu She*	Abode of the *Fu*	4 cun lateral to the anterior midline and 0.7 cun lateral and superior to SP-12	Meeting point with the Liver meridian and *Yin Wei Mai*
SP-14	*Fu Jie*	Abdomen knot	On the midclavicular line, slightly more than a thumbwidth inferior to the umbilicus (Ren-7)	Meeting point with the *Yin Wei Mai*
SP-15	*Da Heng*	Great horizontal	On the midclavicular line, at the level of the umbilicus (Ren-8)	Meeting point with the *Yin Wei Mai*
SP-16	*Fu Ai*	Abdomen sorrow	On the midclavicular line, 3 cun superior to the umbilicus, at the same level as Ren-11	Meeting point with the *Yin Wei Mai*
SP-17	*Shi Dou*	Food cavity	6 cun lateral to the midline, in the 5th ICS	
SP-18	*Tian Xi*	Heavenly stream	6 cun lateral to the midline, in the 4th ICS, level with Ren-17 and the nipples	
SP-19	*Xiong Xiang*	Chest village	6 cun lateral to the midline, in the 3rd ICS, level with Ren-18	
SP-20	*Zhou Rong*	Encircling glory	6 cun lateral to the midline, in the 2nd ICS	
SP-21	*Da Bao*	Great wrapping	On the midaxillary line, 6 cun inferior to the axilla, midway between the free end of the 11th rib and the axilla [Bi: 5th ICS, anterior axillary line, identical with G.B.-24]	

Point	Pinyin	Translation	Location	Action
Heart meridian				
HE-1	*Ji Quan*	Summit spring	In the centre of the axilla, medial to the axillary artery [Bi: 3rd ICS, anterior axillary line]	
HE-2	*Qing Ling*	Green Spirit	With the elbow flexed, 3 cun superior to the cubital crease (HE-3)	
HE-3	*Shao Hai*	Lesser sea	With the elbow fully flexed, between the medial end of the cubital crease and the medial epicondyle	• *He*-sea point • European master point: depression
HE-4	*Ling Dao*	Spirit path	1.5 cun proximal to the palmar wrist crease, radial to the tendon of the flexor carpi radialis	*Jing*-river point
HE-5	*Tong Li*	Penetrating the Interior	1 cun proximal to HE-7	*Luo*-connecting point (to S.I.-4)
HE-6	*Yin Xi*	*Yin* cleft	0.5 cun proximal to HE-7	*Xi*-cleft point

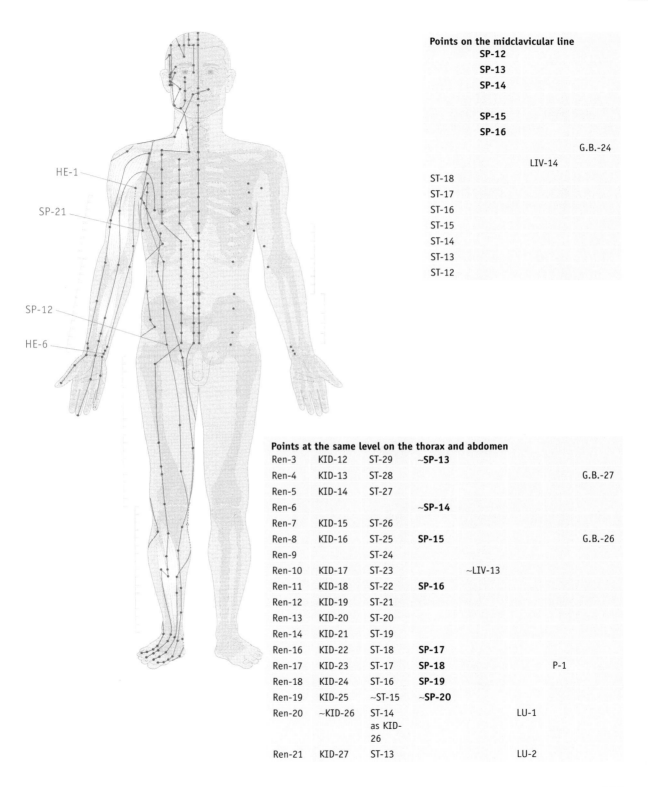

HE-1

SP-21

SP-12

HE-6

Points on the midclavicular line

SP-12				
SP-13				
SP-14				
SP-15				
SP-16				
				G.B.-24
			LIV-14	
ST-18				
ST-17				
ST-16				
ST-15				
ST-14				
ST-13				
ST-12				

Points at the same level on the thorax and abdomen

Ren-3	KID-12	ST-29	~SP-13			
Ren-4	KID-13	ST-28				G.B.-27
Ren-5	KID-14	ST-27				
Ren-6			~SP-14			
Ren-7	KID-15	ST-26				
Ren-8	KID-16	ST-25	SP-15			G.B.-26
Ren-9		ST-24				
Ren-10	KID-17	ST-23		~LIV-13		
Ren-11	KID-18	ST-22	SP-16			
Ren-12	KID-19	ST-21				
Ren-13	KID-20	ST-20				
Ren-14	KID-21	ST-19				
Ren-16	KID-22	ST-18	SP-17			
Ren-17	KID-23	ST-17	SP-18		P-1	
Ren-18	KID-24	ST-16	SP-19			
Ren-19	KID-25	~ST-15	~SP-20			
Ren-20	~KID-26	ST-14 as KID-26			LU-1	
Ren-21	KID-27	ST-13			LU-2	

Point	Pinyin	Translation	Location	Action
Heart meridian				
HE-7	*Shen Men*	Spirit gate	On the ulnar aspect of the wrist crease, on the radial aspect of the pisiform bone	• *Yuan*-source point • *Shu*-stream point • Sedation point
HE-8	*Shao Fu*	Lesser palace	On the palm, between the 4th and 5th metacarpal bones. When a fist is made, the tip of the little finger points to HE-8	*Ying*-spring point
HE-9	*Shao Chong*	Lesser rushing	On the little finger, next to the radial corner of the nail	*Jing*-well point
Small Intestine meridian				
S.I.-1	*Shao Ze*	Lesser marsh	On the little finger, next to the ulnar corner of the nail	*Jing*-well point
S.I.-2	*Qian Gu*	Front valley	When a loose fist is made, distal to the crease over the metacarpophalangeal joint of the little finger, at the junction of the red and white skin	*Ying*-spring point
S.I.-3	*Hou Xi*	Back stream	When a fist is made, on the dorsum of the hand, in the depression at the end of the most distal palmar crease	• *Shu*-stream point • Tonification point • Opening point of the *Du Mai*
S.I.-4	*Wan Gu*	Wrist bone	On the ulnar aspect of the hand, at the junction of the red and white skin, in the space between the base of the 5th metatarsal and the hamate bone	*Yuan*-source point
S.I.-5	*Yang Gu*	*Yang* valley	On the ulnar aspect of the wrist crease, distal to the styloid process of the ulna and proximal to the triquetrum bone	• *Jing*-river point • Fire point
S.I.-6	*Yang Lao*	Support the aged	In a depression just proximal and radial to the styloid process of the ulna	*Xi*-cleft point
S.I.-7	*Zhi Zheng*	Branch of the upright	On the dorsolateral aspect of the forearm, 5 cun proximal to S.I.-5, on a line connecting S.I.-5 and S.I.-8	*Luo*-connecting point (to HE-7)
S.I.-8	*Xiao Hai*	Small sea	With the elbow flexed in the depression between the olecranon process of the ulna and the medial epicondyle of the humerus, 0.5 cun from the tip of the olecranon	• Sedation point • *He*-sea point
S.I.-9	*Jian Zhen*	True shoulder	With the arm adducted 1 cun superior to the end of the posterior axillary fold	
S.I.-10	*Nao Shu*	Upper arm *Shu*	On the lower border of the scapular spine, perpendicularly superior to S.I.-9	Meeting point with the *Yang Qiao Mai* and *Yang Wei Mai*
S.I.-11	*Tian Zong*	Heavenly gathering	In the centre of the infraspinous fossa, at the level of the spinous process of T5	

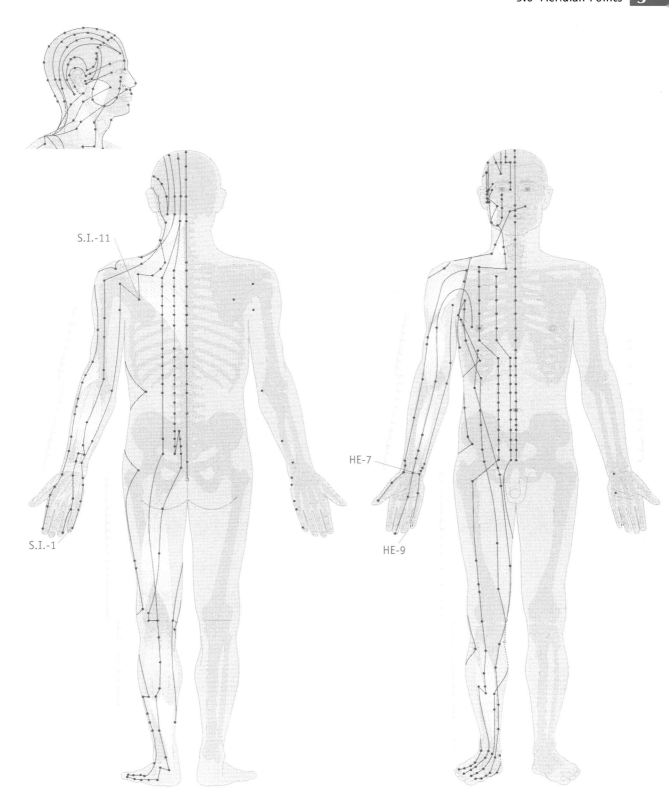

S.I.-11

S.I.-1

HE-7

HE-9

Point	Pinyin	Translation	Location	Action
Small Intestine meridian				
S.I.-12	*Bing Feng*	Grasping the Wind	With the arm abducted in a depression in the centre of the suprascapular fossa	Meeting point with the Large Intestine, Triple Burner, Gall Bladder meridians
S.I.-13	*Qu Yuan*	Crooked wall	On the medial section of the supraspinous fossa, where the scapular spine curves upwards (hence the name); at the midpoint of the distance between S.I.-10 (on the lower border of the scapular spine, perpendicularly superior to the axillary fold) and the spinous process of T2	
S.I.-14	*Jian Wei Shu*	Outer shoulder *Shu*	On the upper part of the scapula; 3 cun lateral to the lower border of the spinous process of T1, level with Du-13 and BL-11	Outer-*Shu* point of the shoulder
S.I.-15	*Jian Zhong Zhu*	Middle shoulder *Shu*	2 cun lateral to the spinous process of C7, at the same level as Du-14 [Bi: Du-13]	*Shu* point of the middle shoulder region
S.I.-16	*Tian Chuang*	Heavenly window	On the posterior border of the sternocleido-mastoid, at the level of the upper border of the thyroid cartilage, at the same level as L.I.-18 and ST-9; posterior and slightly inferior to the mandibular angle	
S.I.-17	*Tian Rong*	Heavenly appearance	Posterior to the mandibular angle, on the anterior border of the sternocleidomastoid, inferior to the earlobe	Meeting point with the Gall Bladder meridian
S.I.-18	*Quan Liao*	Cheek bone crevice	On the anterior border of the insertion of the masseter on the maxilla. Ask the patient to clench their teeth and/or open their mouth	• A branch ascends from here to BL-1 • Meeting point with the Gall Bladder meridian • European master point: trismus
S.I.-19	*Ting Gong*	Palace of hearing	With the mouth open, in the depression between the tragus and temporomandibular joint; T.B.-21 is located superior, G.B.-21 inferior to S.I.-19	Meeting point with the Triple Burner and Gall Bladder meridians
Point	Pinyin	Translation	Location	Action
Bladder meridian				
BL-1	*Jing Ming*	Bright eyes	At the inner canthus of the eye – where glasses rest on the nose!	Meeting point of the Bladder, Small Intestine/Stomach meridians and with the *Yang Qiao Mai* and *Yin Qiao Mai*
BL-2	*Zan Zhu*	Gathered bamboo	At the junction of the vertical line through the medial end of the eyebrow (inner canthus) and the supraorbital foramen	
BL-3	*Mei Chong*	Eyebrow's pouring	Perpendicularly superior to BL-2, 0.5 cun within the anterior hairline	

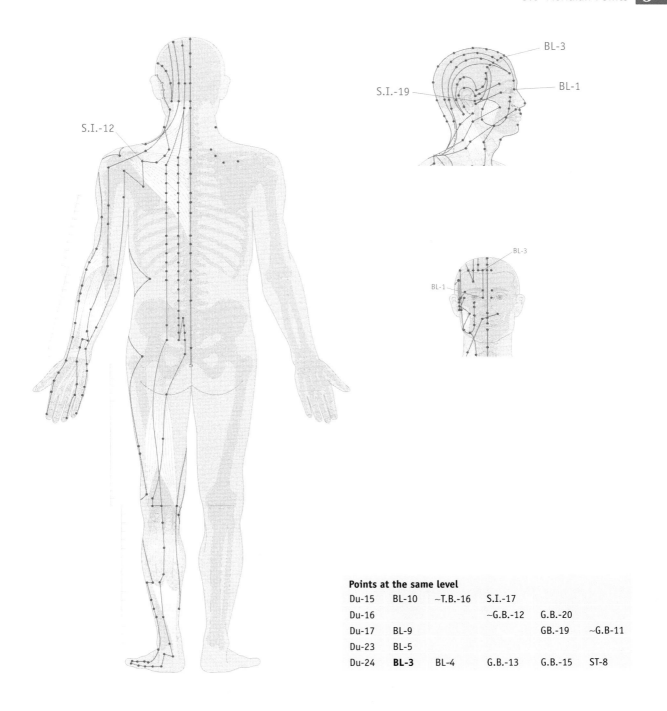

S.I.-12

BL-3

S.I.-19

BL-1

BL-3

BL-1

Points at the same level

Du-15	BL-10	~T.B.-16	S.I.-17		
Du-16			~G.B.-12	G.B.-20	
Du-17	BL-9			GB.-19	~G.B-11
Du-23	BL-5				
Du-24	**BL-3**	BL-4	G.B.-13	G.B.-15	ST-8

Point	Pinyin	Translation	Location	Action
Bladder meridian				
BL-4	*Qu Chai*	Crooked curve	Lateral to BL-3, 0.5 cun within anterior hairline, 1.5 cun lateral to the midline	
BL-5	*Wu Chu*	Fifth place	1 cun within the anterior hairline, 1.5 cun lateral to the midline (Du-23)	
BL-6	*Cheng Guang*	Receiving light	2.5 cun within the anterior hairline, 1.5 cun lateral to the midline	
BL-7	*Tong Tian*	Heavenly connection	1.5 cun lateral to the highest point of the vertex (Du-20)	
BL-8	*Luo Que*	Declining connection	1.5 cun posterior to BL-7	
BL-9	*Yu Zhen*	Jade pillow	1.5 cun lateral to the posterior midline, at the level of the upper border of the external occipital protuberance, at the same level as Du-17	
BL-10	*Tian Zhu*	Celestial pillar	At the external occipital protuberance, on the lateral aspect of the trapezius insertion	Sea of *Qi* point
BL-11	*Da Zhu*	Great shuttle	1.5 cun lateral to the lower border of the spinous process of T1	*Hui*-meeting point of the bones
BL-12	*Feng Men*	Wind gate	1.5 cun lateral to the lower border of the spinous process of T2	
BL-13	*Fei Shu*	Lung *Shu*	1.5 cun lateral to the lower border of the spinous process of T3	Back-*Shu* point of the Lung
BL-14	*Jue Yin Shu*	*Jueyin Shu*	1.5 cun lateral to the lower border of the spinous process of T4	Back-*Shu* point of the Pericardium
BL-15	*Xin Shu*	Heart *Shu*	1.5 cun lateral to the lower border of the spinous process of T5	Back-*Shu* point of the Heart
BL-16	*Du Shu*	Governor *Shu*	1.5 cun lateral to the lower border of the spinous process of T6	Back-*Shu* point of the *Du Mai*
BL-17	*Ge Shu*	Diaphragm *Shu*	1.5 cun lateral to the lower border of the spinous process of T7	Back-*Shu* point of the diaphragm
BL-18	*Gan Shu*	Liver *Shu*	2 cun lateral to the lower border of the spinous process of T9	Back-*Shu* point of the Liver
BL-19	*Dan Shu*	Gall Bladder *Shu*	1.5 cun lateral to the lower border of the spinous process of T10	Back-*Shu* point of the Gall Bladder
BL-20	*Pi Shu*	Spleen *Shu*	1.5 cun lateral to the lower border of the spinous process of T11	Back-*Shu* point of the Spleen
BL-21	*Wei Shu*	Stomach *Shu*	1.5 cun lateral to the lower border of the spinous process of T12	• Back-*Shu* point of the Stomach • European master point of the Stomach
BL-22	*San Jiao Shu*	*Sanjiao Shu*	1.5 cun lateral to the lower border of the spinous process of L1	Back-*Shu* point of the Triple Burner

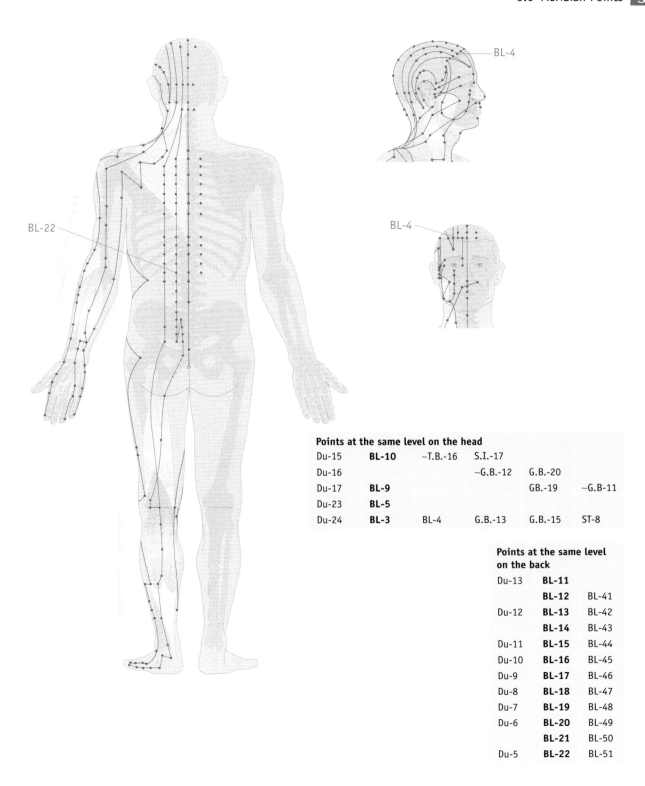

BL-4

BL-4

BL-22

Points at the same level on the head

Du-15	**BL-10**	~T.B.-16	S.I.-17		
Du-16			~G.B.-12	G.B.-20	
Du-17	**BL-9**			GB.-19	~G.B-11
Du-23	**BL-5**				
Du-24	**BL-3**	BL-4	G.B.-13	G.B.-15	ST-8

Points at the same level on the back

Du-13	**BL-11**	
	BL-12	BL-41
Du-12	**BL-13**	BL-42
	BL-14	BL-43
Du-11	**BL-15**	BL-44
Du-10	**BL-16**	BL-45
Du-9	**BL-17**	BL-46
Du-8	**BL-18**	BL-47
Du-7	**BL-19**	BL-48
Du-6	**BL-20**	BL-49
	BL-21	BL-50
Du-5	**BL-22**	BL-51

Point	Pinyin	Translation	Location	Action
Bladder meridian				
BL-23	*Shen Shu*	Kidney *Shu*	1.5 cun lateral to the lower border of the spinous process of L2	Back-*Shu* point of the Kidneys
BL-24	*Qi Hai Shu*	Sea of *Qi Shu*	1.5 cun lateral to the lower border of the spinous process of L3	Back-*Shu* point of Ren-6
BL-25	*Da Chang Shu*	Large Intestine *Shu*	1.5 cun lateral to the lower border of the spinous process of L4	Back-*Shu* point of the Large Intestine
BL-26	*Guan Yuan Shu*	Gate of origin *Shu*	1.5 cun lateral to the lower border of the spinous process of L5	Back-*Shu* point of Ren-4
BL-27	*Xiao Chang Shu*	Small Intestine *Shu*	1.5 cun lateral to the posterior midline, at the level of the 1st sacral foramen	Back-*Shu* point of the Small Intestine
BL-28	*Pang Guang Shu*	Bladder *Shu*	1.5 cun lateral to the posterior midline, at the level of the 2nd sacral foramen	Back-*Shu* point of the Bladder
BL-29	*Zhong Lu Shu*	Mid-spine *Shu*	1.5 cun lateral to the posterior midline, at the level of the 3rd sacral foramen	Back-*Shu* point of the mid-spine
BL-30	*Bai Huan Shu*	White ring *Shu*	1.5 cun lateral to the posterior midline, at the level of the 4th sacral foramen	Back-*Shu* point of the Perineum
BL-31	*Shang Liao*	Upper crevice	Over the 1st sacral foramen	European master point for the menopause
BL-32	*Ci Liao*	Second crevice	Over the 2nd sacral foramen (at the same level as BL-28, back *Shu* point of the Bladder)	
BL-33	*Zhong Liao*	Middle crevice	Over the 3rd sacral foramen	
BL-34	*Xia Liao*	Lower crevice	Over the 4th sacral foramen	
BL-35	*Hui Yang*	Meeting of *Yang*	0.5 cun lateral to the tip of the coccyx	
BL-36 [Bi: BL-50]	*Cheng Fu*	Hold and support	In the centre of the transverse gluteal crease	
BL-37 [Bi: BL-51]	*Yin Men*	Gate of abundance	On the back of the thigh, 6 cun inferior to BL-36, on a line connecting BL-36 and BL-40	
BL-38 [Bi: BL-52]	*Fu Xi*	Floating cleft	1 cun superior to the lateral end of the popliteal crease, on the medial side of the tendon of the biceps femoris	
BL-39 [Bi: BL-53]	*Wei Yang*	Outside of the crook	Lateral (*Yang*) to *Weizhong*, at the medial side of the tendon of the biceps femoris	Lower *He*-sea point of the Triple Burner

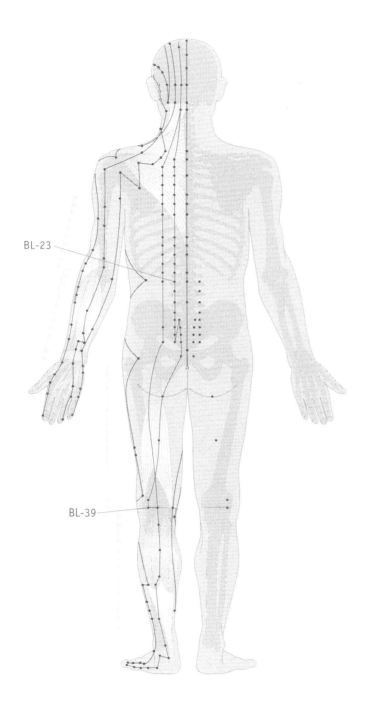

BL-23

BL-39

Points at the same level on the back

Du-4		**BL-23**	BL-52
Du-3		**BL-25**	
	BL-31	**BL-27**	
	BL-32	**BL-28**	BL-53
	BL-33	**BL-29**	
	BL-34	**BL-30**	
Du-2			BL-54

Point	Pinyin	Translation	Location	Action
Bladder meridian				
BL-40 [Bi: BL-54]	*Wei Zhong*	Middle of the crook	In the centre of the popliteal crease, between the tendons of the semitendinosus and biceps femoris	• *He*-sea point • Metabolic point • Painful disorders of the knee joint • European master point for skin disorders
BL-41 [Bi: BL-36]	*Fu Fen*	Attached branch	3 cun lateral to the spinous process of T2, lateral to BL-12, at the medial border of the scapula	Meeting point with the Small Intestine
BL-42 [Bi: BL-37]	*Po Hu*	Door of the corporeal soul	3 cun lateral to the spinous process of T3, lateral to BL-13 (back-*Shu* point of the LU), at the medial border of the scapula	
BL-43 [Bi: BL-38]	*Gao Huang*[a]	Vital region *Shu*	3 cun lateral to the spinous process of T4, lateral to BL-14 (back-*Shu* point of the P), at the medial border of the scapula	Back-*Shu* point of the vital region
BL-44 [Bi: BL-39]	*Shen Tang*	Hall of the Spirit	3 cun lateral to the spinous process of T5, lateral to BL-15 (back-*Shu* point of the HE), at the medial border of the scapula	
BL-45 [Bi: BL-40]	*Yi Xi*	*Yi Xi*	3 cun lateral to the spinous process of T6 (Du-10), lateral to BL-16 (back-*Shu* point of the S.I.), at the medial border of the scapula	
BL-46 [Bi: BL-41]	*Ge Guan*	Diaphragm gate	3 cun lateral to the spinous process of T7, at the level of the inferior angle of the scapula, lateral to BL-17 (back-*Shu* point of the diaphragm)	
BL-47 [Bi: BL-42]	*Hun Men*	Gate of the ethereal soul	3 cun lateral to the spinous process of T9, lateral to BL-18 (back-*Shu* point of the LIV)	
BL-48 [Bi: BL-43]	*Yang Gang*	*Yang*'s key link	3 cun lateral to the spinous process of T10, lateral to BL-19 (back-*Shu* point of the G.B.)	
BL-49 [Bi: BL-44]	*Yi She*	Abode of thought	3 cun lateral to the spinous process of T11, lateral to BL-20 (back-*Shu* point of the SP)	
BL-50 [Bi: BL-45]	*Wei Cang*	Stomach granary	3 cun lateral to the spinous process of T12, lateral to BL-21 (back-*Shu* point of the ST)	

[a]*Gao* is the fat at the apex of the Heart, and *Huang* is the space between the apex of the Heart and the diaphragm – therefore a place that is hardly accessible for treatment. *Xin Hua Ci Dian*

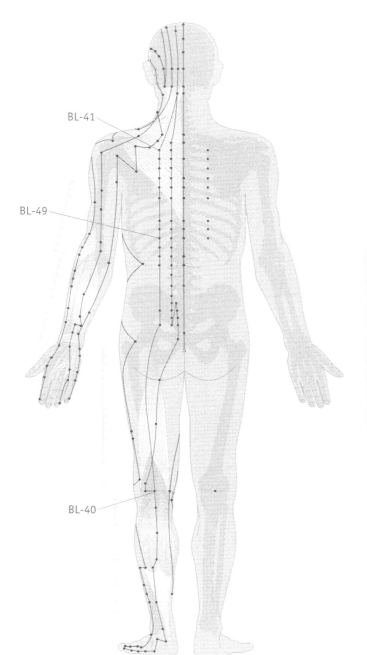

BL-41

BL-49

BL-40

Points at the same level on the back

Du-13	BL-11	
	BL-12	**BL-41**
Du-12	BL-13	**BL-42**
	BL-14	**BL-43**
Du-11	BL-15	**BL-44**
Du-10	BL-16	**BL-45**
Du-9	BL-17	**BL-46**
Du-8	BL-18	**BL-47**
Du-7	BL-19	**BL-48**
Du-6	BL-20	**BL-49**

Point	Pinyin	Translation	Location	Action
Bladder meridian				
BL-51 [Bi: BL-46]	*Huang Men*	Vitals gate	3 cun lateral to the spinous process of L1, lateral to BL-22 (back-*Shu* point of the T.B.)	
BL-52 [Bi: BL-47]	*Zhi Shi*	Residence of the will	3 cun lateral to the spinous process of L2, lateral to BL-23 (back-*Shu* point of the KID)	
BL-53 [Bi: BL-48]	*Bao Huang*	Bladder's vitals	3 cun lateral to the posterior midline, at the level of the spinous process of S2, lateral to BL-28 (back-*Shu* point of the BL)	
BL-54 [Bi: BL-49]	*Zhi Bian*	Order's limit	3 cun lateral to the posterior midline, at the level of the spinous process of S4, lateral to BL-30 and BL-34	
BL-55	*He Yang*	Confluence of *Yang*	2 cun inferior to the popliteal crease, below BL-40	
BL-56	*Cheng Jin*	Support the sinews	4 cun inferior to BL-40; midway between BL-55 and BL-57	
BL-57	*Cheng Shan/Yu Fu*	Support the mountain/ fish belly (gastrocnemius)	In the depression below the two bellies of the gastrocnemius (on tiptoes); midway between BL-40 and BL-60	
BL-58	*Fei Yang*	Soaring upwards	1 cun distal and lateral to BL-57, on the lateral border of the gastrocnemius, on the m. soleus. On a cross-section through the lower leg at 7.30 and 4.30 respectively	• *Luo*-connecting point (to KID-3) • Metabolic point
BL-59	*Fu Yang*	Instep *Yang*	3 cun superior and slightly posterior to the lateral malleolus, perpendicularly above BL-60	
BL-60	*Kun Lun*	Kunlun mountains	In the depression between the Achilles tendon and the lateral malleolus	• *Jing*-river point • European master point for pain along the course of the meridian
BL-61	*Pu Can*	Servant's respect	1.5 cun inferior to BL-60	
BL-62	*Shen Mai*	Extending vessel	Below the prominence of the lateral malleolus	• Opening point of the *Yang Qiao Mai* • European master point for insomnia and for pain that cannot be localized
BL-63	*Jin Men*	Golden gate	In the depression between the calcaneus and cuboid bones, approx. 1 cun anterior and inferior to BL-62	• Meeting point with the *Yang Wei Mai* • *Xi*-cleft point

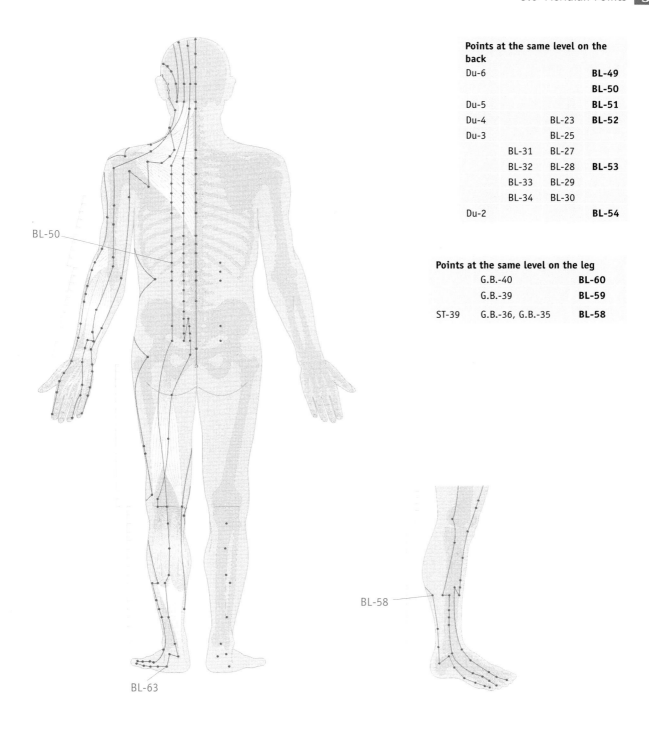

Points at the same level on the back

Du-6		**BL-49**
		BL-50
Du-5		**BL-51**
Du-4	BL-23	**BL-52**
Du-3	BL-25	
	BL-31	BL-27	
	BL-32	BL-28	**BL-53**
	BL-33	BL-29	
	BL-34	BL-30	
Du-2		**BL-54**

Points at the same level on the leg

	G.B.-40	**BL-60**
	G.B.-39	**BL-59**
ST-39	G.B.-36, G.B.-35	**BL-58**

BL-50

BL-63

BL-58

Point	Pinyin	Translation	Location	Action
Bladder meridian				
BL-64	*Jing Ju*	Capital bone	On the lateral aspect of the foot, posterior to the tuberosity of the 5th metatarsal bone, at the junction of the red and white skin	*Yuan*-source point
BL-65	*Shu Gu*	Restraining bone	On the lateral aspect of the foot, with plantar flexion proximal to the metatarsophalangeal joint of the 5th toe, at the junction of the red and white skin	• Sedation point • *Shu*-stream point
BL-66	*Zu Tong Gu*	Foot connecting valley	On the lateral aspect of the foot, with plantar flexion over the joint space of the metatarsophalangeal joint of the 5th toe, at the junction of the red and white skin	*Ying*-spring point
BL-67	*Zhi Yin*	Reaching *Yin*	On the 5th toe, at the lateral corner of the nail	*Jing*-well point
Kidney meridian				
KID-1	*Yang Quan*	Gushing spring	Where the two pads of the toes meet, in the depression formed with plantar flexion	• *Jing*-well point • Shock point • Sedation point
KID-2	*Ran Gu*	Blazing valley	On the medial aspect of the foot, in the depression below the navicular tuberosity	*Ying*-spring point
KID-3	*Tai Xi*	Supreme stream	Between the highest prominence of the medial malleolus and the Achilles tendon	• *Yuan*-source point • *Shu*-stream point
KID-4	*Da Zhang*	Great bell	On the upper border of the calcaneus, half a fingerwidth posterior to the medial malleolus	*Luo*-connecting point
KID-5	*Shui Quan*	Water spring	1 cun inferior to KID-3	*Xi*-cleft point
KID-6	*Zhao Hai*	Shining sea	Below the prominence of the medial malleolus	• Opening point of the *Yin Qiao Mai* • Metabolic point • With BL-62, master point for insomnia and pain that cannot be localized
KID-7	*Fu Liu*	Returning current	On the anterior border of the Achilles tendon, posterior to the flexor digitorum longus, 2 cun superior to the highest prominence of the medial malleolus (=2 cun superior to KID-3)	• Tonification point • *Jing*-river point
KID-8	*Jiao Xin*	Exchange belief	2 cun superior to the highest prominence of the medical malleolus, anterior to KID-7	• *Xi*-cleft point of the *Yin Qiao Mai* • Meeting point of the 3 *Yin* meridians of the leg (KID, LIV, SP)

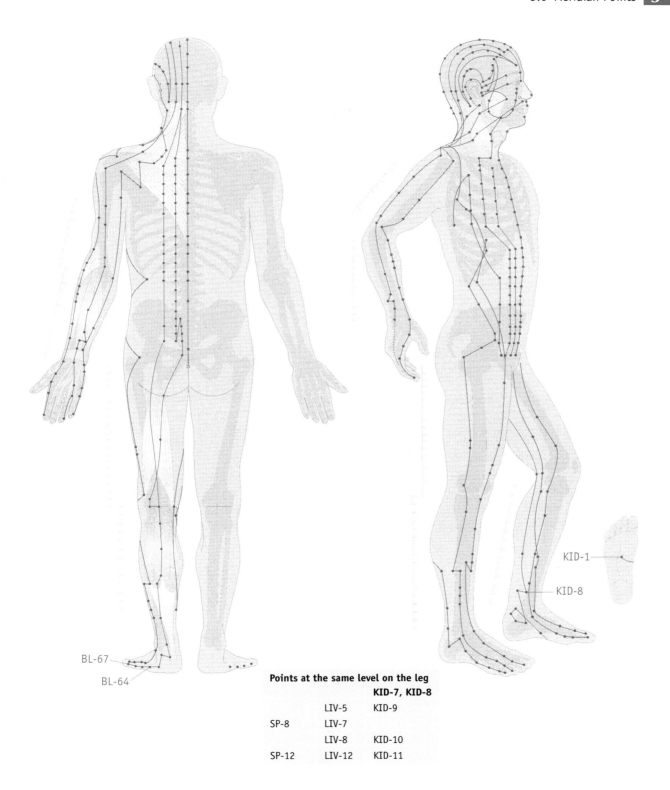

BL-67
BL-64

KID-1
KID-8

Points at the same level on the leg

		KID-7, KID-8
	LIV-5	KID-9
SP-8	LIV-7	
	LIV-8	KID-10
SP-12	LIV-12	KID-11

Point	Pinyin	Translation	Location	Action
Kidney meridian				
KID-9	*Zhu Bin*	Guest house	6 cun superior to the medial malleolus, 1.5 cun posterior to the medial crest of the tibia, on the tibial border of the medial belly of the gastrocnemius	*Xi*-cleft point of the *Yin Wei Mai*
KID-10	*Yin Gu*	*Yin* valley	With the knee flexed, at the medial end of the popliteal crease, between the tendons of the semitendinosus and semimembranosus	*He*-sea point
KID-11	*Heng Gu*	Pubic bone	On the upper border of the pubic symphysis, approx. 0.5 cun lateral to the midline (Ren-2)	Meeting point with the *Chong Mai*
KID-12	*Da He*	Great luminance	0.5 cun [Bi: 1.5 cun] lateral to the midline, 1 cun superior to the pubic symphysis or 1/5 of the distance between the pubic symphysis and the umbilicus, at the level of Ren-3	Meeting point with the *Chong Mai*
KID-13	*Qi Xue*	*Qi* cave	0.5 cun [Bi: 1.5 cun] lateral to the midline, 2 cun superior to the pubic symphysis or 2/5 of the distance between the pubic symphysis and the umbilicus, at the level of Ren-4	Meeting point with the *Chong Mai*
KID-14	*Si Man*	Four fullnesses (4th point superior to the symphysis)	0.5 cun [Bi: 1.5 cun] lateral to the midline, 3 cun superior to the pubic symphysis or 3/5 of the distance between the pubic symphysis and the umbilicus, at the level of Ren-5	Meeting point with the *Chong Mai*
KID-15	*Zhong Zhu*	Middle flow	0.5 cun [Bi: 1.5 cun] lateral to the midline, 4 cun superior to the pubic symphysis or 4/5 of the distance between the pubic symphysis and the umbilicus, at the level of Ren-7	Meeting point with the *Chong Mai*
KID-16	*Huang Shu*	Vitals *Shu* (*Shu* point of the intestines)	0.5 cun [Bi: 1.5 cun] lateral to the midline, at the level of the umbilicus (Ren-8)	
KID-17	*Shang Qu*	Shang bend (Large Intestine bend, impaired digestion)	2/8 of the distance between the umbilicus and the xiphoid process, lateral to Ren-10, 0.5 cun [Bi: 1.5 cun] lateral to the midline	Meeting point with the *Chong Mai*
KID-18	*Shi Guan*	Stone pass	Superior to the umbilicus, 3/8 of the distance between the umbilicus and the xiphoid process, lateral to Ren-11, 0.5 cun [Bi: 1.5 cun] lateral to the midline	Meeting point with the *Chong Mai*
KID-19	*Yin Du*	*Yin* metropolis	At the midpoint of the distance between the umbilicus and the xiphoid process, lateral to Ren-12, 0.5 cun [Bi: 1.5 cun] lateral to the midline	Meeting point with the *Chong Mai*

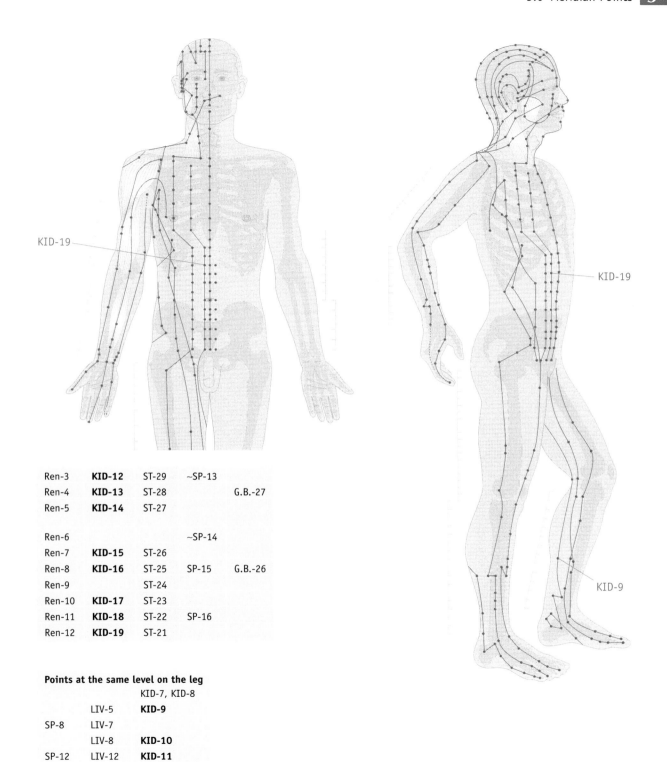

KID-19

KID-19

KID-9

Ren-3	**KID-12**	ST-29	~SP-13	
Ren-4	**KID-13**	ST-28		G.B.-27
Ren-5	**KID-14**	ST-27		
Ren-6			~SP-14	
Ren-7	**KID-15**	ST-26		
Ren-8	**KID-16**	ST-25	SP-15	G.B.-26
Ren-9		ST-24		
Ren-10	**KID-17**	ST-23		
Ren-11	**KID-18**	ST-22	SP-16	
Ren-12	**KID-19**	ST-21		

Points at the same level on the leg

		KID-7, KID-8
	LIV-5	**KID-9**
SP-8	LIV-7	
	LIV-8	**KID-10**
SP-12	LIV-12	**KID-11**

Point	Pinyin	Translation	Location	Action
Kidney meridian				
KID-20	*Fu Tong Gu*	Abdomen connecting valley	Superior to the umbilicus, 5/8 of the distance between the umbilicus and the xiphoid process, lateral to Ren-13, 0.5 cun [Bì: 1.5 cun] lateral to the midline	Meeting point with the *Chong Mai*
KID-21	*You Men*	Hidden gate	Superior to the umbilicus, 6/8 of the distance between the umbilicus and the xiphoid process [Bì: 6th ICS, in the angle between the 6th/7th ICS], lateral to Ren-14, 0.5 cun lateral to the midline	Meeting point with the *Chong Mai*
KID-22	*Bu Lang*	Walking corridor	In the 5th ICS, 2 cun lateral to the midline, at the level of Ren-16	
KID-23	*Shen Feng*	Spirit seal	In the 4th ICS, 2 cun lateral to the midline, at the level of Ren-17 (between the nipples)	
KID-24	*Ling Xu*	Spirit ruin	In the 3rd ICS, 2 cun lateral to the midline, at the level of Ren-18	
KID-25	*Shen Cang*	Spirit storehouse	In the 2nd ICS, 2 cun lateral to the midline, at the level of Ren-19	
KID-26	*Yu Zhong*	Comfortable chest	In the 1st ICS, 2 cun lateral to the midline, at the level of Ren-20	
KID-27	*Shu Fu*	*Shu* mansion	On the lower border of the sternoclavicular joint	
Pericardium meridian				
P-1	*Tian Chi*	Heavenly pool	In the 4th ICS, 1 cun lateral to the midclavicular line or the nipple	
P-2	*Tian Quan*	Heavenly spring	On the upper arm, 2 cun distal to the anterior axillary fold, between the two heads of the biceps	
P-3	*Qu Ze*	Marsh at the crook	On the cubital crease, on the ulnar side of the tendon of the biceps (LU-5 is located radial to the tendon). Locate with elbow flexed	*He*-sea point
P-4	*Xi Men*	*Xi*-cleft gate	On the anterior aspect of the forearm, 5 cun proximal to the midpoint of the wrist crease, between the tendons of the flexor carpi radialis and palmaris longus	*Xi*-cleft point
P-5	*Jian Shi*	Intermediate messenger	On the anterior aspect of the forearm, 3 cun proximal to the midpoint of the wrist crease, between the tendons of the flexor carpi radialis and palmaris longus	• *Jing*-river point • Group *Luo*-connecting point of the 3 *Yin* meridians of the arm

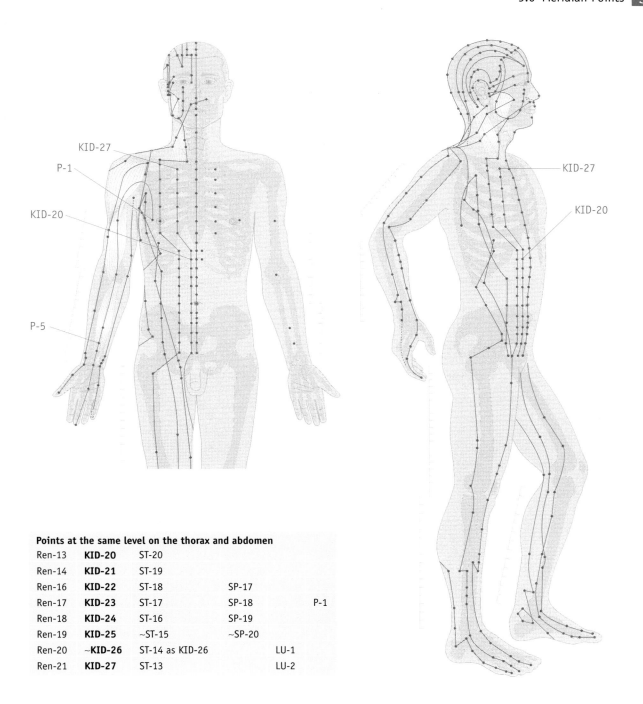

Points at the same level on the thorax and abdomen

Ren-13	**KID-20**	ST-20		
Ren-14	**KID-21**	ST-19		
Ren-16	**KID-22**	ST-18	SP-17	
Ren-17	**KID-23**	ST-17	SP-18	P-1
Ren-18	**KID-24**	ST-16	SP-19	
Ren-19	**KID-25**	~ST-15	~SP-20	
Ren-20	~**KID-26**	ST-14 as KID-26		LU-1
Ren-21	**KID-27**	ST-13		LU-2

Point	Pinyin	Translation	Location	Action
Pericardium meridian				
P-6	*Nei Guan*	Inner pass	On the anterior aspect of the forearm, 2 cun proximal to the midpoint of the wrist crease, between the tendons of the flexor carpi radialis and palmaris longus	• Opening point of the *Yin Wei Mai* • *Luo*-connecting point (to T.B.-4) • European master point for vomiting
P-7	*Da Ling*	Great mound	On the anterior aspect of the wrist joint, between the tendons of the flexor carpi radialis and palmaris longus	• *Yuan*-source point • Sedation point • *Shu*-stream point
P-8	*Lao Gong*	Palace of toil	When a fist is made, the tip of the middle finger will be pointing to P-8, between the distal and medial transverse crease, between the 2nd and 3rd metacarpal bones	*Ying*-spring point
P-9	*Zhon Chong*	Middle rushing	In the centre of the tip of the middle finger [Bi: on the middle finger, next to the radial corner of the nail]	• *Jing*-well point • Shock point
Triple Burner meridian				
T.B.-1	*Guan Chong*	Rushing pass	On the ring finger, next to the ulnar corner of the nail	*Jing*-well point
T.B.-2	*Ye Men*	Fluid gate	Between the 4th and 5th fingers, proximal to the margin of the web	*Ying*-spring point
T.B.-3	*Zhong Zhu*	Central islet	On the dorsum of the hand, between the 4th and 5th metacarpal bones, in the depression proximal to the metacarpophalangeal joints. Locate with the hand formed to a loose fist	• *Shu* stream point • Tonification point
T.B.-4	*Yang Chi*	*Yang* pool	On the wrist crease, in the depression lateral to the tendon of the extensor digitorum longus [Bi: on the dorsum of the hand, in the depression above the space between the 4th metacarpal and the hamate bone]	• *Yuan*-source point • European master point for vasomotor headaches
T.B.-5	*Wai Guan*	Outer pass	2 cun proximal to the midpoint of the dorsal wrist crease, opposite P-6	• *Luo*-connecting point (to T.B.-4) • Opening point of the *Yang Wei Mai* • European master point of the small joints
T.B.-6	*Zhi Gou*	Branch ditch	3 cun proximal to the midpoint of the dorsal wrist crease	*Jing*-river point
T.B.-7	*Hui Zong*	Ancestral meeting	At the same level as T.B.-6, but ulnar to T.B.-6, on the radial aspect of the ulna	*Xi*-cleft point

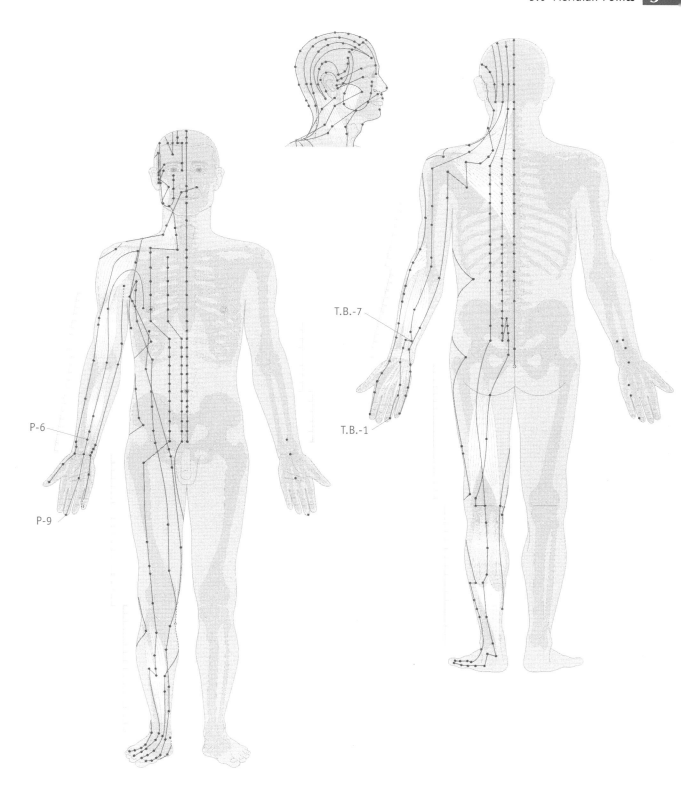

P-6

P-9

T.B.-7

T.B.-1

Point	Pinyin	Translation	Location	Action
Triple Burner meridian				
T.B.-8	*San Yang Luo*	Three *Yang Luo*	4 cun proximal to the midpoint of the dorsal wrist crease	Group *Luo*-connecting point of the 3 *Yang* meridians of the arm (L.I., S.I., T.B.)
T.B.-9	*Si Du*	Four rivers	On a line connecting the midpoint of the dorsal wrist crease and the olecranon, 5 cun distal to the olecranon	
T.B.-10	*Tian Jing*	Heavenly well	With the elbow slightly flexed, in the depression 1 cun superior to the olecranon	*He*-sea point
T.B.-11	*Qing Leng Yuan*	Clear cold abyss	1 cun proximal to T.B.-10, on a line connecting T.B.-10 (in the depression 1 cun superior to the olecranon) and T.B.-14 (in the depression posterior and inferior to the acromion)	
T.B.-12	*Xiao Luo*	Dispersing *Luo* river	At the midpoint of a line connecting T.B.-10 (in the depression 1 cun superior to the olecranon) and T.B.-14 (in the depression posterior and inferior to the acromion) or 4 cun distal to the posterior axillary fold, on the posteromedial aspect of the upper arm	
T.B.-13	*Nao Hui*	Upper arm meeting	On a line connecting T.B.-10 (in the depression 1 cun superior to the olecranon) and T.B.-14 (in the depression posterior and inferior to the acromion), on the posterior border of the deltoid, level with the end of the posterior axillary fold	Meeting point with the *Yang Wei Mai*
T.B.-14	*Jian Liao*	Shoulder crevice	With the arm abducted in the depression posterior and inferior to the acromion, between the medial and posterior fibres of the deltoid (L.I.-15 lies anterior to T.B.-14)	
T.B.-15	*Tian Liao*	Heavenly crevice	In the suprascapular fossa, in the depression midway between G.B.-21 (highest point on the shoulder, midway between the acromion and the spinous process of C7) and S.I.-13 (at the medial and of the supraspinous fossa, at the curved medial end of the scapular spine) [Bi: in the centre of the shoulder, at the border of the trapezius, variable location, sometimes located more inferiorly]	• Meeting point with the *Yang Wei Mai* • European master point for the upper extremities
T.B.-16	*Tian You*	Window of heaven	On the posterior border of the sternocleidomastoid, at the level of the mandibular angle, inferior to T.B.-17 [Bi: where the trapezius forms a kink, identical to G.B.-21, S.I.-15]	

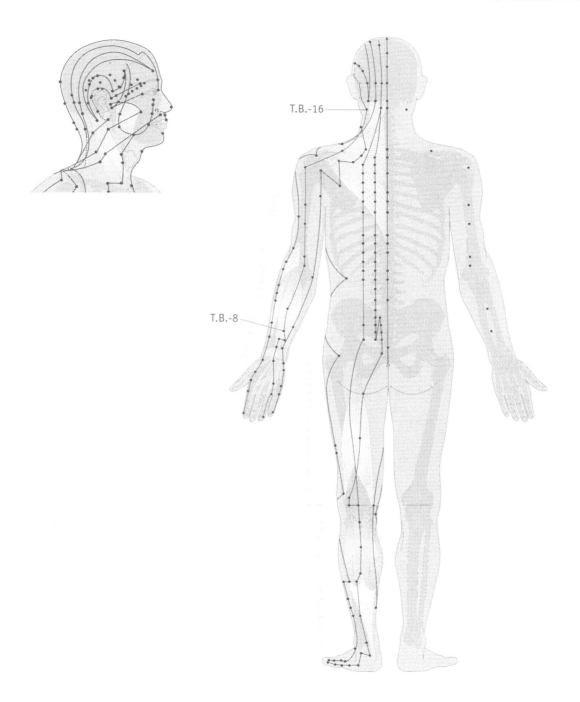

T.B.-16

T.B.-8

Point	Pinyin	Translation	Location	Action
Triple Burner meridian				
T.B.-17	*Yi Feng*	Wind screen	On the anterior border of the mastoid	Meeting point with the G.B. meridian
T.B.-18	*Qi Mai, Ti Mai Zi Mai*	Spasm vessel, body vessel, supporting vessel	In the centre of the mastoid process	
T.B.-19	*Lu Xi*	Skull's rest	1 cun superior to the centre of the mastoid process (T.B.-18)	
T.B.-20	*Jiao Sun*	Minute angle	Directly superior to the apex of the ear, on the hairline	Meeting point with the S.I. and G.B. meridians
T.B.-21	*Er Men*	Ear gate	At the level of the supratragic incisure, with the mouth open in the depression superior to the condyloid process of the mandible	European master point for the ear
T.B.-22	*Er He Liao*	Ear harmony crevice	Anterior and superior to T.B.-21, anterior to the root of the ear, within the temporal hairline, posterior to the temporal artery [Bi: identical to G.B.-3]	Meeting point with the S.I. and G.B. meridians
T.B.-23	*Si Zhu Kong*	Silken bamboo hollow	In a depression at the lateral end of the eyebrow	Meeting point with the G.B. meridian
Gall Bladder meridian				
G.B.-1	*Tong Zi Liao*	Pupil crevice	0.5 cun lateral to the outer canthus of the eye, in the depression lateral to the orbit	Meeting point with the T.B. and S.I. meridians
G.B.-2	*Ting Hui*	Meeting of hearing	With the mouth open, in the depression anterior to the antitragic notch, posterior to the condyoloid process of the mandible	Meeting point with the T.B. meridian
G.B.-3	*Shang Guan*	Above the joint	On the upper border of the zygomatic arch, directly superior to ST-7 (in a depression below the zygomatic arch, anterior to the condyloid process of the mandible) [Bi: identical with T.B.-22]	Meeting point with the T.B. meridian
G.B.-4	*Han Yan*	Jaw serenity	Within the temporal hairline, on the anterior portion of the temporalis muscle, which can be felt with a chewing motion	Meeting point with the T.B., ST and L.I. meridians
G.B.-5	*Xuan Lu*	Suspensed skull	At the level of the parietal suture, 1 cun inferior to G.B.-4, slightly within the hairline	Meeting point with the T.B., ST and L.I. meridians
G.B.-6	*Xuan Li*	Suspensed hair	Where the frontoparietal, frontosphenoidal and sphenoparietal sutures meet, between G.B.-4 and G.B.-7	
G.B.-7	*Qu Bin*	Crook of the temple	At the junction of a horizontal line through the apex of the ear and a vertical line through the anterior border of the auricle, within the circumauricular hairline	Meeting point with the T.B., S.I. and BL meridians

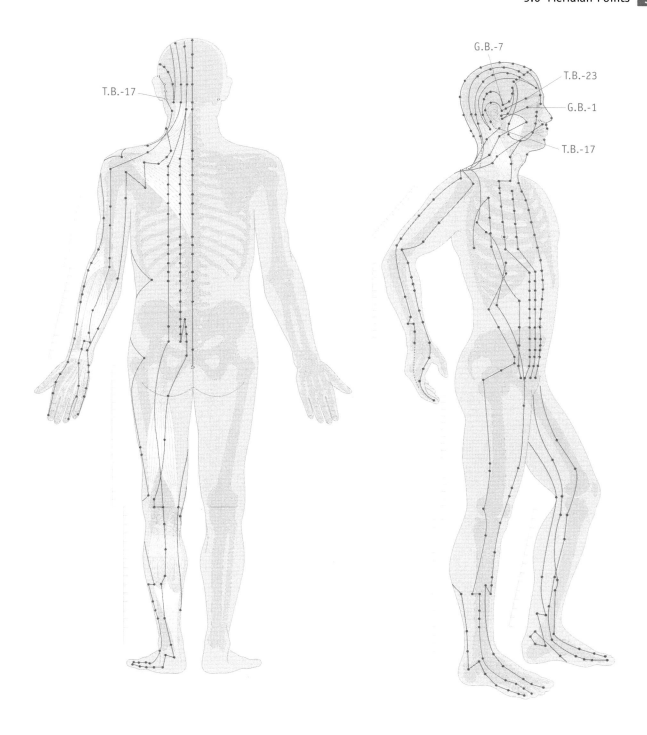

T.B.-17

G.B.-7

T.B.-23

G.B.-1

T.B.-17

Point	Pinyin	Translation	Location	Action
Gall Bladder meridian				
G.B.-8	*Shuai Gu*	Leading valley	1.5 cun superior to the apex of the ear [Bi: 1 cun superior and 1.5 cun posterior to the apex of the ear]	Meeting point with the T.B., ST and L.I. meridians and the *Yang Wei Mai*
G.B.-9	*Tian Chong*	Heavenly rushing	1.5 cun superior to and 0.5 cun posterior to the apex of the ear	
G.B.-10	*Fu Bai*	Floating white	Posterior to the auricle, superior and posterior to the mastoid process, at the junction of a horizontal line through the eyebrow and a vertical line through the posterior border of the mastoid	Meeting point with the T.B. and BL meridians
G.B.-11	*Tou Qiao Yin*	*Yin* portals of the head	Between G.B.-12 (locate first) and G.B.-10	Meeting point with the T.B. and S.I. meridians
G.B.-12	*Wan Gu*	Mastoid process	Posterior and inferior to the mastoid, insertion of the sternocleidomastoid; ask the patient to rotate their head contralaterally	Meeting point with the BL and S.I. meridians
G.B.-13	*Ben Shen*	Root of the Spirit	0.5 cun within the hairline, directly superior to the outer canthus of the eye (3 cun lateral to Du-24)	Meeting point with the *Yang Wei Mai*
G.B.-14	*Yang Bai*	*Yang* white	1 cun superior to the midpoint of the eyebrow, on the pupil line	Meeting point with the T.B., ST and L.I. meridians and the *Yang Wei Mai*
G.B.-15	*Tou Lin Qi*	Head governor of tears	On the pupil line, 0.5 cun within the anterior hairline	Meeting point with the T.B. and BL meridians and the *Yang Wei Mai*
G.B.-16	*Mu Chuang*	Window of the eye	2 cun within the anterior hairline, on a line connecting G.B.-15 (on the pupil line, 0.5 cun within the anterior hairline) and G.B.-20 (posterior to the mastoid); 1.5 cun within the hairline	Meeting point with *Yang Wei Mai*
G.B.-17	*Zheng Ying*	Upright nutrition	At the level of the anterior border of the auricle, on a line connecting G.B.-15 (on the pupil line, 0.5 cun within the anterior hairline) and G.B.-20 (posterior to the mastoid)	Meeting point with *Yang Wei Mai*
G.B.-18	*Cheng Ling*	Support Spirit	At the level of the parietal tuber, on a line connecting G.B.-15 (on the pupil line, 0.5 cun within the anterior hairline) and G.B.-20 (posterior to the mastoid)	Meeting point with *Yang Wei Mai*
G.B.-19	*Nao Kong*	Brain hollow	1.5 cun superior to G.B.-20 (posterior to the mastoid, between the trapezius and sternocleidomastoid, on the lower border of the occiput)	

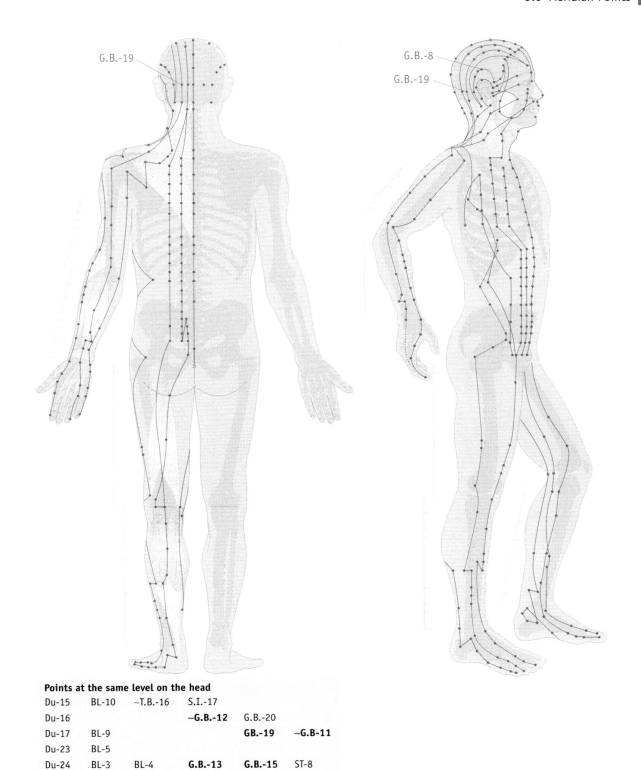

G.B.-19

G.B.-8
G.B.-19

Points at the same level on the head

Du-15	BL-10	~T.B.-16	S.I.-17		
Du-16			~**G.B.-12**	G.B.-20	
Du-17	BL-9		**GB.-19**	~**G.B-11**	
Du-23	BL-5				
Du-24	BL-3	BL-4	**G.B.-13**	**G.B.-15**	ST-8

139

Point	Pinyin	Translation	Location	Action
Gall Bladder meridian				
G.B.-20	*Feng Chi*	Wind pool	Posterior to the mastoid, between the trapezius and sternocleidomastoid, on the lower border of the occiput	Meeting point with the T.B. meridian and the *Yang Wei Mai*
G.B.-21	*Jian Jing*	Shoulder well	On the highest point of the shoulder, midway between the acromion and the spinous process of C7	Meeting point with the ST and T.B. meridians and the *Yang Wei Mai*
			[Bi: on the lateral aspect of the neck, at the 'trapezius kink']	
G.B.-22	*Yuan Ye*	Armpit abyss	With the arm abducted on the midaxillary line, in the 4th ICS (= 3 cun inferior to the apex of the axilla)	
G.B.-23	*Zhe Jin*	Flank sinews	On the pre-axillary line, in the 4th ICS; 1 cun anterior and slightly inferior to G.B.-22	Meeting point with the BL meridian
G.B.-24	*Ri Yue*	Sun and moon	On the midclavicular line, in the 7th ICS [Bi: anterior axillary line, 5th ICS]	• Front-*Mu* point of the Gall Bladder • Meeting point with the SP meridian and the *Yang Wei Mai*
G.B.-25	*Jing Men*	Capital gate	On the lower border of the free end of the 12th rib	
G.B.-26	*Dai Mai*	Girdling vessel	On the anterior axillary line, anterior to the highest point of the anterior superior iliac spine (ASIS), level with the umbilicus	
G.B.-27	*Wu Shu*	Five pivots	3 cun inferior to the umbilicus (level with Ren-4), anterior to the ASIS	
			[Bi: On the ASIS, between G.B.-27 and G.B.-29]	
G.B.-28	*Wei Dao*	Linking path	0.5 cun inferior to the ASIS [G.B.-27 Bi]	Meeting point with the *Dai Mai*
G.B.-29	*Ju Liao*	Stationary crevice	In the depression at the midpoint of a line connecting the ASIS and the highest prominence of the greater trochanter; with the hip flexed at the lateral end of the inguinal crease	Meeting point with the *Yang Wei Mai*
G.B.-30	*Huan Tiao*	Jumping circle	On a line connecting the greater trochanter and the sacral hiatus, at the junction of the lateral and medial third [Bi: posterior to the trochanter; when standing slightly more posterior; closer to the trochanter than the Chinese location]	• Meeting point with the BL meridian • European master point for sciatica and pareses of the lower extremities

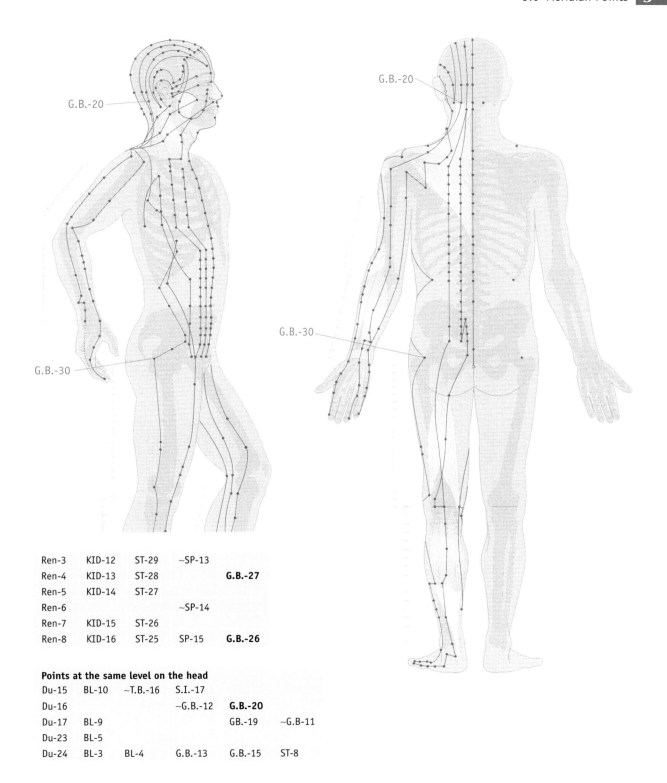

G.B.-20

G.B.-20

G.B.-30

G.B.-30

Ren-3	KID-12	ST-29	~SP-13	
Ren-4	KID-13	ST-28		**G.B.-27**
Ren-5	KID-14	ST-27		
Ren-6			~SP-14	
Ren-7	KID-15	ST-26		
Ren-8	KID-16	ST-25	SP-15	**G.B.-26**

Points at the same level on the head

Du-15	BL-10	~T.B.-16	S.I.-17		
Du-16			~G.B.-12	**G.B.-20**	
Du-17	BL-9			GB.-19	~G.B-11
Du-23	BL-5				
Du-24	BL-3	BL-4	G.B.-13	G.B.-15	ST-8

Point	Pinyin	Translation	Location	Action
Gall Bladder meridian				
G.B.-31	*Feng Shi*	Wind market	On the lateral aspect of the thigh where the trouser seam would be. With the arms hanging down, the middle finger will rest on this point	
G.B.-32	*Zhong Du*	Middle ditch	1 cun inferior to G.B.-31 [Bi: midway between G.B.-30 [Bi] and G.B.-34]	
G.B.-33	*Xi Yang Guan*	Knee *Yang* centre	With the knee flexed in the depression superior to the lateral condyle of the femur, 1 cun superior to the knee joint space, 3 cun superior to G.B.-34	
G.B.-34	*Yang Ling Quan*	*Yang* mound spring	With the knee flexed, in the depression anterior and inferior to the head of the fibula	• *He*-sea point of the Gall Bladder • *Hui*-meeting point of the tendons • European master point for the musculature
G.B.-35	*Yang Jiao*	*Yang* intersection	On the posterior border of the fibula, 7 cun (1 handwidth and 4 fingerwidths) superior to the lateral malleolus. In Chinese literature the locations of G.B.-35 and G.B.-36 are sometimes exchanged!	• *Xi*-cleft point of the *Yang Wei Mai* • Meeting point with the *Yang Wei Mai*
G.B.-36	*Wai Qiu*	Outer hill	At the same level as G.B.-35, but on the anterior border of the fibula, 1 cun anterior to G.B.-35	
G.B.-37	*Guang Ming*	Bright light	5 cun superior to the lateral malleolus, on the anterior border of the fibula	*Luo*-connecting point (connects with LIV-3)
G.B.-38	*Yang Fu*	*Yang* assistance	4 cun superior to the lateral malleolus, on the anterior border of the fibula	• *Jing*-river point • Sedation point
G.B.-39	*Xuan Zhong*	Suspended bell	3 cun superior to the lateral malleolus, on the posterior border of the fibula	• *Hui*-meeting point of the marrow (bone marrow and spinal cord) • Group *Luo*-connecting point of the 3 *Yang* meridians of the leg (ST, G.B., BL)
G.B.-40	*Qiu Xu*	Mound of ruins	On the junction of a horizontal line through the prominence of the lateral malleolus and a vertical line through the greatest circumference of the lateral malleolus, on the calcaneocuboidal joint	*Yuan*-source point
G.B.-41	*Zu Lin Qi*	Foot governor of tears	In the depression distal to the junction of the 4th and 5th metatarsal bones	• *Shu*-stream point • Opening point of the *Dai Mai* • Master point for the big joints

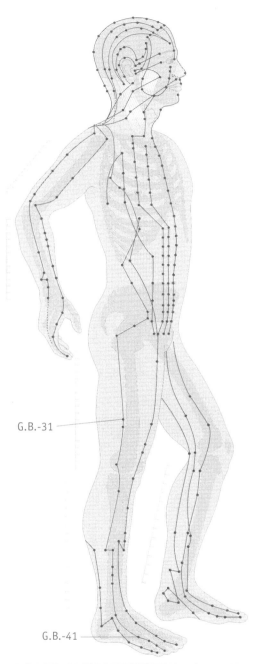

G.B.-31

G.B.-41

G.B.-31

G.B.-41

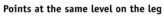

Points at the same level on the leg

	G.B.-40	BL-60
	G.B.-39	BL-59
ST-39	**G.B.-36, G.B.-35**	BL-58
ST-38, ST-40		
		BL-39, BL-40

143

Point	Pinyin	Translation	Location	Action
Gall Bladder meridian				
G.B.-42	*Di Wu Hui*	Earth five meetings	Between the 4th and 5th metatarsal bones, 0.5 cun distal to G.B.-41	
G.B.-43	*Xia Xi*	Clamped stream	Between the 4th and 5th toes, proximal to the margin of the web, closer to the metatarsophalangeal joint of the 4th toe	• *Ying*-spring point • Tonification point
G.B.-44	*Zu Qiao Yin*	*Yin* portals of the foot	On the 4th toe, next to the lateral corner of the nail	*Jing*-well point
Liver meridian				
LIV-1	*Da Dun*	Big mound	On the big toe, next to the lateral corner of the nail	*Jing*-well point
LIV-2	*Xing Jian*	Moving between	Between the 1st and 2nd toes, proximal to the margin of the web, at the lateral aspect of the metatarsophalangeal joint of the 1st toe	• *Ying*-spring point • Sedation point
LIV-3	*Tai Chong*	Great rushing	On the dorsum of the foot, in the depression distal to the junction of the 1st and 2nd metatarsal bones	• *Shu*-stream point • *Yuan*-source point
LIV-4	*Zhong Feng*	Middle seal	1 cun anterior to the medial malleolus, midway between SP-5 and ST-41, in the depression medial to the tendon of the tibialis anterior	*Jing*-river point
LIV-5	*Li Gou*	Woodworm canal	On the medial border of the tibia, 5 cun superior to the medial malleolus [Bi: on the medial border of the tibia, 1.5 cun inferior to the midpoint of the distance between the medial malleolus and upper border of the tibia]	*Luo*-connecting point (connects with G.B.-40)
LIV-6	*Zhong Du*	Central capital	7 cun superior to the medial malleolus, slightly posterior to the medial border of the tibia	*Xi*-cleft point
LIV-7	*Xi Guan*	Knee joint	Posterior and inferior to the medial condyle of the tibia, 1 cun posterior to SP-9	
LIV-8	*Qu Quan*	Spring at the crook	With the knee flexed, in the depression anterior to the medial end of the popliteal crease	*He*-sea point
LIV-9	*Yin Bao*	*Yin* wrapping	4 cun (1 handwidth) superior to the medial epicondyle of the femur, between the gracilis and sartorius muscles	
LIV-10	*Zu Wu Li*	Leg five miles	2 cun lateral and 3 cun inferior to the midpoint of the pubic symphysis, on the lateral border of the abductor longus	
LIV-11	*Yin Lian*	*Yin* corner	2 cun lateral and 2 cun inferior to the midpoint of the pubic symphysis, on the lateral border of the abductor longus	

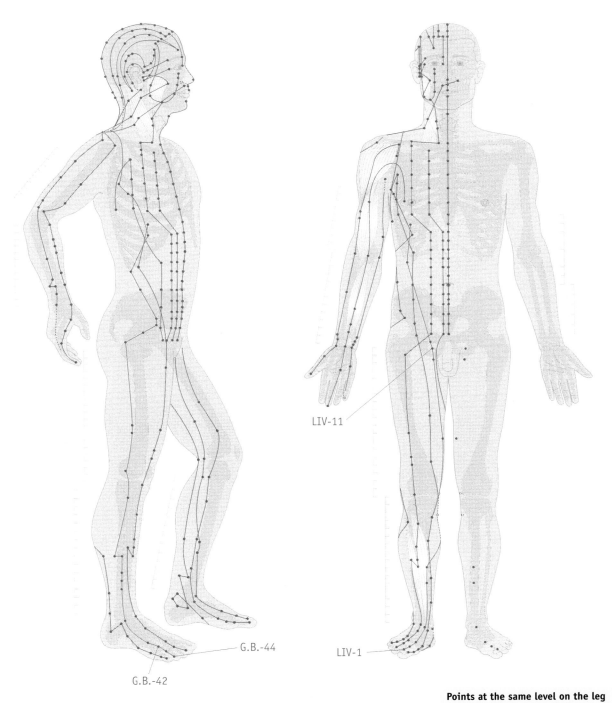

G.B.-44

G.B.-42

LIV-11

LIV-1

Points at the same level on the leg

	LIV-5	KID-9
SP-8	**LIV-7**	
	LIV-8	KID-10

145

Point	Pinyin	Translation	Location	Action
Liver meridian				
LIV-12	*Ji Mai*	Urgent pulse	2.5 cun lateral to the anterior midline, anterior and inferior to the pubic crest	
LIV-13	*Zhang Men*	Completion gate	On the lower border of the free end of the 11th rib	• Metabolic point • Front-*Mu* point of the Spleen • *Hui*-meeting point of the *Zang* organs • Meeting point with the G.B. meridian
LIV-14	*Qi Men*	Cycle gate	On the midclavicular line, in the 6th ICS, directly below the nipple	• Front-*Mu* point of the Liver • Meeting point with the Spleen meridian • Special point: sea sickness, hyperemesis
Du Mai				
Du-1	*Chang Qiang*	Long strong	Between the coccyx and the anus	
Du-2	*Yao Shu*	Lumbar *Shu*	In the sacral hiatus	Back-*Shu* point of the lumbar region
Du-3	*Yao Yang Guan*	Lumbar *Yang* gate	Below the spinous process of L4. By influencing the lower spine, it also has an effect on the opposite (cranial) aspect of the spine	
Du-4	*Ming Men*	Gate of life	Below the spinous process of L2, level with BL-23 and BL-52 [Bi: BL-47]	
Du-5	*Xuan Shu*	Suspended pivot	Below the spinous process of L1, level with BL-22	
Du-6	*Ji Zhong*	Centre of the spine	Below the spinous process of T12, level with BL-20	
Du-7	*Zhong Shu*	Central pivot	Below the spinous process of T10, level with BL-19	
Du-8	*Jin Suo*	Sinew contraction	Below the spinous process of T9, level with BL-18	
Du-9	*Zhi Yang*	Reaching *Yang*	Below the spinous process of T7, level with BL-17	
Du-10	*Ling Tai*	Spirit tower	Below the spinous process of T6, level with BL-16	

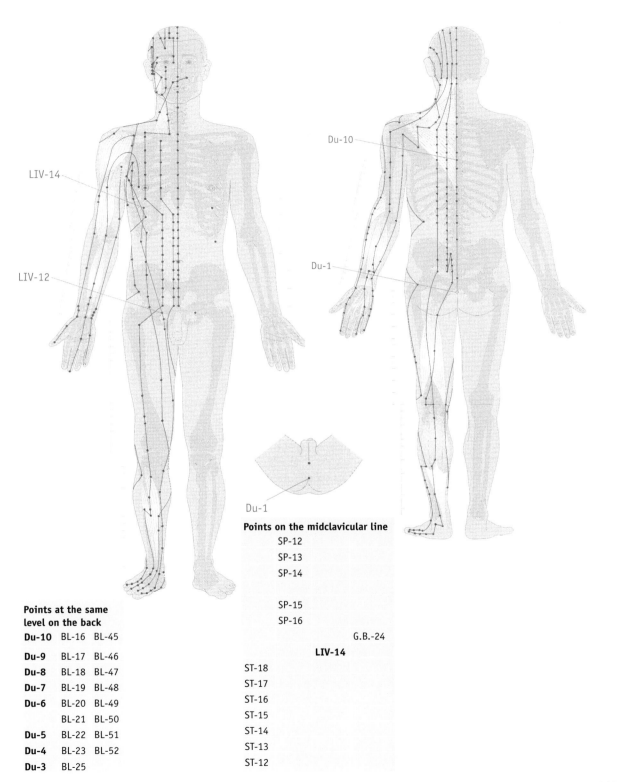

LIV-14

LIV-12

Du-10

Du-1

Du-1

Points on the midclavicular line
SP-12

SP-13

SP-14

SP-15

SP-16

G.B.-24

LIV-14

ST-18

ST-17

ST-16

ST-15

ST-14

ST-13

ST-12

Points at the same level on the back

Du-10	BL-16	BL-45
Du-9	BL-17	BL-46
Du-8	BL-18	BL-47
Du-7	BL-19	BL-48
Du-6	BL-20	BL-49
	BL-21	BL-50
Du-5	BL-22	BL-51
Du-4	BL-23	BL-52
Du-3	BL-25	

Point	Pinyin	Translation	Location	Action
Du Mai				
Du-11	*Shen Dao*	Spirit pathway	Below the spinous process of T5, level with BL-15	
Du-12	*Shen Zhu*	Body pillar	Below the spinous process of T3, level with BL-13	
Du-13	*Tao Dao*	Path of change/ way to the kiln[a]/way of happiness[b]	Below the spinous process of T1	
Du-14	*Da Zhui*	Great vertebra	Below the spinous process of C7	Meeting point of all *Yang* meridians
Du-15	*Ya Men*	Gate of muteness	0.5 cun within the posterior hairline	
Du-16	*Feng Fu*	Palace of Wind	1 cun within the posterior hairline, in the depression inferior to the external occipital protuberance	Meeting point with the Bladder meridian and the *Yang Wei Mai*
Du-17	*Nao Hu*	Brain's door	2.5 cun within the posterior hairline, superior to the external occipital protuberance	
Du-18	*Qiang Jian*	Unyielding space	4 cun within the posterior hairline, midway between Du-16 (1 cun within the posterior hairline) and Du-20 (7 cun superior the posterior hairline)	
Du-19	*Hou Ding*	Behind the crown	5.5 cun superior to the posterior hairline	
Du-20	*Bai Hui*	Hundred meetings	On a line connecting the apices of the ears, 7 cun superior the posterior hairline	Universal meeting point, meeting point of all divergent meridians
Du-21	*Qian Ding*	In front of the crown	1.5 cun anterior to the vertex	
Du-22	*Xin Hui*	Fontanelle meeting	2 cun within the anterior hairline, 9 cun anterior to the posterior hairline, 3 cun anterior to Du-20	
Du-23	*Shang Xing*	Upper star	1 cun within the anterior hairline	Meeting point with the Bladder meridian
Du-24	*Shen Ting*	Courtyard of the Spirit	On the midline, 0.5 cun within the anterior hairline	
Du-25	*Su Liao*	White crevice	On the tip of the nose	
Du-26	*Shui Guo* or *Ren Zhong*	Water groove or man's middle	At the junction of the upper and middle third of the philtrum	Meeting point with the *Yang Ming* meridians (ST, L.I.); emergency and analgesia point
Du-27	*Dui Duan*	Extremity of the mouth	On the midline, at the margin of the upper lip and the philtrum	
Du-28	*Yi Jiao*	Gum intersection	At the labial and of the frenulum	

[a]Maciocia 1989a (p. 470)
[b]Ding 1991 (p. 232)

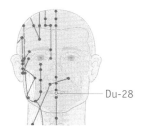

Du-28

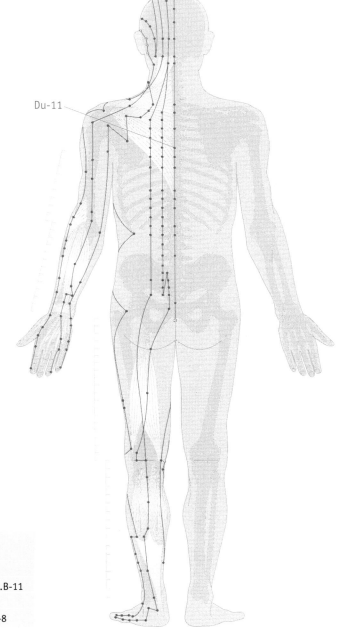

Du-11

Points at the same level on the back

DU-13	BL-11	
	BL-12	BL-41
Du-12	BL-13	BL-42
	BL-14	BL-43
DU-11	BL-15	BL-44

Points at the same level on the head

Du-15	BL-10	~T.B.-16	S.I.-17		
Du-16			~G.B.-12	G.B.-20	
Du-17	BL-9			GB.-19	~G.B-11
Du-23	BL-5				
Du-24	BL-3	BL-4	G.B.-13	G.B.-15	ST-8

Point	Pinyin	Translation	Location	Action
Ren Mai				
Ren-1	*Hui Yin*	Meeting of *Yin*	At the perineum, between the anus and the scrotum and posterior labial commissure respectively	Meeting point with the *Du Mai* and *Chong Mai*
Ren-2	*Qu Gu*	Curved bone	On the midline, at the upper border of the pubic symphysis, in the skin crease that forms when bending forward; level with KID-11, SP-12, ST-30	Meeting point with the Liver meridian
Ren-3	*Zhong Ji*	Middle pole	1 cun superior to the upper border of the pubic symphysis (1/5 of the distance between the symphysis and the umbilicus)	• Meeting point with the 3 *Yin* meridians of the leg (SP, LIV, KID) • Front-*Mu* point of the Bladder
Ren-4	*Guan Yuan*	Gate of the source	2 cun superior to the upper border of the pubic symphysis (2/5 of the distance between the symphysis and the umbilicus)	• Internal meeting point of the 3 *Yin* meridians of the leg (SP, LIV, KID) • Front-*Mu* point of the Small Intestine
Ren-5	*Shi Men*	Stone gate	2 cun inferior to the umbilicus	Main front-*Mu* point of the Triple Burner
Ren-6	*Qi Hai*	Sea of *Qi*	1.5 cun inferior to the umbilicus	
Ren-7	*Yin Jiao*	*Yin* intersection	1 cun inferior to the umbilicus	Meeting point with the *Chong Mai*
Ren-8	*Shen Que*	Spirit gateway	In the centre of the umbilicus	
Ren-9	*Shui Fen*	Water separation	1 cun superior to the umbilicus	
Ren-10	*Xia Wan*	Lower cavity	2 cun superior to the umbilicus	Meeting point with the Spleen meridian
Ren-11	*Jian Li*	Strengthen the interior	3 cun superior to the umbilicus	
Ren-12	*Zhong Wan*	Middle cavity	Midway between the umbilicus and the xiphoid process	• *Hui*-meeting point of the *Fu* organs • Meeting point with the Small Intestine and Triple Burner meridians
Ren-13	*Shang Wan*	Upper cavity	5 cun (1 handwidth and 1 thumbwidth) superior to the umbilicus (5/8 of the distance between the umbilicus and the xiphoid process)	Meeting point with the Stomach and Small Intestine meridians

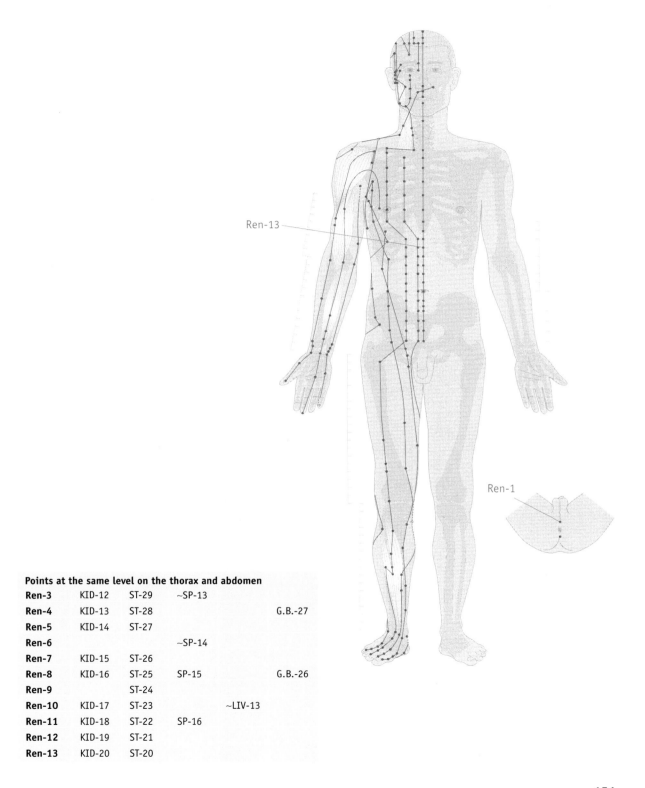

Ren-13

Ren-1

Points at the same level on the thorax and abdomen

Ren-3	KID-12	ST-29	~SP-13		
Ren-4	KID-13	ST-28			G.B.-27
Ren-5	KID-14	ST-27			
Ren-6			~SP-14		
Ren-7	KID-15	ST-26			
Ren-8	KID-16	ST-25	SP-15		G.B.-26
Ren-9		ST-24			
Ren-10	KID-17	ST-23		~LIV-13	
Ren-11	KID-18	ST-22	SP-16		
Ren-12	KID-19	ST-21			
Ren-13	KID-20	ST-20			

Point	Pinyin	Translation	Location	Action
Ren Mai				
Ren-14	*Ju Que*	Great gateway	2 cun inferior to the xiphoid process [Bi: 1 cun inferior to the xiphoid process]	Front-*Mu* point of the Heart
Ren-15	*Jiu Wei*	Turtledove tail	1 cun inferior to the xiphoid process [Bi: directly inferior to the tip of the xiphoid process]	Together with Du-20, the 'Bellergal' of acupuncture (Bachmann)
Ren-16	*Zhong Ting*	Central courtyard	On the midline of the sternum, at the level of the 5th ICS	
Ren-17	*Dan Zhong* (*Shao Zhong*)	Chest centre	On the midline of the sternum, at the level of the 4th ICS, in men between the nipples	• Front-*Mu* point of the Pericardium • Respiratory front-*Mu* point of the Triple Burner • *Hui*-meeting point of the respiratory system • Meeting point with the Spleen, Kidney, Small Intestine and Triple Burner meridians
Ren-18	*Yu Tang*	Jade hall	On the midline of the sternum, at the level of the 3rd ICS	
Ren-19	*Zi Gong*	Purple palace	On the midline of the sternum, at the level of the 2nd ICS	
Ren-20	*Hua Gai*	Magnificent canopy	On the midline of the sternum, at the level of the 1st ICS	
Ren-21	*Xuan Ji*	Jade pivot	On the midline of the sternum, 1 cun below the jugulum (Ren-22)	Meeting point with the *Yin Wei Mai*
Ren-22	*Tian Tu*	Heavenly prominence	In the centre of the jugulum	Meeting point with the *Yin Wei Mai*
Ren-23	*Lian Quan*	Corner spring	Superior to the larynx, above the hyoid bone, at the junction of the neck and the chin [Bi: at the level of the thyroid cartilage]	Meeting point with the *Yin Wei Mai*
Ren-24	*Cheng Jiang*	Container of fluids	In the centre of the mentolabial groove	Meeting point with the Stomach and Large Intestine Meridians, and with the *Du Mai*

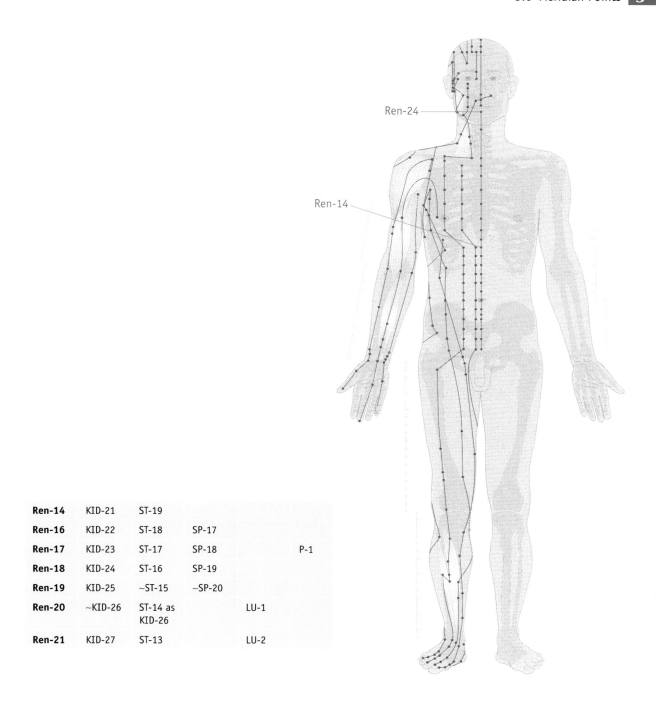

Ren-24

Ren-14

Ren-14	KID-21	ST-19			
Ren-16	KID-22	ST-18	SP-17		
Ren-17	KID-23	ST-17	SP-18		P-1
Ren-18	KID-24	ST-16	SP-19		
Ren-19	KID-25	~ST-15	~SP-20		
Ren-20	~KID-26	ST-14 as KID-26		LU-1	
Ren-21	KID-27	ST-13		LU-2	

5.7 Acupuncture points at the same anatomical level

Points at the same level on the head

		S.I.-17	~T.B.-16	BL-10	Du-15	BL-10	~T.B.-16	S.I.-17		
	G.B.-20	~G.B.-12			Du-16				G.B.-12	~G.B.-20
~G.B.-11	G.B.-19			BL-9	Du-17	BL-9			G.B.-19	~G.B.-11
				BL-3	Du-23	BL-3				
ST-8	G.B.-15	G.B.-13	BL-4	BL-3	Du-24	BL-3	BL-4	G.B.-13	G.B.-15	ST-8

Points at the same level on the thorax and abdomen

		LU-2			ST-13	KID-27	Ren-21	KID-27	ST-13			LU-2		
		LU-1			ST-14	~KID-26	Ren-20	~KID-26	ST-14			LU-1		
				As KID-26						As KID-26				
				~SP-20	~ST-15	KID-25	Ren-19	KID-25	~ST-15	~SP-20				
				SP-19	ST-16	KID-24	Ren-18	KID-24	ST-16	SP-19				
	P-1			SP-18	ST-17	KID-23	Ren-17	KID-23	ST-17	SP-18			P-1	
				SP-17	ST-18	KID-22	Ren-16	KID-22	ST-18	SP-17				
					ST-19	KID-21	Ren-14	KID-21	ST-19					
					ST-20	KID-20	Ren-13	KID-20	ST-20					
					ST-21	KID-19	Ren-12	KID-19	ST-21					
				SP-16	ST-22	KID-18	Ren-11	KID-18	ST-22	SP-16				
			~LIV-13		ST-23	KID-17	Ren-10	KID-17	ST-23		~LIV-13			
					ST-24		Ren-9		ST-24					
G.B.-26				SP-15	ST-25	KID-16	Ren-8	KID-16	ST-25	SP-15				G.B.-26
					ST-26	KID-15	Ren-7	KID-15	ST-26					
				SP-14			Ren-6			SP-14				
					ST-27	KID-14	Ren-5	KID-14	ST-27					
G.B.-27					ST-28	KID-13	Ren-4	KID-13	ST-28					G.B.-27
				SP-13	ST-29	KID-12	Ren-3	KID-12	ST-29	SP-13				

Points on the midclavicular line

- SP-12
- SP-13
- SP-14
- SP-15
- SP-16
- G.B.-24
- LIV-14
- ST-18
- ST-17
- ST-16
- ST-15
- ST-14
- ST-13
- ST-12

Points at the same level on the back

	BL-11		Du-13		BL-11	
BL-41	BL-12				BL-12	BL-41
BL-42	BL-13		Du-12		BL-13	BL-42
BL-43	BL-14				BL-14	BL-43
BL-44	BL-15		Du-11		BL-15	BL-44
BL-45	BL-16		Du-10		BL-16	BL-45
BL-46	BL-17		Du-9		BL-17	BL-46
BL-47	BL-18		Du-8		BL-18	BL-47
BL-48	BL-19		Du-7		BL-19	BL-48
BL-49	BL-20		Du-6		BL-20	BL-49
BL-50	BL-21				BL-21	BL-50
BL-51	BL-22		Du-5		BL-22	BL-51
BL-52	BL-23		Du-4		BL-23	BL-52
	BL-25		Du-3		BL-25	
	BL-27	BL-31		BL-31	BL-27	
BL-53	BL-28	BL-32		BL-32	BL-28	BL-53
	BL-29	BL-33		BL-33	BL-29	
	BL-30	BL-34		BL-34	BL-30	
BL-54			Du-2			BL-54

Points at the same level on the leg (*Yang*)

	G.B.-40	BL-60
	G.B.-39	BL-59
ST-39	G.B.-36, G.B.-35	BL-58
ST-38, ST-40		
		BL-39, BL-40

Points at the same level on the leg (*Yin*)

		KID-7, KID-8
	LIV-5	KID-9
SP-8	LIV-7	
	LIV-8	KID-10
SP-12	LIV-12	KID-11

6

Indications and individual point combinations

6.1 Introduction

G. Kubiena, B. Sommer

One of the central aspects of holistic therapies such as acupuncture are treatment protocols that take the unique make-up of the patient into account.

Translating the findings of a TCM differential diagnosis into a point prescription is a process that, although a challenging task for the beginner, can certainly be learnt over time.

When the translated original literature is compared with both older and more recent publications by Western authors, it is noticeable that the recommended point prescriptions are often quite similar.

We believe that, for practitioners trained in Western medicine, the best and most user-friendly way to design individual treatments is to be familiar with the most important points for a particular indication and to complement these points according to the individual signs and symptoms in each case.

The point combinations described in this chapter are the result of these considerations and are based on existing literature as well as our own clinical experience.

The **basic point combinations** list the most important points for each indication.

The **individual point combinations** take the individual pattern of the patient into account.

Commentaries are added where considered necessary for a deeper understanding of the point prescription. They explain the individual indications of the relevant points as well as more general TCM theories and concepts.

Information on techniques is added when needling and stimulation techniques other than the standard ones are required.

We have limited the point prescriptions to the most important points and techniques which most acupuncturists will be familiar with, in order to make the book as accessible and user-friendly as possible.

The extraordinary points, auricular points and hand points mentioned in this chapter are described on pages 91–101.

6.2 Cardiovascular disorders

D. Bergfeld, B. Sommer

Acupuncture tends to produce good results in the treatment of functional heart disorders as well as problems caused by disorders of the autonomic nervous system. Acupuncture should always be accompanied by Western treatments. The heart muscle, valves and conduction system can, of course, not be influenced. The beginning stages of coronary heart disease without any advanced narrowing of the coronary arteries are well suited for acupuncture.

TCM

In TCM, the head and the upper thorax are associated with the Heart. As well as cardiovascular disorders, organ-specific symptoms attributed to the Heart are loss of memory, insomnia and psychosomatic problems, as well as speech disorders. In TCM, the Heart plays such a central role that any disorder affecting the Heart will also affect other organs, and vice versa.

6.2.1 Peripheral circulatory disorders

Generally, the blood vessels respond very well to acupuncture. As already mentioned, this relates only to functional disorders; advanced vascular sclerosis cannot be treated with acupuncture.

Although Raynaud's syndrome responds well to TENS, it can also be treated with the point combination for the treatment of the upper extremity.

Basic point combination

SP-6, BL-58.
Strong stimulation.

Individual point combination

Circulatory disorder of the upper extremity

LU-9, L.I.-4, L.I.-11, P-6, P-8, Ex-UE-9 (*Ba Xie*).

Acrocyanosis of the hand

L.I.-4, S.I.-3, T.B.-4.
Local points on the palmar aspect of the fingers.

Circulatory disorders of the lower extremity

G.B.-34, Ex-LE-10 (*Ba Feng*).

Intermittent claudication

BL-60, BL-62.
Ear points: leg, foot [Bi: acupuncture will, within a short period of time, improve walking performance and reduce onset of fatigue].

Acupuncture points

BL-58 **Location:** 1 cun distal and lateral to BL-57, on the lateral border of the gastrocnemius, on the soleus.
Notes: *Luo*-connecting point; resolves stagnations (according to TCM circulation disorders correspond to *Qi* and Blood (*Xue*) stagnation).

BL-60 **Location:** in the depression between the Achilles tendon and the lateral malleolus.
Notes: *Jing*-river point, master point for any pain along the course of the meridian.

BL-62 **Location:** below the prominence of the lateral malleolus.
Notes: Opening point of the *Yang Qiao Mai*, which regulates agility and movement.

Ex-UE-9 **Location:** when a loose fist is made, 4 points on the dorsum of each hand, slightly proximal to the margins of the webs between the heads of the 1st to 5th metacarpal bones.
Notes: promotes circulation, expels external pathogens (use bloodletting).

Ex-LE-10 **Location:** 4 points on the dorsum of the foot, 0.5 cun proximal to the interdigital folds.
Notes: promotes circulation, expels external pathogens (let bleed).

G.B.-34 **Location:** with the knee flexed, in the depression anterior and inferior to the head of the fibula.
Notes: *He*-sea point, direct action on the organ; strongly moves *Qi*.

L.I.-4 **Location:** on the dorsum of the hand, at the highest point of the muscle bulge between the 1st and 2nd metacarpal bones.
Notes: *Yuan*-source point; moves *Qi*, removes obstructions in the meridian.

L.I.-11 **Location:** with the arm in maximum flexion, at the radial end of the cubital crease.
Notes: *He*-sea point.

LU-9 **Location:** on the wrist crease, radial to the radial artery.
Notes: *Shu*-stream point, *Hui*-meeting point of the blood vessels.

P-6 **Location:** 2 cun proximal to the midpoint of the palmar wrist crease, between the tendons of the flexor carpi radialis and palmaris longus.
Notes: opening point of the *Yin Wei Mai*, strong general effect on the vessels and cardiovascular system.

P-8 **Location:** when a fist is made, the tip of the middle finger points to P-8, between the distal and medial transverse crease, between the 2nd and 3rd metacarpal bones.
Notes: *Ying*-spring point, local point.

S.I.-3 **Location:** when a fist is made, on the dorsum of the hand, in the depression at the end of the most distal palmar crease.
Notes: *Shu*-stream point, tonification point; spasmolytic.

SP-6 **Location:** 3 cun superior to the highest prominence of the medial malleolus, on the posterior border of the tibia.
Notes: group *Luo*-connecting point of the 3 *Yin* meridians of the leg (SP, KID, LIV); balancing effect on the cardiovascular system, invigorates *Qi* and Blood (*Xue*) circulation and lymphatic flow.

T.B.-4 **Location:** on the wrist crease, in the depression lateral to the tendon of the extensor digitorum longus.
Notes: *Yuan*-source point; eliminates obstructions in the meridian.

S.I.-3 **Location:** when a fist is made, on the dorsum of the hand, in the depression at the end of the most distal palmar crease.
Notes: *Shu*-stream point, tonification point; spasmolytic.

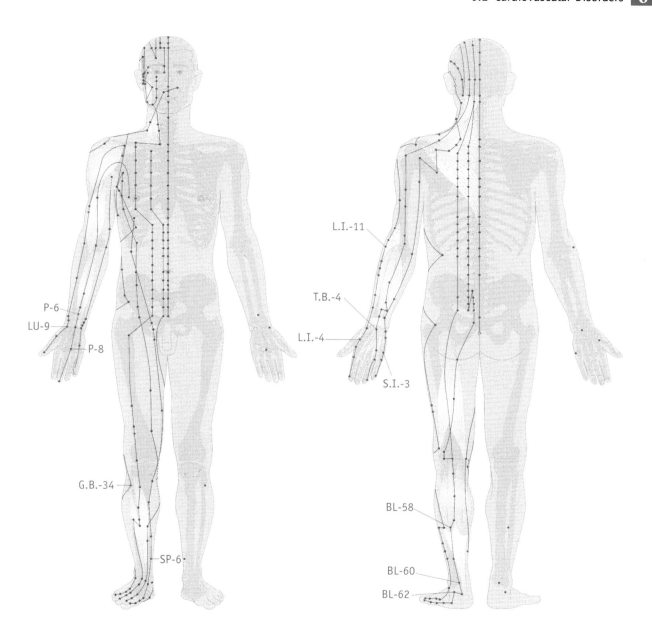

P-6

LU-9

P-8

G.B.-34

SP-6

L.I.-11

T.B.-4

L.I.-4

S.I.-3

BL-58

BL-60

BL-62

6.2.2 Functional disorders

Functional heart disorders tend to respond well to acupuncture. Although common risk factors, as well as other criteria of Western medicine, have to be taken into consideration, medication can often be reduced as a result of acupuncture treatments.

Basic point combination

SP-4, HE-7, BL-15, Ren-17.
Ear points: 21 Heart organ, 51 autonomic nervous system, 100 Heart.

Individual point combination

Angina pectoris

P-6.

Tachycardia

Ex-B-2 (*Hua Tuo Jiaji*) at the relevant level.

Bradycardia

HE-5, Du-25 [Du-24 Bi].

Heart disorders with tendency to oedema

LU-7.

Heart disorders accompanied by dyspnoea

BL-17.

Heart disorders, patient in overall poor condition

ST-36, SP-6, Ren-6.

Cardiac neurosis

HE-3.

Acupuncture points

BL-15 **Location:** 1.5 cun lateral to the spinous process of T5.
Notes: back-*Shu* point of the Heart, invigorates the Blood.

BL-17 **Location:** 1.5 cun lateral to the spinous process of T7, approximately level with the inferior angle of the scapula.
Notes: back-*Shu* point of the diaphragm, improves diaphragmatic motility, *Hui*-meeting point of the Blood, unbinds the chest.

Du-25 **Location:** on the tip of the nose.
Notes: stimulates the autonomic nervous system.

Ex-B-2 **Location:** 17 point pairs, 0.5 cun lateral to the lower borders of the spinous processes of T1 to L5, medial to the inner Bladder line.
Notes: as local points effect on the nerves of the relevant segment.

HE-3 **Location:** with the elbow fully flexed, between the medial end of the cubital crease and the medial epicondyle.
Notes: *He*-sea point, eliminates stagnation in the HE meridian, master point for depression, psychologically uplifting.

HE-5 **Location:** 1 cun proximal to HE-7.
Notes: *Luo*-connecting point, opens the coronary vessels.

HE-7 **Location:** on the ulnar aspect of the wrist crease, on the radial aspect of the pisiform bone.
Notes: *Shu*-stream point, sedation point, calms the Spirit, pacifies the Heart, resolves stagnation of the Heart *Qi* and in the chest.

LU-7 **Location:** 1.5 cun proximal to the wrist crease, at the radial artery.
Notes: *Luo*-connecting point, opening point of the *Ren Mai*, master point for stagnation.

P-6 **Location:** 2 cun proximal to the midpoint of the palmar wrist crease, between the tendons of the flexor carpi radialis and palmaris longus.
Notes: opening point of the *Yin Wei Mai*, has an effect on heart function, strong general effect on the vessels and cardiovascular system.

Ren-6 **Location:** 1.5 cun inferior to the umbilicus.
Notes: tonifies the original *Qi*.

Ren-17 **Location:** on the midline of the sternum, at the level of the 4th intercostal space (ICS), between the nipples (in men).
Notes: front-*Mu* point of the Pericardium, *Hui*-meeting point of the respiratory system, unbinds the chest.

SP-4 **Location:** in the depression at the junction of the base and shaft of the 1st metatarsal bone, at the junction of the red and white skin.
Notes: opening point of the *Chong Mai*, has an effect on heart function.

SP-6 **Location:** 3 cun superior to the highest prominence of the medial malleolus, on the posterior border of the tibia.
Notes: group *Luo*-connecting point of the 3 *Yin* meridians of the leg (SP, KID, LIV); balancing effect on the cardiovascular system, invigorates the *Qi* and Blood (*Xue*) circulation and lymphatic flow.

ST-36 **Location:** 0.5 cun lateral to the anterior crest of the tibia, 1.5 cun inferior to the lower border of the head of the fibula (G.B.-34).
Notes: *He*-sea point.

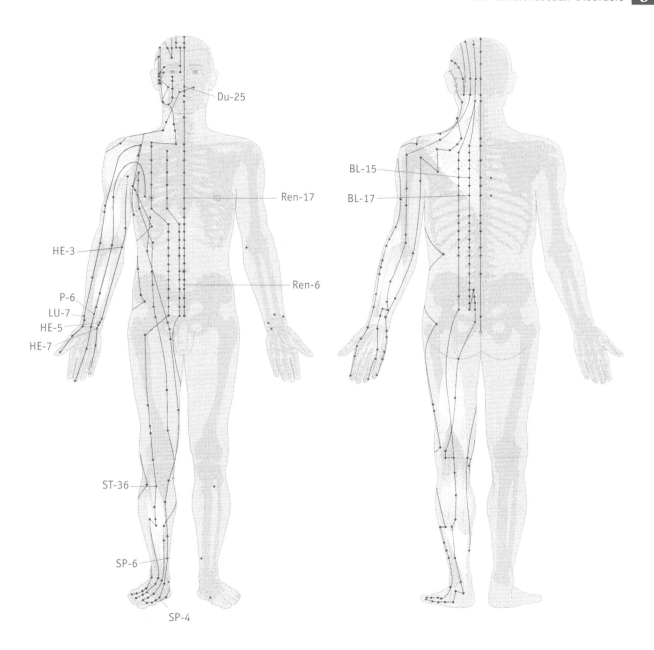

6.2.3 Hypertension

Acupuncture can be used in conjunction with Western medicine to treat essential hypertension and to reduce antihypertensive medication. A chiropractic assessment is important in order to eliminate any blockages of the cervical spine.

TCM

Most commonly Kidney *Yin* deficiency and Liver *Yang* excess.

Basic point combination

ST-36, HE-7, P-6, LIV-2 (during the acute stage), LIV-3 (during remission).
Ear points: 59 (hypertension), 100 (Heart), 105 (blood pressure lowering groove).

Individual point combination

Hypertension with insomnia

HE-5, Du-20, Ex-HN-3 (*Yin Tang*).

Hypertension in patients with an overall poor constitution

L.I.-11, BL-20, Ren-6.

Hypertension accompanied by restlessness, stress

P-7, Du-20.

Acupuncture points

BL-20 **Location:** 1.5 cun lateral to the spinous process of T11.
Notes: back-*Shu* point of the Spleen, tonifies the Spleen and therefore *Qi*.

Du-20 **Location:** on the line connecting the apices of the ears.
Notes: meeting point of all divergent meridians; therefore has a psychosomatic effect, sedating, psychologically harmonizing, stabilizes the autonomic nervous system.

Ex-HN-3 **Location:** at the midpoint between the eyebrows.
Notes: relaxing.

HE-5 **Location:** 1 cun proximal to HE-7.
Notes: clears heat in the Heart, calms the Spirit.

HE-7 **Location:** on the ulnar aspect of the wrist crease, on the radial aspect of the pisiform bone.
Notes: *Yuan*-source point, sedation point, psychologically calming, pacifies the Heart.

L.I.-11 **Location:** with the arm fully flexed at the radial end of the cubital crease.
Noes: *He*-sea point, tonification point.

LIV-2 **Location:** on the web between the 1st and 2nd toes, at the lateral aspect of the metatarsophalangeal joint of the 1st toe.
Notes: sedation point, descends and calms rising Liver Fire.

LIV-3 **Location:** on the dorsum of the foot, in the depression distal to the junction of the 1st and 2nd metatarsal bones.
Notes: *Shu*-stream point, *Yuan*-source point, hypotensive, spasmolytic, harmonizes the Liver *Qi*.

P-6 **Location:** 2 cun proximal to the midpoint of the palmar wrist crease, between the tendons of the flexor carpi radialis and palmaris longus.
Notes: opening point of the *Yin Wei Mai*, has an effect on heart functioning, harmonizes the cardiovascular system.

P-7 **Location:** in the centre of the palmar wrist crease, between the tendons of the flexor carpi radialis and the palmaris longus.
Notes: *Yuan*-source point, sedation point, calms the Spirit, pacifies the Heart.

Ren-6 **Location:** 1.5 cun inferior to the umbilicus.
Notes: tonifies the original *Qi*.

SP-6 **Location:** 3 cun superior to the highest prominence of the medial malleolus, on the posterior border of the tibia.
Notes: group *Luo*-connecting point for the 3 *Yin* of the leg, harmonizes the cardiovascular system.

ST-36 **Location:** 0.5 cun lateral to the anterior crest of the tibia, 1.5 cun inferior to the lower border of the head of the fibula (G.B.-34).
Notes: *He*-sea point, stabilizes, tonifies, psychologically harmonizing.

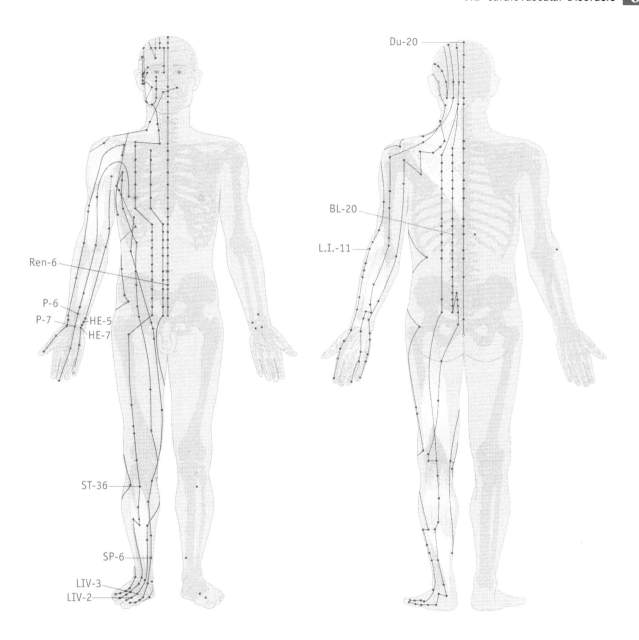

6.2.4 Hypotension

According to most authors, hypotension is more difficult to treat than hypertension. In our experience, small but stable increases in blood pressure can be expected, allowing a significant reduction in medication.

Hypotension often presents with typical symptoms of deficiency such as tiredness, a feeling of weakness, quickly becoming cold, cold hands and feet.

TCM

Qi deficiency, *Yang* deficiency, Blood (*Xue*) deficiency.

Basic point combination

ST-36, KID-7, P-6, Ren-12.
Ear acupuncture: 29 (occiput), 51 (autonomic nervous system), 100 (Heart).
Technique: moxibustion is recommended, tonifying needling technique (little stimulation).

Individual point combination

Hypotension with unstable autonomic nervous system

BL-10, G.B.-20.

Hypotension in patient with psychological stress

HE-3.

Acute hypotension, orthostatic collapse

HE-9, P-9, Du-26.

Acupuncture points

BL-10 **Location:** at the external occipital protuberance, on the lateral aspect of the trapezius insertion.
Notes: combined with G.B.-20, harmonizes the autonomic nervous system.

Du-26 **Location:** at the junction of the upper and middle third of the philtrum.
Notes: emergency point, analgesic point, strong effect on the cardiovascular system.

G.B.-20 **Location:** posterior to the mastoid, between the trapezius and sternocleidomastoid, on the lower border of the occiput.
Notes: together with BL-10 harmonizes the autonomic nervous system, has an effect on the sympathetic nervous system.

HE-3 **Location:** with the elbow fully flexed, between the medial end of the cubital crease and the medial epicondyle.
Notes: *He*-sea point, master point for depression, psychologically uplifting.

HE-9 **Location:** on the little finger, next to the radial corner of the nail.
Notes: tonification point, for collapse.

KID-7 **Location:** on the anterior border of the Achilles tendon, posterior to the flexor digitorum longus, 2 cun superior to the highest prominence of the medial malleolus.
Notes: tonification point, tonifies specifically Kidney *Yang*.

P-6 **Location:** 2 cun proximal to the midpoint of the palmar wrist crease, between the tendons of the flexor carpi radialis and palmaris longus.
Notes: opening point of the *Yin Wei Mai*, has an effect on heart function, also on the vessels and the cardiovascular system.

P-9 **Location:** on the centre of tip of the middle finger.
Notes: shock point.

Ren-12 **Location:** midway between the umbilicus and the xiphoid process.
Notes: front-*Mu* point of the Stomach, together with ST-36 also tonifies the Spleen and therefore *Qi*

ST-36 **Location:** 0.5 cun lateral to the anterior crest of the tibia, 1.5 cun inferior to the lower border of the head of the fibula (G.B.-34).
Notes: *He*-sea point of the Stomach, master point for hormones and blood pressure.

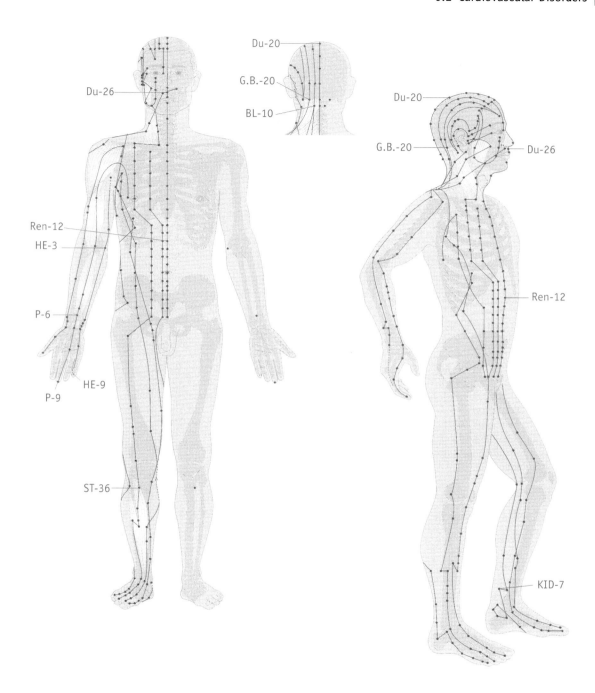

Du-26

Du-20
G.B.-20
BL-10

Du-20
G.B.-20
Du-26

Ren-12
HE-3

P-6

P-9
HE-9

Ren-12

ST-36

KID-7

6.3 Lung disorders

G. Kubiena

6.3.1 Bronchial asthma (1) – Deficiency type

In TCM, 'asthma' is considered a form of dyspnoea caused by a disturbance of the free flow of Lung *Qi*. Deficiency-type asthma is due to Lung or Kidney *Qi* deficiency; excess-type asthma is due to external pathogenic factors, or Phlegm-Heat or Phlegm-Cold.

Basic point combination

LU-9, BL-13, Ren-17 or opening points LU-7 and KID-6. Ear acupuncture: 31 asthma, 101 Lung, 103 trachea.

Individual point combination

General weakness following a prolonged disease, cough

TCM: Lung *Qi* deficiency type.
Symptoms: difficulty breathing in, shortness of breath, weak, deep cough, low voice, sweating upon exertion; **pulse:** forceless; **tongue:** pale.
Treatment principle: tonify the Child (Lung/Metal) by tonifying the Mother (Spleen/Earth).
Points: for tonifying the Lung *Qi*: BL-13, LU-9; for tonifying the Spleen: SP-3, BL-20, Ren-12, ST-36.

Chronic asthma, emphysema, possibly following steroid therapy

TCM: Kidney deficiency type.
Symptoms: similar to above, plus wheezing, contraction of the supraclavicular tissue, tiredness, weakness, cold extremities; pulse: deep, thready.
Points: to tonify the Kidneys: BL-23, KID-3, Du-4 (moxa), Ren-6 (moxa); to regulate breathing: Ren-17, BL-43 (moxa); to tonify the Spleen and resolve phlegm: BL-12, Ren-12, ST-40; to improve the overall condition: BL-43.

Acupuncture points

BL-13 **Location:** 1.5 cun lateral to the spinous process of T3.
Notes: back-*Shu* point of the Lung; regulates Lung *Qi*, promotes the dispersing and descending function of the Lung, together with LU-9 (*Yuan*-source point) particularly effective for chronic Lung disorders.

BL-20 **Location:** 1.5 cun lateral to the spinous process of T11.
Notes: back-*Shu* point of the Spleen; tonifies the Spleen and Stomach, therefore promotes *Qi* production and general wellbeing; eliminates Dampness.

BL-23 **Location:** 1.5 cun lateral to the spinous process of L2.
Notes: back-*Shu* point of the Kidneys; tonifies Kidney *Yin* and *Yang*, corticotrophic.

BL-43 **Location:** 3 cun lateral to the spinous process of T4, level with BL-14 (back-*Shu* point of the Pericardium), on the medial border of the scapula.
Notes: back-*Shu* point of the Vital Region; tonifies *Qi*.

Du-4 **Location:** below the spinous process of L2, level with BL-23 and BL-52.
Notes: tonifies Kidney *Yin*, with moxa tonifies Kidney *Yang*.

KID-3 **Location:** between the highest prominence of the medial malleolus and the Achilles tendon.
Notes: *Yuan*-source point, tonifies the Kidneys, especially with BL-23.

KID-6 **Location:** below the prominence of the medial malleolus.
Notes: metabolic point, unbinds the chest, benefits the throat, disperses heat; opening point of the *Yin Qiao Mai*; combined with LU-7, its coupled opening point, for Lung/Kidney patterns.

LU-7 **Location:** 1.5 cun proximal to the wrist crease, at the radial artery.
Notes: master point for stagnation; moves, descends and disperses Lung *Qi*, expels external pathogens; as opening point of the *Ren Mai* together with its coupled point KID-6 (opening point of the *Yin Qiao Mai*) for combined Lung/Kidney patterns.

LU-9 **Location:** on the wrist crease, radial to the radial artery.
Notes: *Yuan*-source point, tonification point; tonifies Lung *Qi*, thoracic *Qi* and Lung *Yin*; combined with BL-13 (back-*Shu* point of the Lung) particularly effective for chronic Lung disorders.

Ren-6 **Location:** 1.5 cun inferior to the umbilicus.
Notes: tonifies original *Qi*, pulls *Qi* downwards.

Ren-12 **Location:** midway between the umbilicus and the xiphoid process.
Notes: front-*Mu* point of the Stomach; with ST-36 also tonifies the Spleen.

Ren-17 **Location:** on the midline of the sternum, at the level of the 4th ICS, between the nipples (in men).
Notes: front-*Mu* point of the Pericardium, descends counterflow *Qi*, unbinds the chest.

SP-3 **Location:** just proximal to the metatarsophalangeal joint of the big toe, over the tendon of the abductor hallucis longus.
Notes: *Yuan*-source point; tonifies the Spleen, especially in combination with BL-20 (back-*Shu* point of the Spleen); resolves Dampness.

ST-36 **Location:** 0.5 cun lateral to the anterior crest of the tibia, 1.5 cun inferior to the lower border of the head of the fibula (G.B.-34).
Notes: *He*-sea point; tonifies the Spleen and Stomach, thereby promoting the production of *Qi* and Blood (*Xue*); strengthening point, psychologically harmonizing.

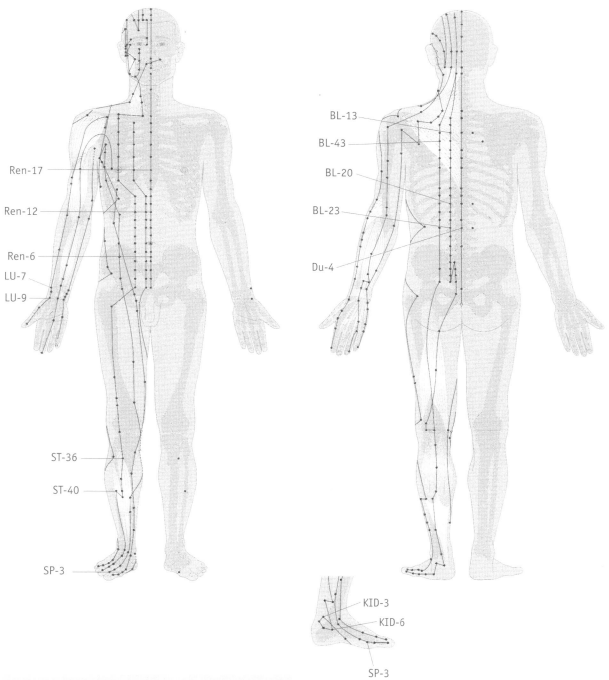

ST-40 **Location:** midway between the medial malleolus
and the knee joint space, 2 cun lateral to the anterior crest
of the tibia.
Notes: *Luo*-connecting point (connects with SP-3).
Phlegm: impaired transformation due to a weak Spleen.

6.3.1 Bronchial asthma (2) – Excess type

TCM

Pathogens obstruct the smooth flow of *Qi*.

Individual point combination

Asthma during onset of cold/flu

TCM: Wind-Cold type.
Cause: the pathogenic factors Wind and Cold obstruct the Lung *Qi* and transform into Heat.
Symptoms: cough with thin expectoration, tachypnoea, chills, fever, no thirst; pulse: floating (Exterior), slow (Cold); **tongue coating:** white (Cold), thin (Exterior).
Points: LU-7, L.I.-4, BL-13, BL-12, Du-14.

Asthma with purulent bronchitis

TCM: Heat-Phlegm type.
Cause: the Spleen's transporting and transforming function is impaired, or excessive Heat in the Lung consumes the Body Fluids, leading to the formation of Phlegm.
Symptoms: tachypnoea, shortness of breath, loud, hoarse voice, cough with yellow, sticky expectoration, fullness of the chest, fever, dry mouth; **pulse:** slippery (Phlegm) and rapid (Heat); **tongue coating:** thick, yellow, sticky, maybe dry.
Points: LU-5, BL-13, Ren-17; Phlegm: ST-40 or P-5 and Ren-22.

Acupuncture points

BL-12 **Location:** 1.5 cun lateral to the spinous process of T2.
Notes: special point for external Wind – use cupping for the first stages of a cold.

BL-13 **Location:** 1.5 cun lateral to the spinous process of T3.
Notes: back-*Shu* point of the Lung; regulates Lung *Qi*, promotes the dispersing and descending function of the Lung, particularly effective if combined with LU-9 (*Yuan*-source point).

Du-14 **Location:** below the spinous process of C7.
Notes: meeting point of all *Yang* meridians; eliminates pathogens from the surface, especially Wind-Cold.

L.I.-4 **Location:** on the dorsum of the hand, at the highest point of the muscle bulge between the 1st and 2nd metacarpal bones.
Notes: *Yuan*-source point of the Large Intestine; releases the surface, moves *Qi*; caution during pregnancy! Expels external Wind, e.g. during the first stages of a cold, strengthens the dispersing function of the Lung.

LU-5 **Location:** on the cubital crease, radial to the tendon of the biceps.
Notes: *He*-sea point, sedation point; clears Heat and Phlegm from the Lung, descends Lung *Qi*.

LU-7 **Location:** 1.5 cun proximal to the wrist crease, at the radial artery.
Notes: master point for stagnation, moves, descends and disperses Lung *Qi*, expels external pathogens, especially in combination with L.I.-4.

P-5 **Location:** 3 cun proximal to the midpoint of the palmar wrist crease, between the tendons of the flexor carpi radialis and palmaris longus.
Notes: resolves Phlegm in the Upper Burner.

Ren-17 **Location:** on the midline of the sternum, at the level of the 4th ICS, between the nipples (in men).
Notes: front-*Mu* point of the Pericardium, descends counterflow *Qi*, unbinds the chest.

Ren-22 **Location:** in the centre of the jugulum.
Notes: promotes the dispersing and descending function of the Lung, combined with P-5 resolves Phlegm in the Upper Burner.

ST-40 **Location:** midway between the medial malleolus and the knee joint space, 2 cun lateral to the anterior crest of the tibia.
Notes: *Luo*-connecting point (connects with SP-3). Phlegm forms if the Spleen's transforming function is impaired; nickname: 'Bisolvon of acupuncture' – expectorant.

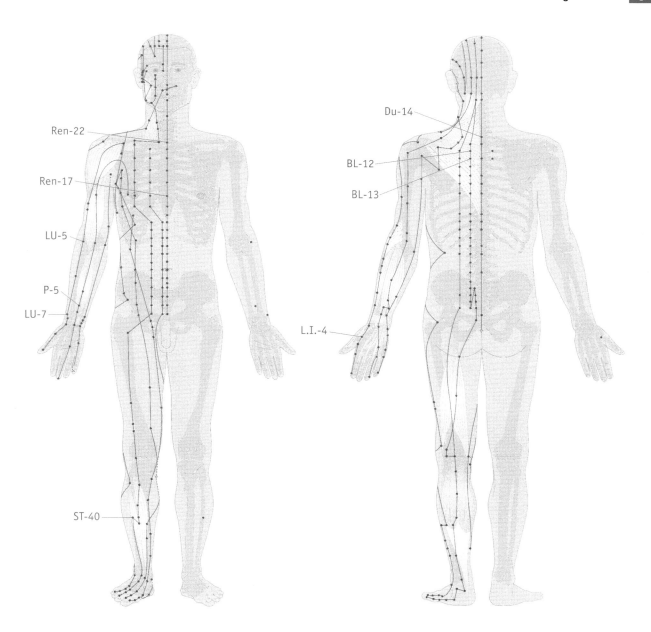

Ren-22

Ren-17

LU-5

P-5

LU-7

ST-40

Du-14

BL-12

BL-13

L.I.-4

6.3.1 Bronchial asthma (3) – according to accompanying signs and symptoms

Individual point combinations

Acute asthma attack

LU-6, Ex-B-1 (*Ding Chuan*), asthma point, for fever.

Sore throat

LU-10 with bloodletting; maybe ST-9.

Allergic asthma

L.I.-4, KID-6 [metabolic point, according to Bischko very effective].
Ear acupuncture: 78 allergy (*Er Jian*, at the tip of the ear).

Impending asthma attack

LU-7, KID-6, ST-36, KID-27, Ren-17.

Phlegm

SP-6, BL-20, ST-40 or Ren-22 and P-5.

Acupuncture points

BL-20 **Location:** 1.5 cun lateral to the spinous process of T11.
Notes: back-*Shu* point of the Spleen; tonifies the Spleen and Stomach, therefore also promotes *Qi* production and overall wellbeing; eliminates Dampness.

Ex-B-1 (Ding Chuan) **Location:** 0.5 cun lateral to the spinous process of C7.
Notes: specific asthma point, together with LU-6 effective for asthma attacks.

KID-6 **Location:** below the prominence of the medial malleolus.
Notes: as metabolic point (after Bischko) effective for allergies, unbinds the chest, benefits the throat, disperses heat; opening point of the *Yin Qiao Mai*; together with LU-7 (its coupled opening point) for Lung/Kidney patterns.

KID-27 **Location:** on the lower border of the sternoclavicular joint.
Notes: fear is the inner pathogenic factor of the Kidneys.

L.I.-4 **Location:** on the dorsum of the hand, at the highest point of the muscle bulge between the 1st and 2nd metacarpal bones.
Notes: *Yuan*-source point, as metabolic point (after Bischko) effective for allergies, moves *Qi*, caution during pregnancy! Expels external Wind (according to TCM this includes, among others, allergens).

LU-6 **Location:** 7 cun proximal to the wrist crease, on a line connecting LU-5 (in the cubital crease, radial to the biceps tendon) and LU-9 (on the wrist crease, at the radial artery).
Notes: *Xi*-cleft point, effective for asthma attacks.

LU-7 **Location:** 1.5 cun proximal to the wrist crease, at the radial artery.
Notes: master point for stagnation; moves, descends and disperses Lung *Qi*, expels external pathogens; as opening point of the *Ren Mai* together with KID-6 (its coupled opening point of the *Yin Qiao Mai*) for Lung/Kidney patterns.

LU-10 **Location:** at the midpoint of the 1st metacarpal bone, at the junction of the red and white skin.
Notes: clears Lung Heat.

P-5 **Location:** 3 cun proximal to the midpoint of the palmar wrist crease, between the tendons of the flexor carpi radialis and palmaris longus.
Notes: combined with Ren-22 transforms Phlegm in the Upper Burner.

Ren-17 **Location:** on the midline of the sternum, at the level of the 4th ICS, between the nipples (in men).
Notes: front-*Mu* point of the Pericardium, descends counterflow *Qi*, unbinds the chest.

Ren-22 **Location:** in the centre of the jugulum.
Notes: together with P-5 transforms Phlegm in the Upper Burner.

SP-6 **Location:** 3 cun superior to the highest prominence of the medial malleolus, on the posterior border of the tibia.
Notes: group *Luo*-connecting point of the 3 *Yin* of the leg (SP, LIV, KID); tonifies the Spleen, eliminates Dampness.

ST-9 **Location:** on the anterior border of the SCM, level with the laryngeal prominence.
Notes: regulates the *Qi* and Blood (*Xue*) circulation, disperses heat.

ST-36 **Location:** 0.5 cun lateral to the anterior crest of the tibia, 1.5 cun inferior to the lower border of the head of the fibula (G.B.-34).
Notes: *He*-sea point; strengthens the Spleen and Stomach, and therefore *Qi* and Blood (*Xue*) production; tonifying, psychologically harmonizing.

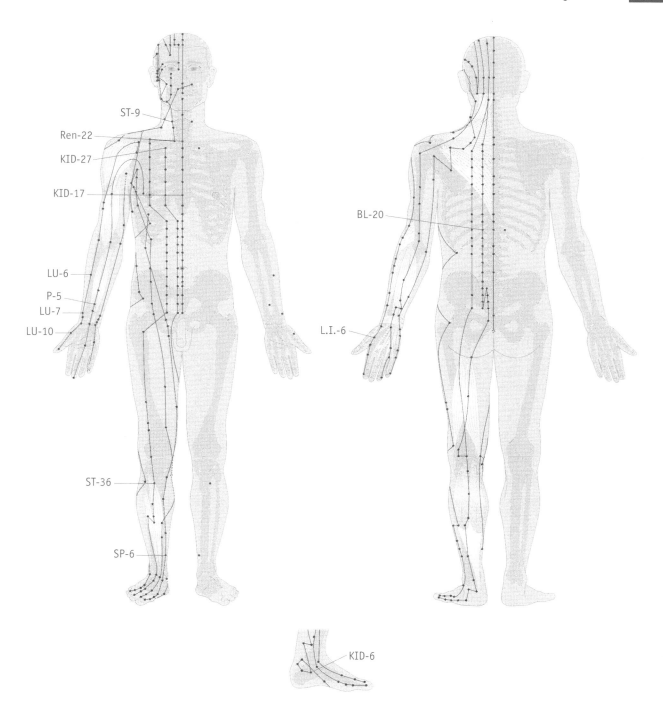

ST-9
Ren-22
KID-27
KID-17
LU-6
P-5
LU-7
LU-10
ST-36
SP-6
BL-20
L.I.-6
KID-6

6.3.2 Cough and bronchitis (1) – acute form

Cough is a symptom with which the Lung reacts to any form of irritation and is considered as 'counterflow Lung *Qi*'. In TCM, the Lungs regulate, disperse and descend the *Qi*. Their proper functioning is based on the harmonious relationship with the other organs, particularly the Spleen and Kidneys. The functions of the Lung can easily be impaired by external pathogenic factors or internal disharmonies.

Basic point combination

L.I.-4, LU-7, BL-13.
Ear acupuncture: 101 Lung, 103 trachea.

Individual point combinations

Wind-Cold: cough at onset of cold

Symptoms: cough, expectoration of white runny mucus, runny nose, nasal congestion, scratchy throat, aversion to cold, fever and chills, headaches, no sweating; **tongue coating:** thin, white; **pulse:** floating.
Points: LU-7, L.I.-4 (moxa), BL-12, BL-13 (moxa), Du-14.

Wind-Heat – purulent bronchitis during highly acute stage of infection

Symptoms: cough with suffocating sensation, yellow, viscous phlegm, thirst, sore throat, headaches, aversion to wind, sweating; tongue coating: thin, yellow; pulse: floating, rapid.
Cause: Wind-Heat injures the Body Fluids, reducing them to thick Phlegm.
Points: LU-7, L.I.-4, BL-13, Du-14, T.B.-5, no moxa!
Sore throat: LU-11 or LU-10 with bloodletting.
Fever: L.I.-4, L.I.-11, Du-14.
Wind/headaches: G.B.-20.

Acupuncture points

BL-12 **Location:** 1.5 cun lateral to the spinous process of T2.
Notes: specific point for external Wind – use cupping for acute colds.

BL-13 **Location:** 1.5 cun lateral to the spinous process of T3.
Notes: back-*Shu* point of the Lung, regulates Lung *Qi*, promotes the dispersing and descending function of the Lung.

Du-14 **Location:** 1 cun inferior to KID-3.
Notes: meeting point of all *Yang* meridians; eliminates pathogens from the surface, especially Wind-Cold; for fever combine with L.I.-4 and L.I.-11.

G.B.-20 **Location:** posterior to the mastoid, between the trapezius and sternocleidomastoid on the lower border of the occiput.
Notes: meeting point with the T.B. meridian and the *Yang Wei Mai*, eliminates external and internal Wind as well as Heat; most important point for headaches due to Wind.

L.I.-4 **Location:** on the dorsum of the hand, at the highest point of the muscle bulge between the 1st and 2nd metacarpal bones.
Notes: *Yuan*-source point, releases the Exterior, moves *Qi*, removes obstructions in the meridians, expels external Wind during the beginning stages of a cold; with L.I.-11 and Du-14 specifically for fever; moves the *Qi*, strengthens the Lungs' dispersing function. Caution during pregnancy!

L.I.-11 **Location:** with the arm fully flexed at the radial end of the cubital crease.
Notes: *He*-sea point, tonification point, expels external Wind, Heat, Dampness; for fever combine with L.I.-4 and Du-14.

LU-7 **Location:** 1.5 cun proximal to the wrist crease, proximal to the radial artery.
Notes: master point for stagnation; moves, descends and disperses Lung *Qi*, expels external pathogens.

LU-10 **Location:** at the midpoint of the 1st metacarpal bone, at the junction of the red and white skin.
Notes: clears Lung-Heat.

LU-11 **Location:** on the thumb, next to the radial corner of the nail.
Notes: master point for throat disorders, clears Lung-Heat.

ST-40 **Location:** midway between the medial malleolus and the knee joint space, 2 cun lateral to the anterior crest of the tibia.
Notes: *Luo*-connecting point, specific action for Phlegm and Dampness, combines well with SP-9.

T.B.-5 **Location:** 2 cun proximal to the midpoint of the dorsal wrist crease, opposite P-6.
Notes: opening point of the *Yang Wei Mai*, releases the Exterior, can expel all external pathogens, but especially Wind-Heat.

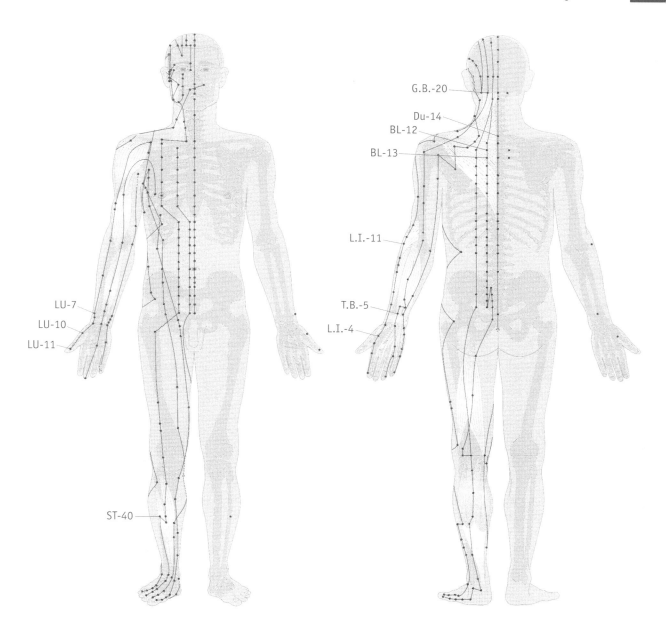

LU-7
LU-10
LU-11

ST-40

G.B.-20
Du-14
BL-12
BL-13

L.I.-11

T.B.-5
L.I.-4

6.3.2 Cough and bronchitis (2) – chronic form

Basic point combination

LU-9, BL-13, ST-40.

Retention of Phlegm in the Lungs – chronic bronchitis

Symptoms: cough with copious, sticky, white mucus, fullness in the chest, no appetite. **Tongue coating:** white, sticky; **pulse:** slippery.
Cause: if the Spleen *Yang* is deficient, the Spleen's transforming function is impaired and leads to the formation of Phlegm, which accumulates in the Lungs.
Points: BL-13, Ren-12, LU-5, ST-36, ST-40.

Yin deficiency with Dryness of the Lungs – dry emphysematous bronchitis, tuberculosis

Symptoms: dry cough with little, possibly blood-tinged, mucus, dry nose and throat, sore throat, afternoon fever, hot flushes; **tongue body:** red; **tongue coating:** thin; pulse: thready, slightly rapid.
Cause: Dryness and/or *Yin* deficiency.
Points: LU-7, KID-6 as opening points; LU-1, BL-13, LU-9. Haemoptysis: LU-6, BL-17. No moxa!

Phlegm

Ren-22 and P-5 or ST-40,SP-4, SP-6, BL-20.

Acupuncture points

BL-13 **Location:** 1.5 cun lateral to the spinous process of T3.
Notes: back-*Shu* point of the Lungs, regulates Lung *Qi*, promotes the dispersing and descending function of the Lung, together with LU-1 (front-*Mu* point) it reaches the Lung organ; combined with LU-9 (*Yuan*-source point) for chronic Lung disorders.

BL-17 **Location:** 1.5 cun lateral to the spinous process of T7.
Notes: *Hui*-meeting point of the Blood, back-*Shu* point of the diaphragm, promotes diaphragmatic breathing, unbinds the chest.

KID-6 **Location:** below the prominence of the medial malleolus.
Notes: metabolic point, unbinds the chest, benefits the throat, disperses Heat; opening point of the *Yin Qiao Mai*; combined with LU-7 (opening point of the *Ren Mai*) for Lung/Kidney patterns.

LU-1 **Location:** find LU-2 first; LU-1 is located directly below in the 1st ICS.
Notes: front-*Mu* point of the Lung, combined with BL-13 (back-*Shu* point of the Lung) reaches the Lung organ.

LU-5 **Location:** on the cubital crease, radial to the tendon of the biceps.
Notes: sedation point, *He*-sea point; clears Heat and Phlegm from the Lung, descends Lung *Qi*.

LU-6 **Location:** 7 cun proximal to the wrist crease, on a line connecting LU-5 (in the cubital crease, radial to the biceps tendon) and LU-9 (on the wrist crease, at the radial artery).
Notes: *Xi*-cleft point, regulates and descends Lung *Qi*, clears Heat, stops bleeding.

LU-9 **Location:** on the wrist crease, radial to the radial artery.
Notes: *Yuan*-source point, tonification point; tonifies the *Qi* of the Lung and chest as well as Lung *Yin*; LU-9 and BL-13 (back-*Shu* point of the Lung) is a very effective combination for chronic Lung disorders.

P-5 **Location:** 3 cun proximal to the midpoint of the palmar wrist crease, between the tendons of the flexor carpi radialis and palmaris longus.
Notes: with Ren-22 resolves Phlegm in the Upper Burner.

Ren-12 **Location:** midway between the umbilicus and the xiphoid process.
Notes: front-*Mu* point of the Stomach; combined with ST-36 also tonifies the Spleen.

Ren-22 **Location:** in the centre of the jugulum.
Notes: together with P-5 resolves Phlegm in the Upper Burner.

SP-4 **Location:** in the depression at the junction of the base and shaft of the 1st metatarsal bone, at the junction of the red and white skin.
Notes: opening point of the *Chong Mai*, tonifies the Stomach and Spleen and therefore indirectly transforms Phlegm.

SP-6 **Location:** 3 cun superior to the highest prominence of the medial malleolus, on the posterior border of the tibia.
Notes: group *Luo*-connecting point of the 3 *Yin* of the leg (SP, KID, LIV); tonifies the Spleen, eliminates Dampness.

ST-36 **Location:** 0.5 cun lateral to the anterior crest of the tibia, 1.5 cun inferior to the lower border of the head of the fibula (G.B.-34).
Notes: *He*-sea point of the Stomach, tonifies Stomach and Spleen and therefore *Qi* and Blood (*Xue*) production; strengthening, psychologically harmonizing.

ST-40 **Location:** midway between the medial malleolus and the knee joint space, 2 cun lateral to the anterior crest of the tibia.
Notes: *Luo*-connecting point (connects with SP-3). If the Spleen is weak, its transforming function is impaired and Phlegm will form; nickname: 'Bisolvon' of acupuncture – expectorant.

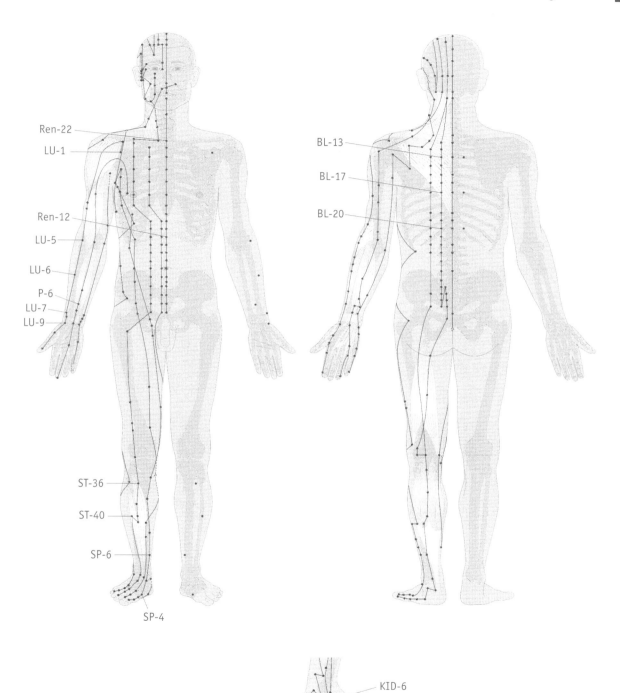

Ren-22
LU-1
Ren-12
LU-5
LU-6
P-6
LU-7
LU-9
ST-36
ST-40
SP-6
SP-4

BL-13
BL-17
BL-20

KID-6

6.4 Gastrointestinal disorders

H. Rausch, B. Sommer

Many functional disorders of the gastrointestinal tract respond well to acupuncture. However, it should be stressed that the disorders described below should be treated with acupuncture only after a Western assessment, as, for example, cancer of the colon often starts with non-specific symptoms. By the same token, stomach ulcers may develop into a malignancy. On the other hand, taking a detailed medical history may pick up minor imbalances, giving the TCM practitioner the chance to discover a malignant disease in its very early stages.

The disorders in this section are described according to Western medicine and clinical considerations. They may partially overlap.

TCM

Patterns are differentiated according to excess syndromes (e.g. acute gastritis) that require a sedating treatment, and deficiency syndromes that are treated in a tonifying manner and, if Cold is present, also with moxibustion.

6.4.1 Nausea and vomiting

Although, by definition, acupuncture can help only with functional disorders, recent research trials (e.g. Dundee et al. 1990) have demonstrated that the point P-6 is also effective in the treatment of postoperative and chemotherapy-related nausea.

Basic point combination

P-6, SP-4, ST-36, LIV-14.
Ear points: 29 occiput.

Individual point combination

Hyperemesis gravidarum

Needle P-6 daily for up to 1 week. Advise the patient to massage this point at home. For more detail and commentary → 6.7.

Altitude sickness

BL-14.

Sea sickness

LIV-13 or LIV-14, KID-21.

Very nervous patient

Ren-13.

Vomiting with stomach cramps

BL-21, Ren-13.

Extra point for resistance to therapy

Ex-B-3 (*Wei Wan Xia Xu*).

Acupuncture points

BL-14 **Location:** 1.5 cun lateral to the spinous process of T4.
Notes: back *Shu* point of the Pericardium, strengthens the cardiovascular system.

BL-21 **Location:** 1.5 cun lateral to the spinous process of T12.
Notes: back *Shu* point and master point of the Stomach, pacifies the Stomach, descends counterflow Stomach *Qi*.

Ex-B-3 **Location:** 1.5 cun lateral to the lower border of the spinous process of T8.
Notes: for epigastric pain.

KID-21 **Location:** superior to the umbilicus, 6/8 of the distance between the umbilicus and the xiphoid process, 0.5 cun lateral to the midline, lateral to Ren-14.
Notes: has a relationship with the cardia.

LIV-13 **Location:** on the lower border of the free end of the 11th rib.
Notes: front-*Mu* point of the Spleen, *Hui* meeting point for the parenchymatous organs (*Zang*), harmonizes the Liver and the Spleen.

LIV-14 **Location:** on the midclavicular line, in the 6th ICS, directly below the nipple.
Notes: front-*Mu* point of the Liver; special point: seasickness, hyperemesis.

P-6 **Location:** 2 cun proximal to the midpoint of the palmar wrist crease, between the tendons of the flexor carpi radialis and palmaris longus.
Notes: master point for vomiting, as opening point of the *Yin Wei Mai* together with SP-4 (opening point of the *Chong Mai*) for heart and digestive problems.

Ren-13 **Location:** 5 cun superior to the umbilicus or 5/8 of the distance between the umbilicus and the xiphoid process.
Notes: controls the fundus of the stomach, descends counterflow Qi, for excess patterns of the Stomach.

SP-4 **Location:** in the depression at the junction of the base and shaft of the 1st metatarsal bone, at the junction of the red and white skin.
Notes: *Luo*-connecting point, opening point of the *Chong Mai*, tonifies the Spleen, calms the Stomach.

ST-36 **Location:** 0.5 cun lateral to the anterior crest of the tibia, 1.5 cun inferior to the lower border of the head of the fibula (G.B.-34).
Notes: *He*-sea point with direct effect on the organ, command point for the abdomen; regulates *Qi*.

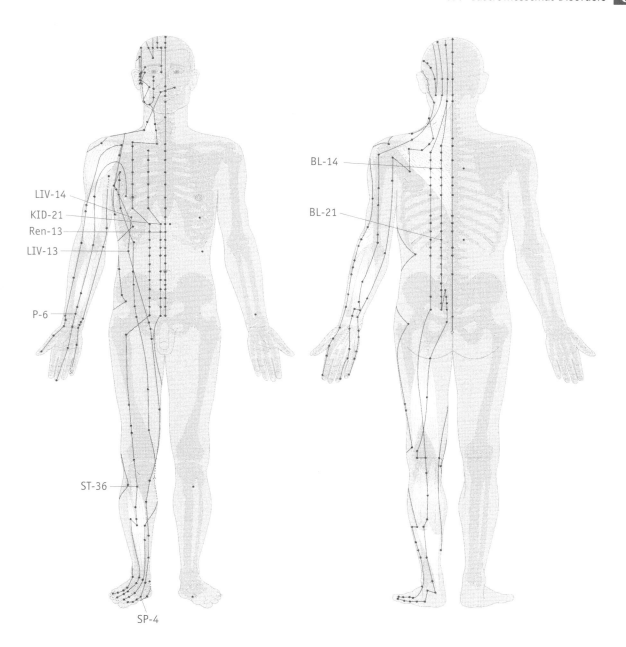

LIV-14
KID-21
Ren-13
LIV-13

P-6

ST-36

SP-4

BL-14

BL-21

6.4.2 Gastritis

Chronic gastritis lends itself well to treatment with acupuncture. However, it is important to explore any psychosomatic component and provide appropriate care.

TCM

Acute cases require treatment with sedating needling techniques (strong stimulation), whereas chronic disorders should be treated with tonifying techniques; if there are signs of Cold (white tongue coating, cold sensations), use moxibustion. For the treatment of internal disorders, dietary advice is essential, possibly also psychotherapy.

Basic point combination

ST-21, ST-36, SP-4, BL-21, Ren-12

Individual point combination

Extra points for all Stomach disorders

Ex-B-3 (*Wei Wan Xia Shu*), Ex-UE-3 (*Zhong Quan*).

Acute gastritis, irritable stomach, diffuse cramping pain

ST-36, Ren-13.

Chronic gastritis, worse with cold food/drinks

TCM: Cold attacks the Stomach with underlying Stomach deficiency Cold.
KID-3, BL-23, Ren-12 **M**, Ren-6 **M**, Ren-13.

With bloating and a sensation of fullness

SP-3, BL-20, SP-4.

Chronic gastritis, reduced appetite, poor overall condition

ST-36, Ren-12, BL-21, LIV-13 **M**, BL-20 **M**.

Chronic, recurring gastritis

ST-36, Du-20; ear points (choose 2 points per treatment): psychotropic zones, frustration point, anti-aggression point (PT 1), antidepression point (PT 3), anxiety point (PT 2).

Condition worse with stress

TCM: Liver attacks the Stomach.
LIV-14, Ren-12, P-6, ST-36, LIV-3.

Acupuncture points

BL-20 **Location:** 1.5 cun lateral to the spinous process of T11.
Notes: back-*Shu* point of the Spleen, tonifies the Spleen, especially in combination with SP-3 (*Yuan*-source point); use moxibustion to eliminate Dampness.

BL-21 **Location:** 1.5 cun lateral to the spinous process of T12.
Notes: back-*Shu* point and master point of the Stomach, regulates and tonifies Stomach *Qi*, eliminates Dampness and food stagnation, pacifies the Stomach, descends counterflow Stomach *Qi* for acid reflux.

BL-23 **Location:** 1.5 cun lateral to the spinous process of L2.
Notes: tonifies *Yin*, *Yang* and Essence (*Jing*) of the Kidneys; use for Kidney symptoms (lower back pain, weakness of the knees, early morning diarrhoea); for *Yang* deficiency use moxa; moxa is contraindicated for *Yin* deficiency. Particularly effective when combined with KID-3 (*Yuan*-source point).

Du-20 **Location:** on a line connecting the apices of the ears, 7 cun superior the posterior hairline.
Notes: harmonizing, lifts the *Qi*.

Ex-B-3 **Location:** 1.5 cun lateral to the lower border of the spinous process of T8.
Notes: for epigastric pain.

Ex-UE-3 **Location:** on the dorsal aspect of the wrist joint, in the depression between the 'anatomical snuffbox' and the midpoint of the wrist crease.
Notes: for haematemesis.

KID-3 **Location:** between the highest prominence of the medial malleolus and the Achilles tendon.
Notes: *Yuan*-source point; tonifies Kidney *Qi* and *Yin*, especially with BL-23 (back-*Shu* point).

LIV-13 **Location:** on the lower border of the free end of the 11th rib.
Notes: front-*Mu* point of the Spleen, *Hui*-meeting point for the parenchymatous organs (*Zang*), harmonizes the Liver and the Spleen, relieves food stagnation.

LIV-14 **Location:** on the midclavicular line, in the 6th ICS, directly below the nipple.
Notes: front-*Mu* point of the Liver. Special point: seasickness, hyperemesis.

Ren-6 **Location:** 1.5 cun inferior to the umbilicus.
Notes: tonifies the Kidneys, original *Qi* and *Yang* (with moxibustion).

Ren-12 **Location:** midway between the umbilicus and the xiphoid process.
Notes: front-*Mu* point of the Stomach; *Hui*-meeting point of the hollow organs (*Fu*); controls the Middle Burner, tonifies the Stomach and Spleen, regulates Stomach *Qi* and the Middle Burner, eliminates Dampness, promotes digestion of stagnant food.

Ren-13 **Location:** 5 cun superior to the umbilicus or 5/8 of the distance between the umbilicus and the xiphoid process.
Notes: controls the fundus of the Stomach, descends counterflow Stomach *Qi*, for excess patterns of the Stomach.

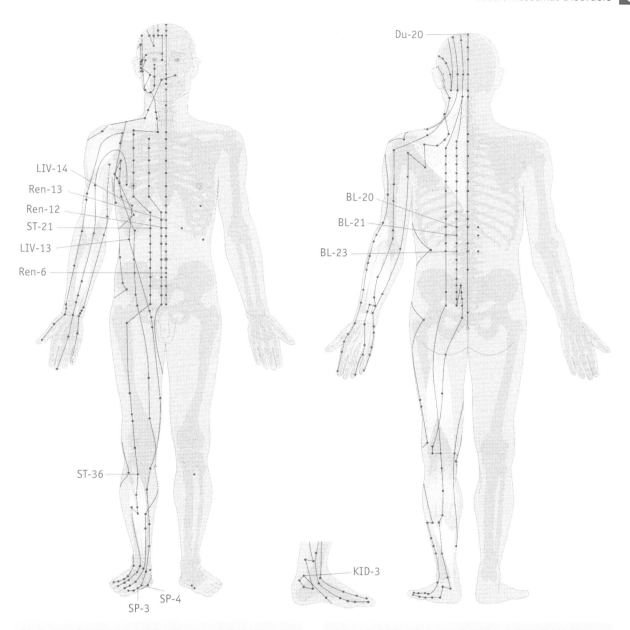

SP-3 **Location:** just proximal to the metatarsophalangeal joint of the big toe, over the tendon of the abductor hallucis longus.
Notes: *Yuan*-source point; tonifies the Spleen, especially with BL-20; eliminates Dampness.

SP-4 **Location:** in the depression at the junction of the base and shaft of the 1st metatarsal bone, at the junction of the red and white skin.
Notes: *Luo*-connecting point, opening point of the *Chong Mai*, master point for diarrhoea, tonifies the Spleen, calms the Stomach.

ST-21 **Location:** 2 cun lateral to the midline, level with Ren-12, at the midpoint of the distance between the umbilicus and the xiphoid process.
Notes: for excess patterns! Regulates the Stomach, suppresses counterflow *Qi*.

ST-36 **Location:** 0.5 cun lateral to the anterior crest of the tibia, 1.5 cun inferior to the lower border of the head of the fibula (G.B.-34).
Notes: *He*-sea point with direct effect on the organ, command point for the abdomen; also tonifies the Spleen, especially when combined with Ren-12 (its front-*Mu* point).

6.4.3 Ventricular/duodenal ulcer

Acupuncture has demonstrated impressive results for ventricular/duodenal ulcers with often rapid improvement of the subjective symptoms. We suggest a series of approximately 15 treatments at regular intervals – initially daily, later fortnightly. Electro-acupuncture at ST-36 has been shown to be effective in reducing gastric acid, even in healthy subjects (Lux et al. 1994).

TCM

The ulcer-related symptoms are caused by stagnation of Blood (*Xue*) and *Qi*. Treatment principle: eliminate stagnation. Acute, colicky pain is often caused by a Liver disharmony. Treatment principle: harmonize the Liver *Qi* (LIV-14, LIV-3).

Basic point combination

BL-21, ST-36, Ren-12; ear points: 51 autonomic nervous system.

Individual point combination

Extra point for any epigastric pain

Ex-B-3 (*Wei Wan Xia Xu*), Ex-UE-3 (*Zhong Quan*).

Strong emotional component

Du-20.

Frequent belching

ST-45, P-6, Ren-22.

Worse after eating, with warmth and pressure, haematemesis (Blood stagnation in the Stomach)

Technique: reducing method; ST-21, SP-10, Ren-10.

Better after eating, with warmth and pressure

TCM: deficiency Cold in the Stomach (*Yang* deficiency). P-6, BL-20 M, ST-36 M, Ren-4 M.

Burning pain, constant thirst and hunger (rising Stomach Fire)

Technique: reducing method; ST-44, SP-6, P-6.

Sudden, colicky pain with epigastric distension caused by emotions

TCM: Liver *Qi* is attacking the Stomach.
Technique: reducing method; LIV-3, P-6, SP-6, BL-18.

180

Acupuncture points

BL-18 **Location:** 2 cun lateral to the spinous process of T9.
Notes: back-*Shu* point of the Liver, eliminates Damp-Heat, moves stagnant *Qi*.

BL-20 **Location:** 1.5 cun lateral to the spinous process of T11.
Notes: back-*Shu* point of the Spleen!

BL-21 **Location:** 1.5 cun lateral to the spinous process of T12.
Notes: back-*Shu* point and master point of the Stomach; regulates and tonifies Stomach *Qi*, eliminates Dampness and food stagnation, pacifies the Stomach and descends Stomach *Qi* for acid reflux.

Du-20 **Location:** on a line connecting the apices of the ears, 7 cun superior the posterior hairline.
Notes: harmonizing.

Ex-B-3 **Location:** 1.5 cun lateral to the lower border of the spinous process of T8.
Notes: for epigastric pain.

Ex-UE-3 **Location:** on the dorsal aspect of the wrist joint, in the depression between the 'anatomical snuffbox' and the midpoint of the wrist crease.
Notes: for haematemesis.

LIV-3 **Location:** on the dorsum of the foot, in the depression distal to the junction of the 1st and 2nd metatarsal bones.
Notes: *Shu*-stream point and *Yuan*-source point; moves the *Qi*, especially together with L.I.-4, promotes the smooth flow of *Qi*, spasmolytic.

LIV-14 **Location:** on the midclavicular line, in the 6th ICS, directly below the nipple.
Notes: front-*Mu* point of the Liver, meeting point with the Spleen, special point for nausea, tonifies the *Yin* aspect of the Liver, harmonizes excess of Liver *Yang*.

P-6 **Location:** 2 cun proximal to the midpoint of the palmar wrist crease, between the tendons of the flexor carpi radialis and palmaris longus.
Notes: opening point of the *Yin Wei Mai*, master point for emesis, harmonizes the Stomach, calms the Spirit.

Ren-4 **Location:** 2 cun superior to the upper border of the pubic symphysis.
Notes: front-*Mu* point of the Small Intestine, meeting point of the 3 *Yin* meridians of the leg; tonifies the *Qi*, *Yang*, *Yin*, Blood (*Xue*) and Kidneys.

Ren-10 **Location:** 2 cun superior to the umbilicus.
Notes: controls the pylorus, promotes the descending of the Stomach *Qi*, tonifies the Spleen.

Ren-12 **Location:** midway between the umbilicus and the xiphoid process.
Notes: front-*Mu* point of the Stomach, controls the mid-section of the Stomach, tonifies the Stomach and Spleen, regulates the Stomach and Middle Burner *Qi*, eliminates Dampness, promotes digestion of stagnant food.

Ren-22 **Location:** in the centre of the jugulum.
Notes: descends counterflow *Qi*.

SP-6 **Location:** 3 cun superior to the highest prominence of the medial malleolus, on the posterior border of the tibia.
Notes: group *Luo*-connecting point of the 3 *Yin* meridians of the leg (SP, LIV, KID); tonifies the Kidneys, Blood (*Xue*) and *Yin*, cools and moves the Blood, promotes the smooth flow of Liver *Qi*, alleviates pain.

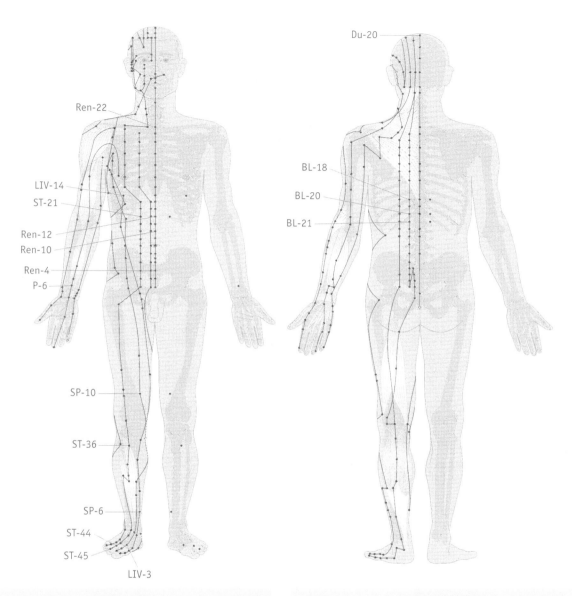

SP-10   **Location:** with the knee flexed, 2 cun superior to the upper patellar border, medial to the vastus medialis.
Notes: name: 'Sea of Blood'; cools and tonifies the Blood (*Xue*), disperses Heat, regulates the flow of *Qi* and Blood (*Xue*).

ST-21   **Location:** 2 cun lateral to the midline, level with Ren-12, at the midpoint of the distance between the umbilicus and the xiphoid process.
Notes: for excess patterns! Regulates the Stomach, descends counterflow *Qi*.

ST-36   **Location:** 0.5 cun lateral to the anterior crest of the tibia, 1.5 cun inferior to the lower border of the head of the fibula (G.B.-34).

Notes: *He*-sea point with direct effect on the organ, command point for the abdomen; also tonifies the Spleen, especially when combined with its front-*Mu* point (Ren-12).

ST-44   **Location:** on the interdigital fold between the 2nd and 3rd toes, near the metatarsophalangeal joint of the 2nd toe.
Notes: eliminates Stomach Heat and Excess, regulates counterflow Stomach *Qi*, alleviates epigastric pain with fever, promotes digestion.

ST-45   **Location:** on the 2nd toe, near the lateral corner of the nail.
Notes: *Jing*-well point, sedation point; resolves food stagnation.

181

6.4.4 Irritable bowel syndrome (IBS)

This syndrome is characterized by changing intestinal symptoms without any structural correlation. As emotional stress often leads to an exacerbation of symptoms, the psychosomatic component of this disorder should be discussed. Non-specific forms of IBS often show good results with acupuncture treatments.

TCM

Excess patterns manifest with acute, colicky pain, acute diarrhoea or spastic constipation; deficiency patterns are typified by chronic constipation or diarrhoea and dull pain.

Basic point combination

ST-25, ST-37, SP-4; ear acupuncture: 51 autonomic nervous system.

Individual point combination

Acute symptoms

BL-25, ST-37 (daily or every other day).

Chronic symptoms, poor general condition

ST-36 (+/M of BL-25 (back-*Shu* point) and ST-25 (front-*Mu* point).

Severe emotional strain

Point selection according to the affected organ/channel and the causes.

Symptoms related to menstruation

SP-6.

Acupuncture points

BL-25 **Location:** 1.5 cun lateral to the spinous process of L4.
Notes: back-*Shu* point of the Large Intestine, promotes the functioning of the Large Intestine.

KID-15 **Location:** 0.5 cun lateral to the midline, 4 cun superior to the pubic symphysis or 4/5 of the distance pubic symphysis/umbilicus, at the level of Ren-7.
Notes: local point.

Ren-6 **Location:** 1.5 cun inferior to the umbilicus.
Notes: tonifies the Kidneys, original *Qi*, Lower Burner *Qi* and *Yang* (with moxa).

Ren-12 **Location:** midway between the umbilicus and the xiphoid process.
Notes: front-*Mu* point of the Stomach, *Hui*-meeting point of the *Fu* (hollow organs); controls the mid-section of the Stomach, tonifies the Stomach and Spleen, regulates the Stomach and Middle Burner *Qi*, eliminates Dampness, promotes digestion of stagnant food.

SP-4 **Location:** in the depression at the junction of the base and shaft of the 1st metatarsal bone, at the junction of the red and white skin.
Notes: *Luo*-connecting point, opening point of the *Chong Mai*, master point for diarrhoea, tonifies the Spleen, calms the Stomach.

SP-6 **Location:** 3 cun superior to the highest prominence of the medial malleolus, on the posterior border of the tibia.
Notes: group *Luo*-connecting point of the 3 *Yin* meridians of the leg (SP, LIV, KID); tonifies the Spleen, Kidneys, Blood (*Xue*) and *Yin*, cools and moves the Blood, promotes the smooth flow of Liver *Qi* for irritability, eliminates Blood stagnation, regulates the uterus and menstruation.

ST-25 **Location:** 2 cun lateral to the centre of the umbilicus (Ren-8).
Notes: front-*Mu* point of the Large Intestine; regulates the intestines, especially with ST-37 (lower *He*-sea point of the Large Intestine).

ST-36 **Location:** 0.5 cun lateral to the anterior crest of the tibia, 1.5 cun inferior to the lower border of the head of the fibula (G.B.-34).
Notes: *He*-sea point with direct action on the Stomach organ; command point of the Stomach; also tonifies the Spleen; particularly effective when combined with Ren-12 (front-*Mu* point of the ST); tonifying, harmonizing.

ST-37 **Location:** 1 cun lateral to the anterior crest of the tibia, 4 cun inferior to the lower border of the head of the fibula or 3 cun inferior to ST-36.
Notes: lower *He*-sea point of the Large Intestine; regulates the Stomach and intestines, especially with ST-25 (front-*Mu* point of the Large Intestine).

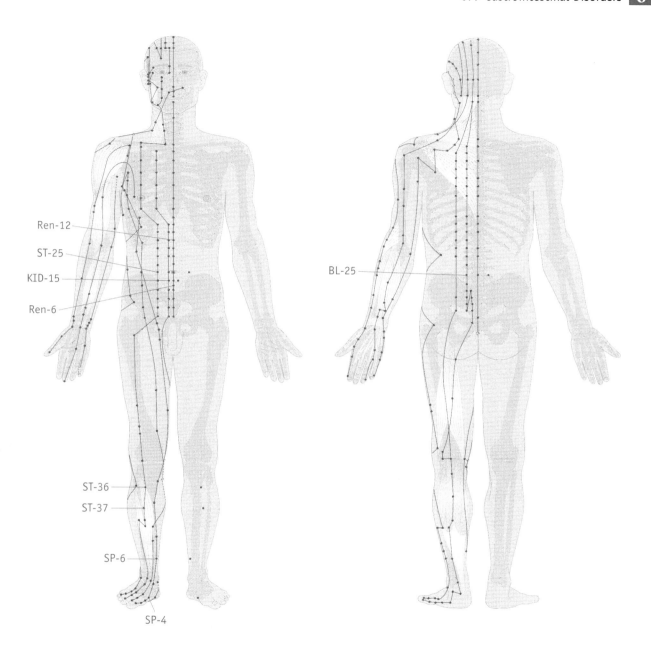

Ren-12

ST-25

KID-15

Ren-6

BL-25

ST-36

ST-37

SP-6

SP-4

6.4.5 Ulcerative colitis and Crohn's disease

Acupuncture presents a genuine alternative in the treatment of these chronic inflammatory disorders, particularly as long-term Western treatment with sulfonamides and steroids or surgical interventions generally does not lead to a proper cure. Depending on the patient and the stage of the disorder, acupuncture can lead to longer symptom-free intervals. In addition, Western medication seems to be more effective in conjunction with acupuncture, allowing a decrease in the dosage.

Ulcerative colitis and Crohn's disease are best treated with acupuncture during remission or the subacute stage.

Basic point combination

ST-25, BL-25, SP-4, ST-37 or ST-36

Individual point combination

Strong emotional component

HE-3, Ren-15, Du-20.

Severe pain

L.I.-4, LIV-3.

Overall poor condition, cold sensations

SP-6, Ren-6 M, BL-52 [BL-47 Bi].

Spasms

S.I.-3, Ren-3, G.B.-34.

Crohn's disease

L.I.-4, LIV-13.

Acupuncture points

BL-25 **Location:** 1.5 cun lateral to the spinous process of L4.
Notes: back-*Shu* point of the Large Intestine.
BL-52 **Location:** 3 cun lateral to the spinous process of L2, lateral to BL-23 (back-*Shu* point of the KID).
Notes: corticotrophic point.
Du-20 **Location:** on a line connecting the apices of the ears, 7 cun superior the posterior hairline.

G.B.-34 **Location:** with the knee flexed, in the depression anterior and inferior to the head of the fibula.
Notes: *He*-sea point, direct effect on the organ; strongly moves *Qi*.
HE-3 **Location:** with the elbow fully flexed, between the medial end of the cubital crease and the medial epicondyle.
Notes: *He*-sea point, master point for depression.
L.I.-4 **Location:** on the dorsum of the hand, at the highest point of the muscle bulge between the 1st and 2nd metacarpal bones.
Notes: *Yuan*-source point, moves the *Qi*, especially when combined with LIV-3.
Notes: harmonizing point, lifts the *Qi*, with Ren-15 calming (like bromazepam).
LIV-3 **Location:** on the dorsum of the foot, in the depression distal to the junction of the 1st and 2nd metatarsal bones.
Notes: *Shu*-stream point and *Yuan*-source point; moves the *Qi*, especially together with L.I.-4, promotes the smooth flow of *Qi*, spasmolytic.
LIV-13 **Location:** on the lower border of the free end of the 11th rib.
Notes: metabolic point, front-*Mu* point of the Spleen, *Hui*-meeting point of the parenchymatous organs (*Zang*); harmonizes the Liver and Spleen.
Ren-3 **Location:** 1 cun superior to the upper border of the pubic symphysis (1/5 of the distance between the symphysis and the umbilicus).
Notes: front-*Mu* point of the Bladder, meeting point of the 3 *Yin* meridians of the leg, local point.
Ren-6 **Location:** 1.5 cun inferior to the umbilicus.
Notes: 'Sea of *Qi*'; tonifies the Kidneys, original *Qi* and the Lower Burner *Qi*, with moxa also Kidney *Yang*.
Ren-15 **Location:** 1 cun inferior to the xiphoid process.
Notes: calms the Spirit, benefits the original *Qi*; with Du-20 calming as bromazepam.
S.I.-3 **Location:** when a fist is made, on the dorsum of the hand, in the depression at the end of the most distal palmar crease.
Notes: tonification point, opening point of the *Du Mai*, master point for the mucous membranes, spasmolytic point.
SP-4 **Location:** in the depression at the junction of the base and shaft of the 1st metatarsal bone, at the junction of the red and white skin.
Notes: *Luo*-connecting point, opening point of the *Chong Mai*, master point for diarrhoea, tonifies the Spleen, calms the Stomach.
SP-6 **Location:** 3 cun superior to the highest prominence of the medial malleolus, on the posterior border of the tibia.
Notes: group *Luo*-connecting point of the 3 *Yin* meridians of the leg (SP, LIV, KID); tonifies the Kidneys, Blood (*Xue*) and *Yin*, cools and moves the Blood, promotes the

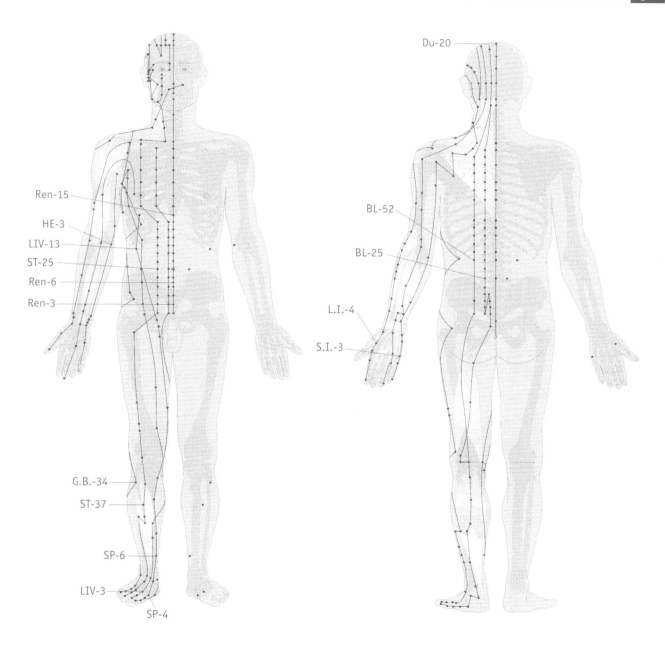

Ren-15
HE-3
LIV-13
ST-25
Ren-6
Ren-3
G.B.-34
ST-37
SP-6
LIV-3
SP-4

Du-20
BL-52
BL-25
L.I.-4
S.I.-3

smooth flow of Liver *Qi*, eliminates Blood stagnation, regulates the uterus and menstruation.

ST-25   **Location:** 2 cun lateral to the centre of the umbilicus (Ren-8).
Notes: front-*Mu* point of the Large Intestine, regulates the intestines, especially with ST-37 (lower *He*-sea point of the L.I.).

ST-37   **Location:** 1 cun lateral to the anterior crest of the tibia, 4 cun inferior to the lower border of the head of the fibula or 3 cun inferior to ST-36.
Notes: lower *He*-sea point of the Large Intestine; regulates the Stomach and intestines, especially together with ST-25 (front-*Mu* point of the Large Intestine), clears Damp-Heat, for diarrhoea.

185

6.4.6 Diarrhoea

Acupuncture is used mainly as an adjunctive therapy, which can, for example, quickly alleviate painful tenesmus.

TCM

From the viewpoint of TCM, the Spleen represents the digestive tract, so that points on the Spleen meridian are commonly used in the treatment of diarrhoea. Excess patterns with fullness and acute pain are often caused by external pathogens such as contaminated food, Summer-Heat but also Cold. Chronic diarrhoea is mainly caused by deficiency patterns due to Spleen and possibly also Kidney deficiency.

Basic point combination

SP-4, ST-25, ST-37, BL-25, Ren-4 or Ren-6.

Individual point combination

Acute symptoms with nausea

Sudden onset, watery and/or foul-smelling stools, pressure pain: P-6, SP-9.

Accompanied by raised temperature

L.I.-11.

With cardiovascular symptoms

P-6, ST-36.

To relieve spasms

LIV-3, S.I.-3.

With pain

Ex-UE-8 (*Wai Lao Gong*).

For chronic disorders – Spleen deficiency or Spleen/Kidney deficiency

Loose stools, better with warmth and pressure, sensitive to cold.
SP-9, BL-23 **M**, KID-3, SP-4, Ren-12 **M**, Ren-6 **M**, ST-36.

Acupuncture points

BL-23   **Location:** 1.5 cun lateral to the spinous process of L2.
Notes: back-*Shu* point of the Kidneys; tonifies the Kidney *Yin* and Essence (*Jing*), with moxa also Kidney *Yang*.

BL-25   **Location:** 1.5 cun lateral to the spinous process of L4.
Notes: back-*Shu* point of the Large Intestine.

Ex-UE-8 (*Wai Lao Gong*)   **Location:** on the dorsal aspect of the hand, between the 2nd and 3rd metacarpal bones, 0.5 cun proximal to the metacarpophalangeal joints.
Notes: for dyspepsia, abdominal pain, diarrhoea.

KID-3   **Location:** between the highest prominence of the medial malleolus and the Achilles tendon.
Notes: *Yuan*-source point; tonifies Kidney *Qi* and *Yin*, especially with BL-23 (back-*Shu* point).

L.I.-11   **Location:** with the arm fully flexed at the radial end of the cubital crease.
Notes: *He*-sea point; eliminates Damp-Heat, with L.I.-4 and Du-14 for fever.

LIV-3   **Location:** on the dorsum of the foot, in the depression distal to the junction of the 1st and 2nd metatarsal bones.
Notes: *Shu*-stream point and *Yuan*-source point; promotes the smooth flow of *Qi*, spasmolytic point.

P-6   **Location:** 2 cun proximal to the midpoint of the palmar wrist crease, between the tendons of the flexor carpi radialis and palmaris longus.
Notes: opening point of the *Yin Wei Mai*, master point for vomiting.

Ren-4   **Location:** 2 cun superior to the upper border of the pubic symphysis.
Notes: front-*Mu* point of the Small Intestine, meeting point of the 3 *Yin* meridians of the leg; local point.

Ren-6   **Location:** 1.5 cun inferior to the umbilicus.
Notes: tonifies *Qi*.

Ren-12   **Location:** midway between the umbilicus and the xiphoid process.
Notes: front-*Mu* point of the Stomach, controls the mid-section of the Stomach, tonifies the Stomach and Spleen, regulates the *Qi* of the Stomach and the Middle Burner, eliminates Dampness.

S.I.-3   **Location:** when a fist is made, on the dorsum of the hand, in the depression at the end of the most distal palmar crease.
Notes: master point for the mucous membranes, spasmolytic point.

SP-4   **Location:** in the depression at the junction of the base and shaft of the 1st metatarsal bone, at the junction of the red and white skin.
Notes: *Luo*-connecting point, opening point of the *Chong Mai*, master point for diarrhoea, tonifies the Spleen, calms the Stomach.

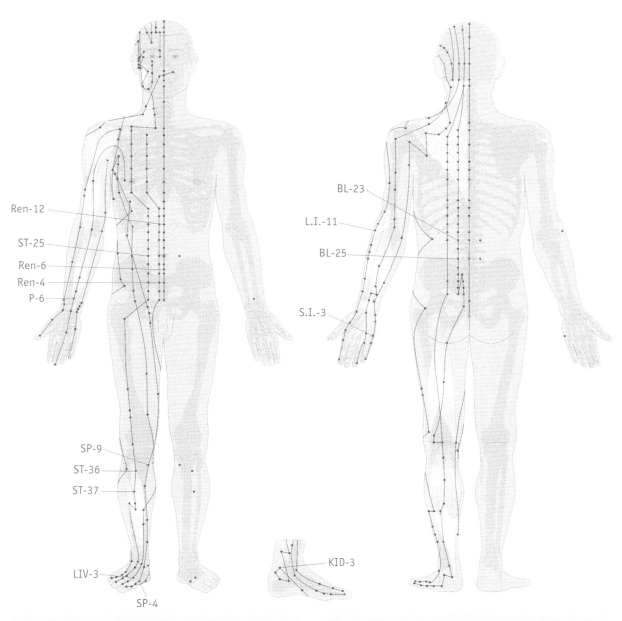

Ren-12

ST-25

Ren-6

Ren-4

P-6

SP-9

ST-36

ST-37

LIV-3

SP-4

BL-23

L.I.-11

BL-25

S.I.-3

KID-3

SP-9 **Location:** with the knee flexed in the depression inferior to the medial condyle of the tibia, at the same level as G.B.-34.
Notes: *He*-sea point, eliminates Damp-Heat from the Lower Burner.

ST-25 **Location:** 2 cun lateral to the centre of the umbilicus (Ren-8).
Notes: front-*Mu* point of the Large Intestine.

ST-36 **Location:** 0.5 cun lateral to the anterior crest of the tibia, 1.5 cun inferior to the lower border of the head of the fibula (G.B.-34).

Notes: *He*-sea point with a direct effect on the organ, also tonifies the Spleen, especially with Ren-12 (front-*Mu* point of the Stomach); command point for the abdomen.

ST-37 **Location:** 1 cun lateral to the anterior crest of the tibia, 4 cun inferior to the lower border of the head of the fibula or 3 cun inferior to ST-36.
Notes: lower *He*-sea point of the Large Intestine; regulates the Stomach and intestines, especially together with ST-25 (front-*Mu* point of the Large Intestine); eliminates Damp-Heat, for diarrhoea.

6.4.7 Constipation

Cause: a drying up of the stools due to heat, fever or unsuitable diet (excess patterns); *Qi* stagnation (spasms) or *Qi* and/or *Yang* deficiency, often accompanied by cold symptoms; deficiency of Blood (*Xue*) and Body Fluids.

Basic point combination

BL-25, ST-25, T.B.-6, KID-6 or KID-5.

Individual point combination

Excess pattern, for instance dry stools, foul-smelling stools (e.g. with fever)

L.I.-11, L.I.-4.

Qi stagnation – abdominal pain

Ren-12, LIV-3.

Deficiency pattern – *Qi* and Blood (*Xue*) deficiency, also abuse of laxatives

BL-20, BL-21, ST-36.

Cold symptoms – 'sluggish bowls' (*Yang* deficiency)

Ren-8 (only moxa, no needling!), Ren-6 **M**.

Acupuncture points

BL-20 Location: 1.5 cun lateral to the spinous process of T11.
Notes: back-*Shu* point of the Spleen, tonifies the Spleen and the Stomach, and thus *Qi* and Blood (*Xue*).
BL-21 Location: 1.5 cun lateral to the spinous process of T12.
Notes: back-*Shu* point of the Stomach, master point for the Stomach, tonifies the Spleen and the Stomach, and thus *Qi* and Blood (*Xue*).

BL-25 Location: 1.5 cun lateral to the spinous process of L4.
Notes: back-*Shu* point of the Large Intestine, together with ST-25 promotes the smooth flow of *Qi* in the Large Intestine.
KID-5 Location: 1 cun inferior to KID-3.
Notes: *Xi*-cleft point of the Kidneys; combined with T.B.-6 often more effective for constipation than the combination with KID-6.
KID-6 Location: below the prominence of the medial malleolus.
Notes: KID-6 and T.B.-6 are a standard combination for constipation.
L.I.-4 Location: on the dorsum of the hand, at the highest point of the muscle bulge between the 1st and 2nd metacarpal bones.
Notes: *Yuan*-source point, eliminates Heat from the Large Intestine.
L.I.-11 Location: with the arm fully flexed, at the radial end of the cubital crease.
Notes: *He*-sea point, eliminates Heat from the Large Intestine.
LIV-3 Location: on the dorsum of the foot, in the depression distal to the junction of the 1st and 2nd metatarsal bones.
Notes: *Shu*-stream point and *Yuan*-source point; promotes the smooth flow of *Qi*, spasmolytic point.
Ren-6 Location: 1.5 cun inferior to the umbilicus.
Notes: tonifies original *Qi*, descends the *Qi*.
Ren-8 Location: in the centre of the umbilicus.
Notes: needling contraindicated! Fill the umbilicus with salt, place a ginger slice on the salt and on top of this a moxa cone: warms and relaxes the intestines.
Ren-12 Location: midway between the umbilicus and the xiphoid process.
Notes: front-*Mu* point of the Stomach, *Hui*-meeting point of the hollow organs (*Fu*); descends the *Qi* of the *Fu* organs.
ST-25 Location: 2 cun lateral to the centre of the umbilicus (Ren-8).
Notes: front-*Mu* point of the Large Intestine, together with BL-25 (back-*Shu* point) promotes the smooth flow of *Qi* in the Large Intestine.
ST-36 Location: 0.5 cun lateral to the anterior crest of the tibia, 1.5 cun inferior to the lower border of the head of the fibula (G.B.-34).
Notes: *He*-sea point with direct effect on the organ, tonifies the Spleen and Stomach, and thus *Qi* and Blood (*Xue*).
T.B.-6 Location: 3 cun proximal to the midpoint of the dorsal wrist crease.
Notes: regulates *Qi*, moistens the stools, especially when combined with KID-3.

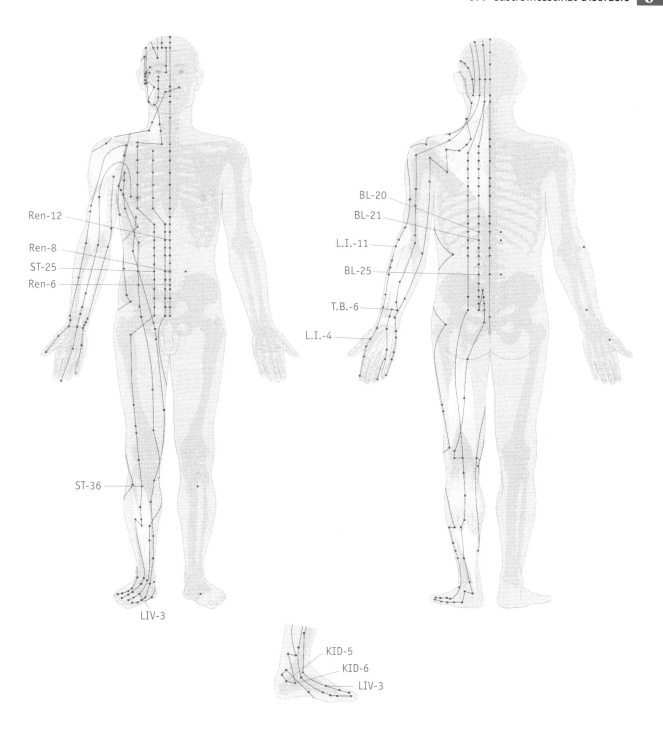

Ren-12

Ren-8

ST-25

Ren-6

ST-36

LIV-3

BL-20

BL-21

L.I.-11

BL-25

T.B.-6

L.I.-4

KID-5

KID-6

LIV-3

6.5 Urinary tract disorders

A. Römer, B. Seybold

6.5.1 Urinary incontinence, retention of urine

According to TCM, the Bladder belongs to the Water element, which also includes the uterus, the ovaries and the Kidneys.

Heavy lifting, difficult birth, and excessive mental or physical work may all result in a weakness of the Bladder.

Post-partum stress incontinence should, besides acupuncture, initially be treated with a sufficient period of rest, followed by specific pelvic floor exercises, ideally administered by midwives or experienced physiotherapists.

> Rule of thumb: Do not lift anything heavier than the weight of the child. Avoid cold, ensure sufficient intake of water (preferably non-carbonated).

TCM

Bladder and Kidney *Qi* deficiency, Essence (*Jing*) deficiency.

Basic point combination

SP-6, BL-23, BL-28, BL-60, Du-20, Ren-3.

Individual point combination

Retention of urine (postoperative or post-partum)

TCM: *Qi* stagnation, Spleen *Yang* deficiency.
BL-39 [BL-53 Bi], BL-58, LIV-2, LIV-3, Ren-4.

Acupuncture points

BL-23 **Location:** 1.5 cun lateral to L2, level with Du-4.
Notes: back-*Shu* point of the Kidneys, has segmental action, tonifies the *Qi*, *Yang*, *Yin* and Essence (*Jing*) of the Kidneys, strengthens the lumbar region and the knees.
BL-28 **Location:** 1.5 cun lateral to the posterior midline, at the level of the 2nd sacral foramen.

Notes: back-*Shu* point of the of the Bladder, has segmental action, eliminates Damp-Heat; opens the Water passages, tonifies Kidney *Yang*.
BL-39 **Location:** on the lateral aspect of the popliteal crease, on the medial border of the tendon of the biceps femoris.
Notes: lower *He*-sea point of the Triple Burner, opens the Water passages.
BL-58 **Location:** 1 cun distal and lateral to BL-57, on the lateral border of the gastrocnemius, on the soleus. On a cross-section through the lower leg at 7.30 and 4.30 respectively.
Notes: *Luo*-connecting point, moves Bladder *Qi*.
BL-60 **Location:** in the depression between the Achilles tendon and the lateral malleolus.
Notes: strengthens the Kidneys and the Bladder.
Du-20 **Location:** on a line connecting the apices of the ears, on the midline, just posterior to the highest point of the head.
Notes: raises the *Qi*; use tonifying needling technique (possibly moxa).
LIV-2 **Location:** on the interdigital web between the 1st and 2nd toes, at the lateral aspect of the metatarsophalangeal joint of the 1st toe.
Notes: *Ying*-spring point, sedation point, eliminates Liver Fire, spasmolytic point.
LIV-3 **Location:** on the dorsum of the foot, in the depression distal to the junction of the 1st and 2nd metatarsal bones.
Notes: *Shu*-stream point, *Yuan*-source point, calms Liver *Yang*, harmonizes the flow of Liver *Qi*, spasmolytic point.
Ren-3 **Location:** 1 cun superior to the upper border of the pubic symphysis (1/5 of the distance between the symphysis and the umbilicus).
Notes: meeting point of the 3 *Yin* meridians of the leg (KID, LIV, SP); as front-*Mu* point, eliminates Damp-Heat from the Bladder.
Ren-4 **Location:** 2 cun superior to the upper border of the pubic symphysis (2/5 of the distance between the symphysis and the umbilicus).
Notes: meeting point of the 3 *Yin* meridians of the leg (KID, LIV, SP), front-*Mu* point of the Small Intestine; tonifying, strengthens the Essence (*Jing*), *Qi*, *Yang*, Blood (*Xue*) and Yin.
SP-6 **Location:** 3 cun superior to the highest prominence of the medial malleolus, on the posterior border of the tibia.
Notes: group *Luo*-connecting point of the 3 *Yin* meridians of the leg; tonifies the Spleen, Liver and Kidneys, tonifies Blood (*Xue*), *Qi* and *Yin*, nourishes and regulates the Blood (*Xue*), distal point for promoting the blood circulation in the lower abdomen, eliminates Dampness from the Lower Burner.

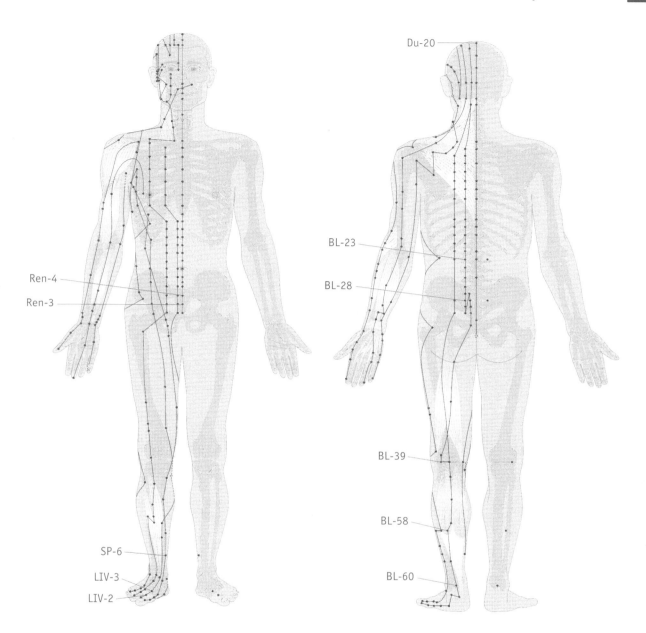

6.5.2 *Urethritis and cystitis*

Urethritis and cystitis are often triggered and sustained by an infection at the entrance of the vagina. Cold, either as an external pathogenic (climatic) factor or as food (cold meals and drinks), may result in an infection becoming chronic.

Women with chronic cystitis should wear warm clothes covering the Bladder and Kidney area, and drink sufficient water. They should also make sure they keep warm after sex and during menstruation, because at these times there is an increased susceptibility for external Cold to penetrate the body. Dampness often has its origin in a diet rich in dairy or cold foods. In the body, Dampness and Cold will, over time, transform into Damp-Heat.

TCM

Usually Dampness or Damp-Heat in the Bladder.

Basic point combination

ST-40, SP-9, BL-28, BL-32, LIV-2, LIV-3, Ren-2, Ren-3; ear points: 92 Bladder, 95 Kidneys.

Individual point combination

Irritable Bladder (responds well to acupuncture)

TCM: Liver *Qi* stagnation, Liver *Yin* deficiency, Kidney *Qi* deficiency, Kidney *Yang* deficiency.
LIV-2, LIV-3; ear acupuncture: 97 Liver.

Neurasthenia

HE-7.

Acupuncture points

BL-28 **Location:** 1.5 cun lateral to the posterior midline, at the level of the 2nd sacral foramen.
Notes: back-*Shu* point of the of the Bladder; has segmental action, eliminates Damp-Heat, opens the Water passages, tonifies Kidney *Yang*.

BL-32 **Location:** over the 2nd sacral foramen.
Notes: has segmental action; combined with Ren-2 and Ren-3, promotes horizontal circulation in the lower abdomen.

HE-7 **Location:** on the ulnar aspect of the wrist crease, on the radial aspect of the pisiform bone.
Notes: *Yuan*-source point, *Shu*-stream point, sedation point, corresponds to the Kidney meridian (*Shao Yin*), calms the Spirit, pacifies the Heart.

LIV-2 **Location:** on the interdigital web between the 1st and 2nd toes, at the lateral aspect of the metatarsophalangeal joint of the 1st toe.
Notes: *Ying*-spring point, sedation point, eliminates Liver Fire, spasmolytic point.

LIV-3 **Location:** on the dorsum of the foot, in the depression distal to the junction of the 1st and 2nd metatarsal bones.
Notes: *Shu*-stream point, *Yuan*-source point, calms Liver *Yang*, harmonizes the flow of Liver *Qi*, spasmolytic point.

Ren-2 **Location:** on the midline, at the upper border of the pubic symphysis, in the skin crease that forms when bending forward; level with KID-11, SP-12, ST-30.
Notes: eliminates Damp-Heat and Deficiency-Fire.

Ren-3 **Location:** 1 cun superior to the upper border of the pubic symphysis (1/5 of the distance between the symphysis and the umbilicus).
Notes: meeting point of the 3 *Yin* meridians of the leg (KID, LIV, SP); as front-*Mu* point, eliminates Damp-Heat from the Bladder.

SP-9 **Location:** with the knee flexed, in the depression inferior to the medial condyle of the tibia, at the same level as G.B.-34.
Notes: *He*-sea point, eliminates Dampness and Heat, regulates the Water passages.

ST-40 **Location:** at the midpoint of the distance between the medial malleolus and the knee joint space, 2 cun lateral to the anterior crest of the tibia.
Notes: *Luo*-connecting point (connects with the Spleen meridian), thus specific point for Phlegm and Dampness.

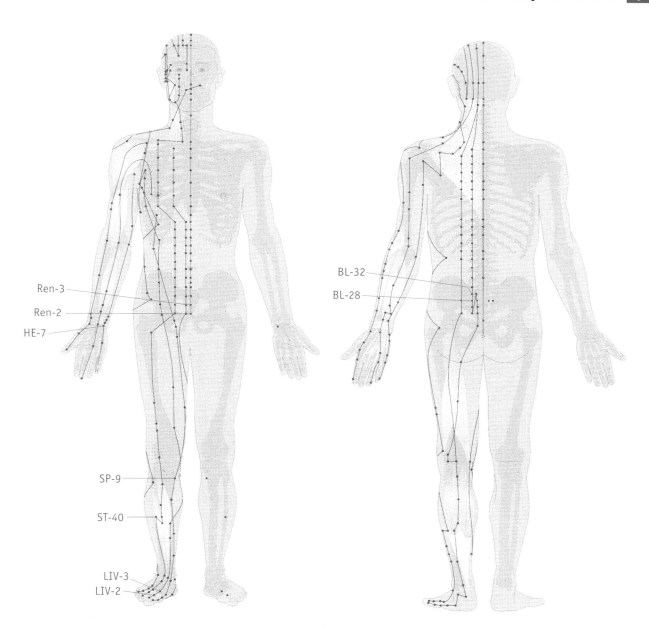

Ren-3
Ren-2
HE-7

BL-32
BL-28

SP-9

ST-40

LIV-3
LIV-2

6.6 Disorders of the male sexual organs

G. Kubiena

6.6.1 Impotence

Impotence is a good indication for acupuncture, improving both functional disorders and semen analysis results. Impotence is often due to a functional disorder (e.g. sexual neurosis).

Basic point combination

HE-7, BL-15, BL-31, KID-12, Ren-3/4/6, Du-4.

Individual point combination

Kidney *Yang* deficiency = reduced *Ming Men* Fire (erectile dysfunction, male infertility)

Symptoms: unable to obtain an erection but also no sexual desire, no or only weak erection, pain and weakness in the lumbar region and knees, cold extremities, frequent urination, blurry vision, dizziness, lethargy.
Tongue body: pale; **pulse:** deep, thready.
Cause: too much sex weakens the Kidney *Yang/Ming Men* Fire and exhausts the Essence (*Jing*); anxiety and worry disturb the *Qi* of the Heart, Spleen and Kidneys.
Treatment principle: tonify the Kidney *Yang*.
BL-23 M, KID-3 M, Du-4 M, Ren-4 M (also for original *Qi* or Ren-6 M; Du-20 raises Kidney *Qi*. Insomnia and palpitations: SP-6, HE-7, BL-15.

Damp-Heat pouring downward – contracture, atrophy

Symptoms: no erection, dark urine, thirst, weakness of the lower extremities, possibly bitter taste in the mouth.
Tongue coating: thick, yellow; **pulse:** soft, rapid.
Cause: cystitis, prostatitis, urethritis, sexually transmitted diseases.
Therapy: ST-36, SP-6, SP-9, Ren-3.

Acupuncture points

BL-15 Location: 1.5 cun lateral to the spinous process of T5.
Notes: back-*Shu* point of the Heart; together with HE-7 psychologically stabilizing; for insomnia and palpitations.

BL-23 Location: 1.5 cun lateral to L2, level with Du-4.
Notes: back-*Shu* point of the Kidneys; use moxa to tonify Kidney *Yang*.
BL-31 Location: over the 1st sacral foramen.
Notes: strongly sexually stimulating point.
Du-4 Location: below the spinous process of L2.
Notes: tonifies particularly Kidney *Yang*, but also Kidney *Yin*; firms the Essence (*Jing*); tonifying point.
Du-20 Location: on a line connecting the apices of the ears, on the midline, just posterior to the highest point of the head.
Notes: meeting point of all divergent meridians; psychosomatic effect; raises the *Qi* (erection).
HE-7 Location: on the ulnar aspect of the wrist crease, on the radial aspect of the pisiform bone.
Notes: *Yuan*-source point, sedation point, psychologically stabilizing; for palpitations and insomnia.
KID-3 Location: between the highest prominence of the medial malleolus and the Achilles tendon.
Notes: *Yuan*-source point and *Shu*-stream point; tonifies the Kidneys, strengthens the lumbar region and the knees; benefits the Essence (*Jing*).
KID-12 Location: 0.5 cun lateral to the midline, 1 cun superior to the pubic symphysis or 1/5 of the distance between the pubic symphysis and the umbilicus, at the level of Ren-3.
Notes: has a particular effect on the male genitalia; for nocturnal emissions.
Ren-3 Location: 1 cun superior to the upper border of the pubic symphysis (1/5 of the distance between the symphysis and the umbilicus).
Notes: meeting point of the 3 *Yin* meridians of the leg (KID, LIV, SP); front-*Mu* point of the Bladder; eliminates Damp-Heat (cystitis).
Ren-4 Location: 2 cun superior to the upper border of the pubic symphysis (2/5 of the distance between the symphysis and the umbilicus).
Notes: meeting point of the 3 *Yin* meridians of the leg, front-*Mu* point of the Small Intestine (paired with the Heart!); tonifies the Kidneys, rescues *Yang Qi*.
Ren-6 Location: 1.5 cun inferior to the umbilicus.
Notes: 'Sea of *Qi*'; activates the *Yang Qi*, stops emissions. [Bi] 'Sea of male fertility'.
SP-6 Location: 3 cun superior to the highest prominence of the medial malleolus, on the posterior border of the tibia.
Notes: group *Luo*-connecting point of the 3 *Yin* meridians of the leg; tonifies the Spleen, eliminates Dampness.
SP-9 Location: with the knee flexed, in the depression inferior to the medial condyle of the tibia, at the same level as G.B.-34.
Notes: *He*-sea point; eliminates Dampness and Heat.
ST-36 Location: 0.5 cun lateral to the anterior crest of the tibia, 1.5 cun inferior to the lower border of the head of the fibula (G.B.-34).
Notes: *He*-sea point, used here to strengthen the Spleen in order to treat Damp-Heat.

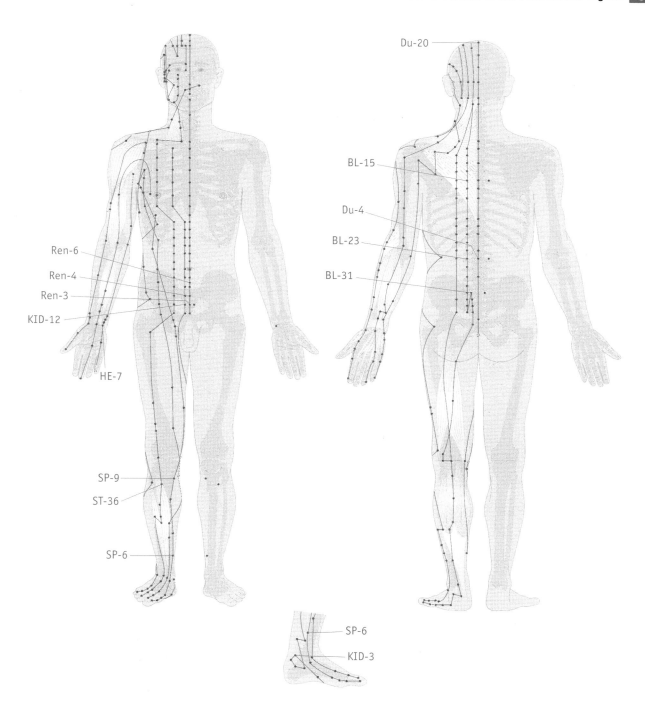

6.6.2 Spermatorrhoea

TCM

The loss of sperm is seen as the loss of Essence (*Jing*), so spermatorrhoea is considered to be of concern (prior to Sigmund Freud, the same idea existed in the West).

Basic point combination

HE-7, BL-15, BL-31, KID-12, Ren-3/4/6, Du-4.

Individual point combination

Spermatorrhoea – involuntary loss of sperm (during day or night)

Symptoms: flow of sperm, particularly if desiring sex, pale, lethargic. **Tongue body**: pale; **pulse:** deep, thready, weak.
Cause: general weakness (during convalescence, due to general overexertion).
SP-6, BL-23, KID-11, KID-12, Ren-4, Ren-6.

Nocturnal emission – 'wet dreams'

Symptoms: dizziness, palpitations, lethargy, scanty yellow urine. **Tongue body:** red; **pulse:** thready, rapid.
Cause: disharmony between the Kidneys and the Heart.
HE-7- and BL-15, KID-3+ and BL-52+.

Acupuncture points

BL-15 **Location:** 1.5 cun lateral to the spinous process of T5.
Notes: back-*Shu* point of the Heart; together with HE-7, psychologically stabilizing effect; for insomnia and palpitations.
BL-23 **Location:** 1.5 cun lateral to L2, level with Du-4.
Notes: back-*Shu* point of the Kidneys; use moxa to tonify Kidney *Yang*.

BL-31 **Location:** over the 1st sacral foramen.
Notes: sexually strongly stimulating point.
BL-52 **Location:** 3 cun lateral to the spinous process of L2, lateral to BL-23.
Notes: firms the Essence (*Jing*) and willpower.
Du-4 **Location:** below the spinous process of L2.
Notes: firms the Essence (*Jing*), tonifies Kidney *Yin* and *Yang*, strengthens the lower back and knees.
HE-7 **Location:** on the ulnar aspect of the wrist crease, on the radial aspect of the pisiform bone.
Notes: *Yuan*-source point, sedation point, psychologically stabilizing; for insomnia and palpitations.
KID-3 **Location:** between the highest prominence of the medial malleolus and the Achilles tendon.
Notes: *Yuan*-source point and *Shu*-stream point; tonifies the Kidneys, strengthens the lumbar region and the knees; benefits the Essence (*Jing*).
KID-11 **Location:** on the upper border of the pubic symphysis, approximately 0.5 cun lateral to the midline (Ren-2).
Notes: has an effect on the external genitalia.
KID-12 **Location:** 0.5 cun lateral to the midline, 1 cun superior to the pubic symphysis or 1/5 of the distance between the pubic symphysis and the umbilicus, at the level of Ren-3.
Notes: has a particular effect on the male genitalia, for nocturnal emissions.
Ren-3 **Location:** 1 cun superior to the upper border of the pubic symphysis (1/5 of the distance between the symphysis and the umbilicus).
Notes: meeting point of the 3 *Yin* meridians of the leg; front-*Mu* point of the Bladder; benefits Bladder *Qi*, eliminates Damp-Heat (cystitis).
Ren-4 **Location:** 2 cun superior to the upper border of the pubic symphysis (2/5 of the distance between the symphysis and the umbilicus).
Notes: meeting point of the 3 *Yin* meridians of the leg, front-*Mu* point of the Small Intestine (paired with the Heart!); tonifies the Kidneys, rescues *Yang Qi*.
Ren-6 **Location:** 1.5 cun inferior to the umbilicus.
Notes: 'Sea of *Qi*'; activates the *Yang Qi*, stops emissions. [Bi] 'Sea of male fertility'.
SP-6 **Location:** 3 cun superior to the highest prominence of the medial malleolus, on the posterior border of the tibia.
Notes: group *Luo*-connecting point of the 3 *Yin* of the leg; tonifies the Spleen, eliminates Dampness.

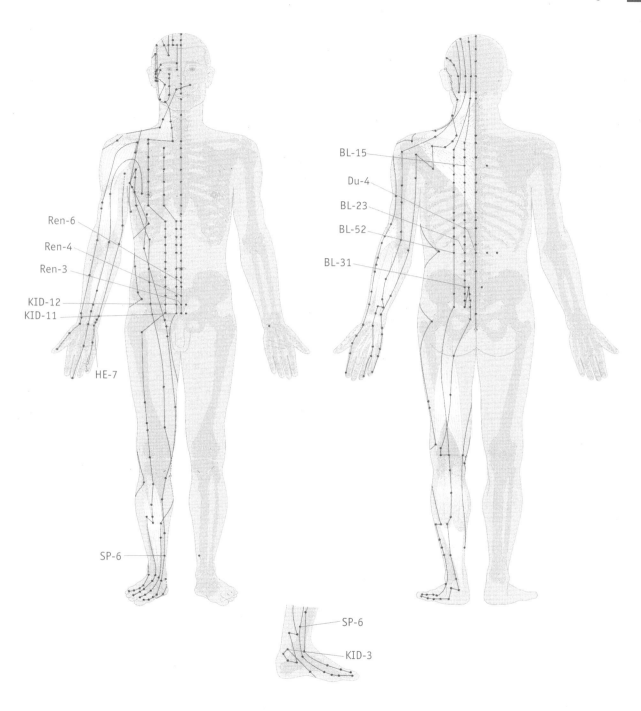

Ren-6
Ren-4
Ren-3
KID-12
KID-11
HE-7
SP-6

BL-15
Du-4
BL-23
BL-52
BL-31

SP-6
KID-3

6.6.3 *Premature ejaculation*

Basic point combination

HE-7, BL-15, BL-23, KID-12, Ren-3/4/6, Du-4.

Individual point combination

Kidney *Yin* deficiency

Symptoms: sexual desire but unable to achieve an erection; premature ejaculation; 'hyper' but no stamina; pain and weakness in the lumbar region. **Tongue body:** bright red; **pulse:** thready, rapid.
Cause: too much sex, 'loss of substance', organic disorders (e.g. tuberculosis).
Therapy: Ren-4+, KID-6+, ST-36+, SP-6+; alternate with Du-4+. BL-23+, BL-44+, BL-52+; disturbed sleep and palpitations: as with Kidney *Yang* deficiency: HE-7-, BL-15, SP-6+.

Acupuncture points

BL-15 **Location:** 1.5 cun lateral to the spinous process of T5.
Notes: back-*Shu* point of the Heart; together with HE-7, psychologically stabilizing effect; for insomnia and palpitations.

BL-23 **Location:** 1.5 cun lateral to L2, level with Du-4.
Notes: back-*Shu* point of the Kidneys; tonifies the Kidneys and the Essence (*Jing*), strengthens the lumbar region.

BL-44 **Location:** 3 cun lateral to the spinous process of T5, lateral to BL-15 (back-*Shu* point of the HE), on the medial border of the scapula.
Notes: calms the *Shen* (mentally calming).

BL-52 **Location:** 3 cun lateral to the spinous process of L2, lateral to BL-23.
Notes: firms the Essence (*Jing*) and the willpower.

Du-4 **Location:** below the spinous process of L2.
Notes: firms the Essence (*Jing*), tonifies Kidney *Yin* and *Yang*, strengthens the lower back and the knees.

HE-7 **Location:** on the ulnar aspect of the wrist crease, on the radial aspect of the pisiform bone.
Notes: *Yuan*-source point of the Heart, *Shu*-stream point, sedation point, calms the Spirit, pacifies the Heart.

KID-6 **Location:** below the prominence of the medial malleolus.
Notes: opening point of the *Yin Qiao Mai*; tonifies *Yin*, cools the Blood (*Xue*), calms the Spirit.

KID-12 **Location:** 0.5 cun lateral to the midline, 1 cun superior to the pubic symphysis or 1/5 of the distance between the pubic symphysis and the umbilicus, at the level of Ren-3.
Notes: has a particular effect on the male genitalia; for nocturnal emissions.

Ren-3 **Location:** 1 cun superior to the upper border of the pubic symphysis (1/5 of the distance between the symphysis and the umbilicus).
Notes: meeting point of the 3 *Yin* meridians of the leg (KID, LIV, SP); as front-*Mu* point, eliminates Dampness from the Bladder.

Ren-4 **Location:** 2 cun superior to the upper border of the pubic symphysis (2/5 of the distance between the symphysis and the umbilicus).
Notes: meeting point of the 3 *Yin* meridians of the leg, front *Mu* point of the Small Intestine (paired with the Heart!); tonifies the Kidneys, rescues *Yang Qi*.

Ren-6 **Location:** 1.5 cun inferior to the umbilicus.
Notes: 'Sea of *Qi*'; activates the *Yang Qi*, stops emissions. [Bi] 'Sea of male fertility'.

SP-6 **Location:** 3 cun superior to the highest prominence of the medial malleolus, on the posterior border of the tibia.
Notes: as group *Luo*-connecting point of the 3 *Yin* of the leg, tonifying effect on the Spleen, Liver and Kidneys; tonifies Blood (*Xue*), *Qi* and *Yin*, nourishes and regulates the Blood (*Xue*); distal point for promoting blood circulation in the lower abdomen; eliminates Dampness.

ST-36 **Location:** 0.5 cun lateral to the anterior crest of the tibia, 1.5 cun inferior to the lower border of the head of the fibula (G.B.-34).
Notes: *He*-sea point; used here to stabilize.

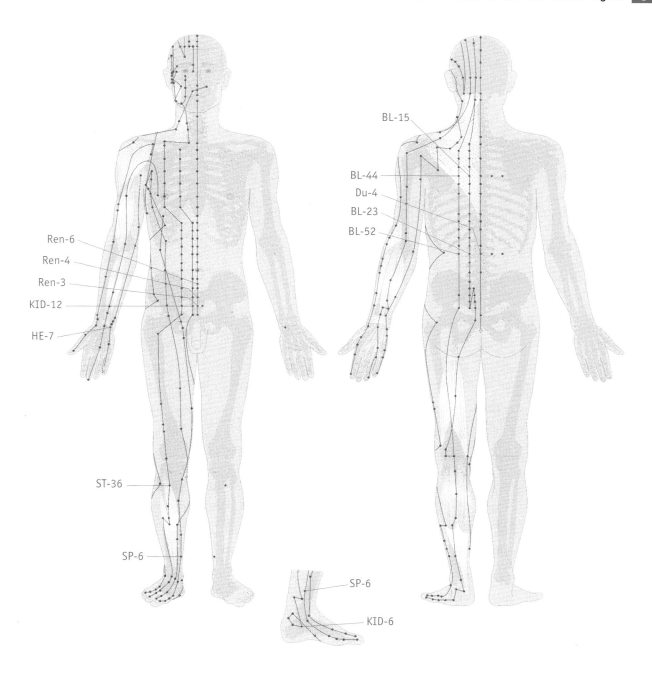

6.6.4 Genital eczema and discharge

Individual point combination

Genital eczema

LIV-1–, LIV-5–, LIV-11–, Ren-3–.

Discharge

SP-9–.

Acupuncture points

LIV-1 **Location:** on the big toe, next to the lateral corner of the nail.
Notes: *Jing*-well point; eliminates Damp-Heat.
LIV-5 **Location:** on the medial border of the tibia, 5 cun superior to the medial malleolus [Bi: on the medial border of the tibia, 1.5 cun inferior to the midpoint of the distance between the medial malleolus and the upper border of the tibia.]
Notes: *Luo*-connecting point; eliminates Damp-Heat, alleviates itching.
LIV-11 **Location:** 2 cun lateral and 2 cun inferior to the midpoint of the pubic symphysis, on the lateral border of the abductor longus.
Notes: eliminates Damp-Heat as well as *Qi* and Blood stagnation in the inguinal groove and the genitalia.
Ren-3 **Location:** 1 cun superior to the upper border of the pubic symphysis (1/5 of the distance between the symphysis and the umbilicus).
Notes: meeting point of the 3 *Yin* meridians of the leg (KID, LIV, SP); as front-*Mu* point, eliminates Dampness from the Bladder.
SP-9 **Location:** with the knee flexed, in the depression inferior to the medial condyle of the tibia, at the same level as G.B.-34.
Notes: *He*-sea point; eliminates Dampness and Heat.

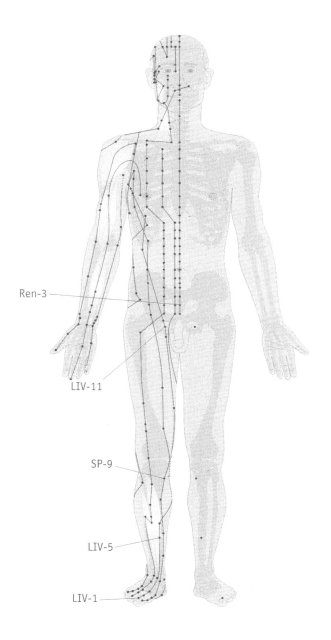

Ren-3

LIV-11

SP-9

LIV-5

LIV-1

6.7 Obstetrics and gynaecology

A. Römer, B. Seybold

Obstetric indications respond well to acupuncture, usually requiring only a few treatments with well-proven point combinations. However, owing to the chronic nature of most other gynaecological disorders, an individual diagnosis is essential in order to achieve satisfactory treatment results.

Generally, patients with gynaecological disorders will be treated for a period of 3–6 menstrual cycles, with 2–4 treatments per cycle. In cases where the TCM pattern is correlated with the phases of the cycle, treatments will be scheduled according to the relevant phase. In other cases, treatments will mostly take place at regular (weekly) intervals.

TCM

The treatment goal is to establish the harmonious balance of *Qi*. After menstruation, the *Qi* migrates to the surface of the body. Following ovulation, the *Qi* courses together with the Blood (*Xue*) towards the lower abdomen in order to fill the uterus with Blood (*Xue*). After ovulation, harmonizing the *Qi* flow and spreading the *Qi* can therefore alleviate many disorders, such as dysmenorrhoea. In the treatment of gynaecological disorders, identifying the constitutional type, taking a detailed menstrual history and determining the TCM syndromes (patterns of disharmony or disturbed *Qi*) are of great importance. A detailed description of these is beyond the scope of this book, so, for complex cases where it seems insufficient simply to state a point prescription, the reader is asked to refer to the relevant textbooks.

> If scars, especially in the genital region, cause discomfort or if acupuncture treatments are not showing any improvement, the scars should be investigated and, if necessary, treated with neural therapy.

6.7.1 Dysmenorrhoea

Determine the precise onset of the dysmenorrhoea; for example, for postoperative onset (horizontal or vertical abdominal scars) clear the scar first with neural therapy; if linked to body piercing, remove the piercing; if it follows the insertion of an IUD ('coil'), discuss alternative methods of contraception.

TCM

Dysmenorrhoea is defined as a monthly, recurring pain, either shortly before menstruation (stagnation syndrome) or during menstruation (Heat syndrome, excess; stagnation of Phlegm, *Qi*, or Blood and *Qi*, etc.). Pain may also be the result of a deficiency syndrome, such as *Qi* or Blood (*Xue*) deficiency.

According to TCM the Liver is responsible for the smooth flow of menstrual Blood (*Xue*) and also for supplying sufficient Blood (*Xue*).

Qi and Blood (*Xue*) stagnation is caused by either a primary Liver *Qi* stagnation (for example due to emotional disturbances), a pathogenic factor (Cold or Heat [inflammation]), or a deficiency of *Qi* or of *Qi* and Blood (*Xue*).

Basic point combination

L.I.-4, SP-6, LIV-3, Ren-4; ear points: 22 endocrine system, 58 uterus.

Individual point combination

Liver *Qi* stagnation

Symptoms: fullness and distension in the chest and abdomen, irritability; **menstrual blood:** may be dark purple and sticky; **tongue:** may have red edges; **points:** P-6, G.B.-37, LIV-14, Du-20.

Cold in the uterus

Symptoms: Cold as internal and external pathogenic factor, cold sensations in the abdomen, abdomen cold to the touch, pain before and during menstruation, better with hot water bottle or hot bath; **menstrual blood:** scanty, dilute; **tongue:** white, moist; **pulse:** slow; **points:** ST-36, BL-23, KID-3, Ren-6; moxa (either 'warming needle' or moxa pole) to warm the points, e.g. on Ren-4, SP-6, ST-36, BL-23.

Liver and Kidney deficiency

Symptoms: exhaustion, tiredness, pale complexion, pain after menstruation; **tongue:** pale, thin.
Points: ST-36, BL-20, BL-23; moxa if no Heat signs are present (with Heat: yellow tongue coating, rapid pulse);

for any discomfort following tubal ligation, use procaine infiltration to clear the scar.

Dysfunctional bleeding in adolescent girls

Ear points: 22 endocrine system, 58 uterus: often 1 or 2 treatments are sufficient for regulating the cycle.

> The more recent the onset of dysmenorrhoea, the shorter the period required for treatment.

Acupuncture points

BL-23   Location: 1.5 cun lateral to the lower border of the spinous process of L2.
Notes: back-*Shu* point of the Kidneys; tonifies the *Qi*, *Yang*, *Yin* and Essence (*Jing*) of the Kidneys, has an effect on the hormones.

Du-20   Location: on a line connecting the apices of the ears, 7 cun superior the posterior hairline.
Notes: meeting point with the Liver meridian and all *Yang* meridians; sedating; complements the effect of LIV-3.

G.B.-37   Location: 5 cun superior to the lateral malleolus.
Notes: *Luo*-connecting point; promotes the *Qi* flow in the network vessels, tonifying for chronic diseases; important point for the Water element.

KID-3   Location: midway between the highest prominence of the medial malleolus and the Achilles tendon.
Notes: *Yuan*-source point, *Shu*-stream point; tonifies the *Yin*, *Yang* and Essence (*Jing*) of the Kidneys, strengthens the lumbar region and the knees; use moxa for Cold patterns.

L-20   Location: 1.5 cun lateral to the lower border of the spinous process of T11.
Notes: back-*Shu* point of the Spleen; tonifies the Spleen and Stomach and therefore *Qi* and Blood (*Xue*) production; eliminates Dampness.

L.I.-4   Location: on the highest point of the adductor pollicis.
Notes: *Yuan*-source point; drains, relieves pain, especially with LIV-3.

LIV-3   Location: in the depression distal to the junction of the 1st and 2nd metatarsal bones.
Notes: *Yuan*-source point, *Shu*-stream point; calms Liver *Yang*, harmonizes the Liver *Qi* flow, spasmolytic.

LIV-14   Location: on the midclavicular line, 6th ICS, directly below the nipple.
Notes: front-*Mu* point of the Liver, meeting point with the SP, special point for nausea.

P-6   Location: 2 cun proximal to the midpoint of the palmar aspect of the wrist crease, between the tendons of the flexor carpi radialis and palmaris longus.
Notes: opening point of the *Yin Wei Mai*; master point nausea; harmonizes the Stomach, regulates Heart *Qi* and Blood, calming, complements the effect of LIV-3.

Ren-4   Location: 2 cun superior to the upper border of the pubic symphysis.
Notes: meeting point of the 3 lower *Yin* (SP, KID, LIV), front-*Mu* point of the Small Intestine; tonifying - strengthens the Essence (*Jing*), *Qi*, *Yang*, Blood and *Yin*.

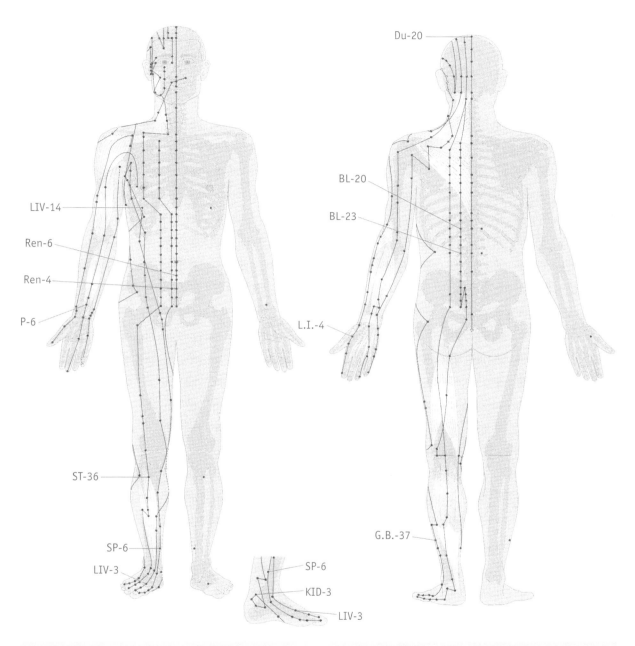

Du-20

BL-20

BL-23

L.I.-4

G.B.-37

SP-6
KID-3
LIV-3

LIV-14

Ren-6

Ren-4

P-6

ST-36

SP-6

LIV-3

Ren-6 **Location:** 1.5 cun inferior to the umbilicus.
Notes: 'Sea of *Qi*' - tonifies the Kidneys, original *Qi* and *Yang Qi*; strengthens and moves *Qi* in the Lower Burner, eliminates Dampness.

SP-6 **Location:** 3 cun superior to the highest prominence of the medial malleolus, on the posterior border of the tibia.
Notes: as group *Luo*-connecting point of the Spleen, Liver and Kidney, it tonifies Blood, *Qi* and *Yin*, and moves the Blood (*Xue*); distal point to promote circulation in the lower abdomen, eliminates Dampness.

ST-36 **Location:** 1 cun lateral to the anterior crest of the tibia, 1.5 cun inferior to the lower border of the head of the fibula (G.B.-34).
Notes: *He*-sea point, master point of hormones; tonifies the Stomach and Spleen, and therefore *Qi* and Blood (*Xue*).

6.7.2 Breast disorders

Acupuncture should be administered only after a thorough investigation by conventional medicine. Acupuncture should resolve any discomfort or pain within a short period of time (only a few treatments).

If there is no improvement with acupuncture, it is essential to refer the patient for further Western medicine tests to investigate the possibility of a tumour.

TCM

Longstanding Liver *Qi* stagnation results in Blood (*Xue*) stagnation and Phlegm (forms from Dampness). This in turn leads to the formation of palpable masses that are not related to the menstrual cycle.

Basic point combination

ST-18, ST-36, P-6, LIV-3, Ren-17.

Individual point combination

Dampness, Phlegm

Symptoms: often in obese patients, tendency to oedema, varicose veins.
Tongue coating: greasy, may be yellow.
Pulse: slippery.
Points: ST-40, SP-9.

Blood (*Xue*) stagnation

Symptoms: often in combination with painful periods with clotting.
Tongue body: bluish due to stagnation.
Pulse: wiry.
Points: SP-6, SP-10, SP-17.

Posterior mastectomy complaints

Local points near the scar.
Ear points: 22 endocrine system, 42 thorax, 58 uterus.

Acupuncture points

BL-17 Location: 1.5 cun lateral to the spinous process of T7.
Notes: *Hui*-meeting point of the Blood; tonifies and invigorates Blood; back-*Shu* point of the diaphragm.

LIV-3 Location: in the depression distal to the junction of the 1st and 2nd metatarsal bones.
Notes: *Yuan*-source point, *Shu*-stream point; calms Liver *Yang*, harmonizes Liver *Qi*, spasmolytic.

P-6 Location: 2 cun proximal to the midpoint of the palmar aspect of the wrist crease, between the tendons of the flexor carpi radialis and palmaris longus.
Notes: opening point of the *Yin Wei Mai*, master point for nausea; harmonizes the Stomach, regulates Heart *Qi* and Blood, calming; distal point for the breasts.

Ren-17 Location: on the midline of the sternum, level with the 4th ICS, between the nipples.
Notes: front-*Mu* point of the Pericardium; unbinds the chest, promotes lactation, regulates *Qi* in the Upper Burner; local point.

SP-6 Location: 3 cun superior to the highest prominence of the medial malleolus, on the posterior border of the tibia.
Notes: meeting point of the 3 *Yin* meridians of the leg; tonifies and moves Blood (*Xue*).

SP-9 Location: in the depression on the lower border of the medial condyle of the tibia.
Notes: *He*-sea point; eliminates Dampness.

SP-10 Location: 2 cun superior to the upper medial patellar border.
Notes: clears Heat from the Blood (*Xue*), 'cleanses' and moves Blood (*Xue*).

ST-18 Location: in the 5th ICS, on the lower border of the breast, on the midclavicular line.
Notes: regulates the function of the breasts.

ST-36 Location: 1 cun lateral to the anterior crest of the tibia, 1.5 cun inferior to the lower border of the head of the fibula (G.B.-34).
Notes: moves and tonifies Blood (*Xue*) and *Qi*; most important distal point on the Stomach meridian, distal point for the breast.

ST-40 Location: at the midpoint of the lower leg, 2 cun lateral to the anterior crest of the tibia.
Notes: *Luo*-connecting point; transforms Phlegm; good in combination with SP-9.

Local points in the scar region Notes: increase the circulation and immune activity and therefore speed up the healing process; use short needles with shallow insertions, do not needle into the scar.
Laser: good results with posterior surgical scar pain, several treatments necessary; oedema fluid will also be absorbed quicker and the contralateral breast will become soft and free of pain.

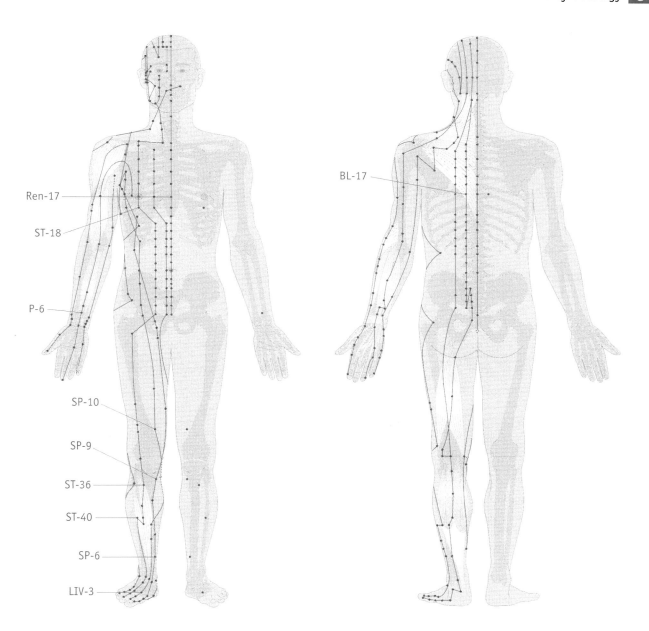

Ren-17

ST-18

P-6

SP-10

SP-9

ST-36

ST-40

SP-6

LIV-3

BL-17

6.7.3 Infertility in women (1)

The causes of infertility tend to be complex, so that after a biomedical investigation treatments should be based on a differential TCM diagnosis.

In secondary infertility, the medical history will often reveal disturbances in the lower abdomen, particularly following dilatation and curettage.

TCM

The ability to conceive is a function of the Water element (kidneys, uterus, ovaries, etc.). This means that a woman requires sufficient Kidney energy in order to produce eggs, to menstruate and to conceive. She further needs sufficient Blood (*Xue*). To hold the fetus beyond the first trimester, the Spleen energy has to be sufficient. If the uterus is 'blocked', for example due to Phlegm, Cold or Blood (*Xue*) stasis, pregnancy may not occur despite sufficient Kidney energy.

Primary infertility:

- Kidney Essence (*Jing*) deficiency: congenital, constitutional; energy deficiency
- Kidney *Yin* deficiency: due to a lifestyle that uses up the body's resources
- Kidney *Yang* deficiency: cold sensations, lethargy, possibly depression
- Phlegm-Dampness: often seen with oligorrhoea, amenorrhoea, in overweight patients, with polycystic ovary syndrome.
- Blood (*Xue*) stagnation: painful periods with blood clots
- Liver *Qi* stagnation: emotional stagnation, abdominal bloating, often premenstrual syndrome, irritability, may have high stress levels
- Liver Blood (*Xue*) deficiency: tiredness as primary symptom, pale, lethargic.

Basic point combination

ST-29, SP-6, BL-23, DU-4, Ex-CA-1 (*Zi Gong*); ear points: 22 endocrine system, 58 uterus.

Individual point combination

Kidney *Yang* deficiency

Symptoms: cold sensations, depression, weakness, may have ear problems, back pain, menstrual irregularities, etc.
Tongue body: pale

Pulse: weak, slow.
Points: KID-3, KID-7, moxa (e.g. KID-3, KID-7, BL-23).

Kidney *Yin* deficiency

Symptoms: back pain, may have night sweats, heat sensations, malar flush, may have tinnitus, menstrual irregularities; **tongue:** red tongue body, no coating; **pulse:** thin, rapid; **points:** -, KID-6, KID-7.

Acupuncture points

BL-23 **Location:** 1.5 cun lateral to the lower border of the spinous process of L2.
Notes: back-*Shu* point of the Kidneys; tonifies the *Qi, Yang, Yin* and Essence (*Jing*) of the Kidneys; strengthens the lumbar region and the knees, strengthens the Water element (receiving = function of the Water element).

Du-4 **Location:** on the posterior midline, below the spinous process of L2.
Notes: *Ming Men* (Gate of Life); activates the original *Qi* for all life-supporting processes.

Ex-CA-1 **Location:** 3 cun lateral to the anterior midline, 3 cun inferior to the umbilicus, lateral to Ren-3 and KID-12.
Notes: for infertility, treat 3–4 times per cycle; best results when the protocol is adapted to the cycle.

KID-3 **Location:** midway between the highest prominence of the medial malleolus and the Achilles tendon.
Notes: *Yuan*-source and *Shu*-stream point; tonifies the Kidney *Yin* and *Yang*, strengthens the lumbar region and the knees, benefits the Essence (*Jing*).

KID-6 **Location:** directly below the medial malleolus, often in a small cleft.
Notes: opening point of the *Yin Qiao Mai*; tonifies Kidney *Yin*.

KID-7 **Location:** 2 cun superior to KID-3 (KID-3: midway between the highest prominence of the medial malleolus and the Achilles tendon).
Notes: *Jing*-river point; with moxa tonifies Kidney *Yang*, needling tonifies Kidney *Yin*.

Ren-4 **Location:** 2 cun superior to the upper border of the pubic symphysis.
Notes: meeting point of the 3 lower *Yin* meridians (SP, KID, LIV), front-*Mu* point of the Small Intestine; tonifying - strengthens the Essence (*Jing*), *Qi, Yang*, Blood and *Yin*.

SP-6 **Location:** 3 cun superior to the highest prominence of the medial malleolus, on the posterior border of the tibia.
Notes: as group *Luo*-connecting point, tonifies the Spleen, Liver and Kidneys; also tonifies Blood (*Xue*), *Qi* and *Yin*, nourishes and moves the Blood (*Xue*); distal point for promoting the Blood circulation in the lower abdomen; eliminates Dampness.

ST-29 **Location:** 2 cun lateral to the midline, 4 cun inferior to the umbilicus, level with Ren-3 and KID-12.
Notes: local point for the ovaries and internal genitalia; removes Blood (*Xue*) stagnation in the uterus; raises the *Qi* (prolapse).

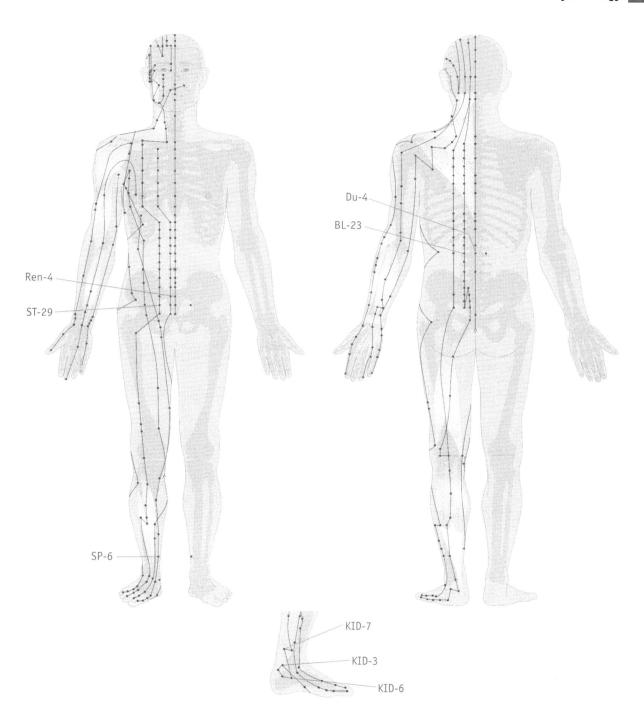

Du-4

BL-23

Ren-4

ST-29

SP-6

KID-7

KID-3

KID-6

6.7.3 Infertility in women (2)

Individual point combination

Phlegm-Dampness

Symptoms: tendency to oedema, often overweight, often menstrual blood with a slippery, stringy coating.
Tongue coating: greasy, may be yellow.
Pulse: slippery.
Points: ST-40, SP-9.

Blood stagnation

Often in combination with painful menstruation with blood clots.
Tongue body: stagnated, bluish.
Pulse: wiry.
Points: SP-6, SP-10, BL-17.

Liver *Qi* stagnation

Symptoms: stressful environment, irritability, often premenstrual syndrome, dysmenorrhoea, especially 1–2 days before onset of menstruation.
Tongue body: may have red edges.
Pulse: wiry.
Points: P-6, LIV-3.

Acupuncture points

BL-17 **Location:** 1.5 cun lateral to the spinous process of T7.
Notes: as the *Hui*-meeting point of the Blood (*Xue*), tonifies and regulates the Blood; back-*Shu* point of the diaphragm.

LIV-3 **Location:** in the depression distal to the junction of the 1st and 2nd metatarsal bones.
Notes: *Yuan*-source and *Shu*-stream point; calms the Liver *Yang*, harmonizes the flow of Liver *Qi*, spasmolytic.

P-6 **Location:** 2 cun proximal to the midpoint of the palmar aspect of the wrist crease, between the tendons of the flexor carpi radialis and palmaris longus.
Notes: opening point of the *Yin Wei Mai*; master point for nausea; harmonizes the Stomach, regulates Heart *Qi* and Blood, calming (connection between the Liver and Pericardium meridians!).

SP-6 **Location:** 3 cun superior to the highest prominence of the medial malleolus, on the posterior border of the tibia.
Notes: as group *Luo*-connecting point, tonifies the Spleen, Liver and Kidneys; also tonifies Blood (*Xue*), *Qi* and *Yin*, nourishes and moves the Blood (*Xue*); distal point for promoting the Blood circulation in the lower abdomen; eliminates Dampness.

SP-9 **Location:** in the depression on the lower border of the medial condyle of the tibia.
Notes: *He*-sea point; moves Dampness.

SP-10 **Location:** 2 cun superior to the upper medial patellar border.
Notes: 'Sea of Blood'; nourishes and cools the Blood (*Xue*), regulates *Qi* and Blood (*Xue*), clears Heat.

ST-40 **Location:** at the midpoint of the lower leg, 2 cun lateral to the anterior crest of the tibia.
Notes: *Luo*-connecting point (connects with the Spleen), therefore specifically for Dampness and Phlegm; combines well with SP-9.

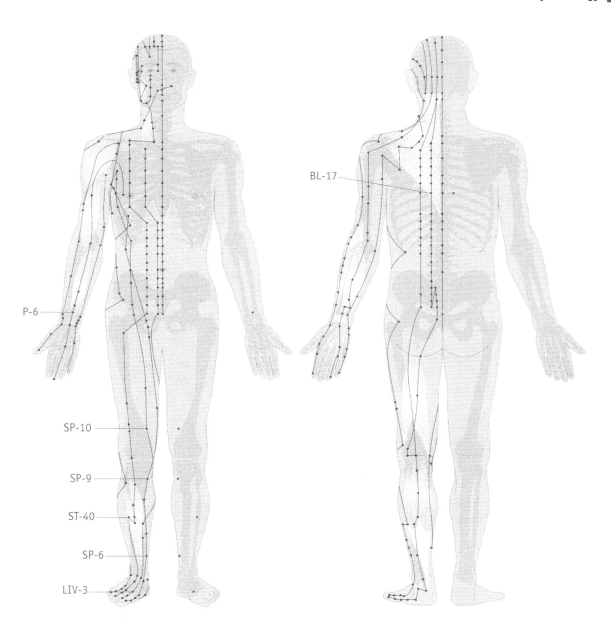

6.7.4 *Morning sickness*

■ Good results with acupuncture treatments!

Basic point combination

P-6, Du-20, daily treatments for up to 1 week; advise the patient to massage these points at home.

Individual point combination

Spleen and Stomach deficiency

Symptoms: tendency to oedema, craving for sweet foods, prone to worrying.
Tongue body: tooth marks, big, generally moist.
Pulse: slippery.
Points: ST-36, ST-44, SP-6, Ren-12.

Liver and Stomach disharmony

Symptoms: symptoms worse with stress, often acid reflux, irritability.
Tongue body: may have red edges.
Pulse: wiry.
Points: ST-36, LIV-3, Ren-12.

Counterflow *Qi* in the *Chong Mai*

No relief with acupuncture at the 'usual' Stomach and Spleen points. Severe nausea, often beyond the first trimester; cold sensations in the legs, heat sensation in the head.
Points: SP-4, ST-30.

Acupuncture points

Du-20 **Location:** on a line connecting the apices of the ears, 7 cun superior the posterior hairline.
Notes: meeting point with the Liver meridian and all *Yang* meridians; sedating.

LIV-3 **Location:** in the depression distal to the junction of the 1st and 2nd metatarsal bones.
Notes: *Yuan*-source and *Shu*-stream point; calms the Liver *Yang*, harmonizes the flow of Liver *Qi*, spasmolytic.

P-6 **Location:** 2 cun proximal to the midpoint of the palmar aspect of the wrist crease, between the tendons of the flexor carpi radialis and palmaris longus.
Notes: opening point of the *Yin Wei Mai*, master point for nausea; harmonizes the Stomach, regulates Heart *Qi* and Blood, calming; most important point for hyperemesis.

Ren-12 **Location:** midway between the umbilicus and the xiphoid process.
Notes: *Hui*-meeting point of the hollow organs (*Fu*), front-*Mu* point of the Stomach; tonifies the Stomach and Spleen, regulates Stomach *Qi*, eliminates Dampness.

SP-4 **Location:** in the depression at the junction of the base and shaft of the 1st metatarsal bone, at the junction of the red and white skin.
Notes: *Luo*-connecting point and opening point of the *Chong Mai*; tonifies the Spleen and calms the Stomach, combines well with P-6 (opening point of the *Yin Wei Mai*); needle SP-4 on one side and P-6 on the other.

SP-6 **Location:** 3 cun superior to the highest prominence of the medial malleolus, on the posterior border of the tibia.
Notes: as group *Luo*-connecting point, tonifies the Spleen, Liver and Kidneys; also tonifies Blood (*Xue*), *Qi* and *Yin*, nourishes and moves the Blood (*Xue*); distal point for promoting the Blood circulation in the lower abdomen; eliminates Dampness, promotes the smooth flow of Liver *Qi*.

ST-30 **Location:** 2 cun lateral to the anterior midline, on the upper border of the pubic symphysis; shallow insertion towards the pubic bone.
Notes: descends counterflow *Qi*.

ST-36 **Location:** 1 cun lateral to the anterior crest of the tibia, 1.5 cun inferior to the lower border of the head of the fibula (G.B.-34).
Notes: *He*-sea point, master point of hormones; tonifies the Stomach and Spleen, and therefore *Qi* and Blood (*Xue*), stabilizing and strengthening, psychologically harmonizing.

ST-44 **Location:** on the interdigital fold between the 2nd and 3rd toes.
Notes: descends counterflow Stomach *Qi*, clears Stomach Heat; for severe vomiting in addition to or instead of ST-36.

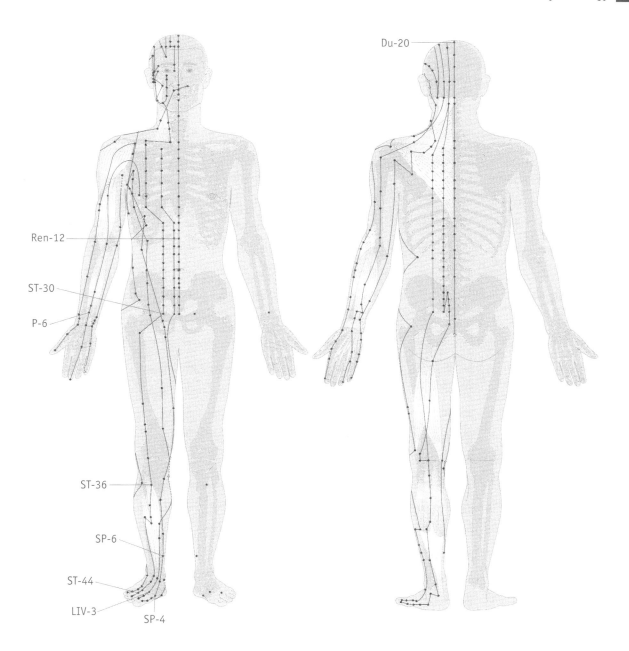

6.7.5 Preparation for labour

Acupuncture according to the 'Mannheim protocol' has decreased labour in primigravidas by an average of 2 hours due to a shortening of the first stage of labour, as demonstrated in a prospective randomized trial by Römer & Seybold (2003). After an average of 3–4 treatments, most women showed a softening and shortening of the cervix but without labour starting earlier. A further effect of acupuncture treatments is seen in the coordinated progression of contractions. Hypofrequent or hyperfrequent contractions, as well as cervical dystocia, occur more rarely.

> Pain relief during labour requires electroacupuncture at specific points (L.I.-4, L.I.-10).

Basic point combination

ST-36, SP-6, BL-67, G.B.-34.

- After the 36th week: G.B.-34, SP-6 and ST-36 weekly, in a sitting or side-lying position
- After the 38th week (3rd treatment): add BL-67, needle retention 20–25 minutes.

> If the term is overdue, continue with weekly treatments until labour begins.

Individual point combination

Oedema during pregnancy

ST-40, SP-9.
In cases of oedema, the intake of dairy products, sweets and greasy fried foods should be reduced.

Breech presentation

BL-67.
Only use moxa for turning a breech presentation if any severe pathology during late pregnancy has been excluded (under developed fetus, bleeding, premature labour, etc.).

> Ideally treatments should start during the 34th or 35th week. No more than four treatments at an interval of 2–3 days. Moxibustion is contraindicated after the 36th week. Moxibustion should be applied only by the practitioner (letting the patient take a moxa pole home is irresponsible).

The patient should be in a knee-elbow position (on a treatment couch, with the practitioner sitting behind the patient). Warm both points BL-67 for a total of 15–20 minutes.

Acupuncture points

BL-67 **Location:** on the little toe, at the lateral corner of the nail.
Notes: *Jing*-well point, tonification point, most tonifying point of the Water element; strengthens the uterus (uterus, Kidneys, Water) and is included for this indication after the 38th week; use bilateral moxibustion for breech presentation.

G.B.-34 **Location:** in a depression anterior and inferior to the head of the fibula.
Notes: *Hui*-meeting point of the muscles and tendons, *He*-sea point; regulates labour.

SP-6 **Location:** 3 cun superior to the highest prominence of the medial malleolus, on the posterior border of the tibia.
Notes: eliminates Dampness.

SP-9 **Location:** in the depression on the lower border of the medial condyle of the tibia.
Notes: *He*-sea point, moves Dampness.

ST-36 **Location:** 1 cun lateral to the anterior crest of the tibia, 1.5 cun inferior to the lower border of the head of the fibula (G.B.-34).
Notes: *He*-sea point; tonifies the Stomach and Spleen, 'Divine Serenity', combined with SP-6 has an effect on the cervix (connective tissue, Earth element).

ST-40 **Location:** at the midpoint of the lower leg, 2 cun lateral to the anterior crest of the tibia.
Notes: *Luo*-connecting point, specific action for Dampness and Phlegm, combines well with SP-9.

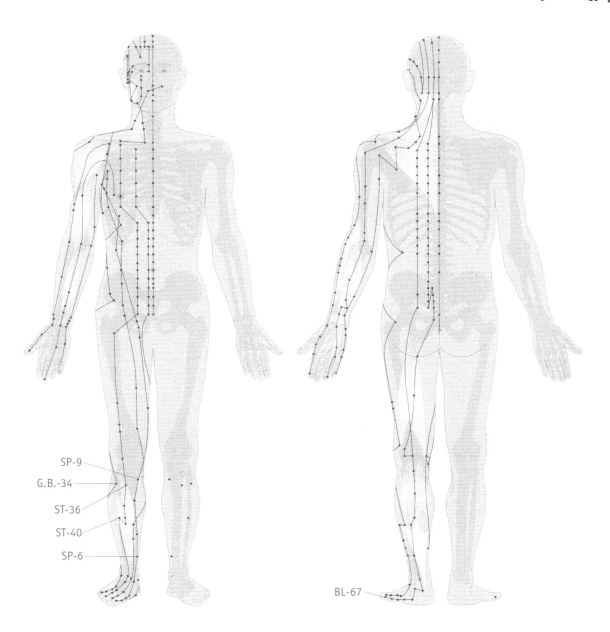

SP-9
G.B.-34
ST-36
ST-40
SP-6

BL-67

6.7.6 *Acupuncture during labour*

Acupuncture during labour can help to alleviate discomfort and pain, as well as making the birth process easier.

Individual point combination

Inducing labour

L.I.-4, BL-67, SP-6.

Regulate contractions

G.B.-34, LIV-3.

First stage of labour, cervical dystocia

ST-36, SP-6.

Second stage of labour

L.I.-4, BL-67.

Retained placenta

TCM: the mother is unable to deliver the placenta due to *Qi* deficiency. *Qi* can be activated by using the following points:
KID-16, SP-6, (G.B.-21).

Analgesia, pain relief during birth

Start treatment as early as possible (as soon as the contractions act on the cervix).

Unilateral acupuncture at L.I.-4 and L.I.-10, simultaneous stimulation of the points with electroacupuncture (20–30 Hz, 30–45 minutes). The intensity should be controlled by the patient. After a break of about 30–45 minutes, repeat electroacupuncture as above. The electrical stimulation triggers the release of β-endorphins, resulting in a higher pain threshold. Electroacupuncture is essential: manual stimulation of the points is not sufficient for the desired effect.

Acupuncture points

BL-67 **Location:** on the little toe, at the lateral corner of the nail.
Notes: *Jing*-well point, tonification point, strengthens the uterus.

G.B.-21 **Location:** on the highest point of the shoulder, midway between the acromion and the spinous process of C7.
Notes: descends the *Qi*; in theory a good point, but not recommended as too dangerous during birthing in hospital.

G.B.-34 **Location:** in a depression anterior and inferior to the head of the fibula.
Notes: *Hui*-meeting point of the muscles and tendons, *He*-sea point, regulates labour.

KID-16 **Location:** 0.5 cun lateral to the centre of the umbilicus (do not needle into the umbilicus, rather needle somewhat more laterally).
Notes: pertains to the Water element; meeting point with the *Chong Mai*, local point, single most important point.

L.I.-4 **Location:** on the highest point of the adductor pollicis.
Notes: *Yuan*-source point; moves the *Qi*, speeds up labour; important analgesic point.

L.I.-10 **Location:** 2 cun distal to L.I.-11, in the direction of L.I.-4.
Notes: tends to be very sensitive to pressure, combines well with L.I.-4 for electroacupuncture.

LIV-3 **Location:** in the depression distal to the junction of the 1st and 2nd metatarsal bones.
Notes: *Yuan*-source and *Shu*-stream point; regulates labour, harmonizes the Liver *Qi*.

SP-6 **Location:** 3 cun superior to the highest prominence of the medial malleolus, on the posterior border of the tibia.
Notes: general distal point for the lower abdomen; promotes blood circulation in the lower abdomen, moves the Blood (*Xue*) and *Qi*, has an effect on the cervix.

ST-36 **Location:** 1 cun lateral to the anterior crest of the tibia, 1.5 cun inferior to the lower border of the head of the fibula (G.B.-34).
Notes: *He*-sea point, master point of hormones and blood pressure; has an effect on the cervix.

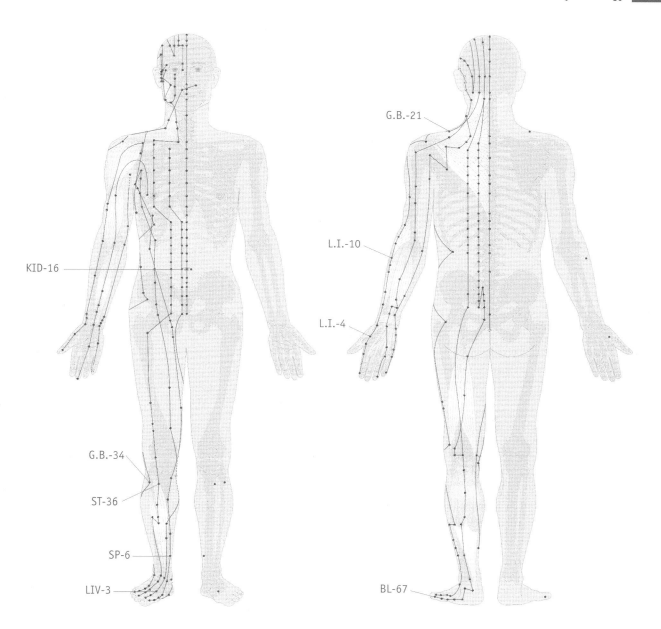

6.7.7 Difficult lactation

Basic point combination

ST-16, ST-18, Ren-17, Ex-preaxillary breast point.
Ear points: 22 endocrine system, 44 breasts.

Individual point combination

Insufficient lactation due to *Yin* deficiency, *Qi* and Blood (*Xue*) deficiency

ST-36, SP-6, S.I.-1, G.B.-41.

Insufficient lactation due to Liver *Qi* stagnation

Symptoms: depression, irritability, reduced appetite.
Tongue body: may be purple, red edges.
Tongue coating: thin, white.
Pulse: wiry.
Points: S.I.-1, P-6, LIV-3.
Commentary: the most important aspect of treatment is to build *Yin*. This can best be achieved by sufficient rest (not too many visitors!), sleep and nourishing food. Of course, there must be sufficient fluid intake (still water, teas that promote lactation).

Galactostasis, painful ejection of milk

L.I.-4, ST-36, LIV-3.
Commentary: results are often impressive! The milk often begins to flow upon needle insertion. Needle once daily.

Onset of mastitis

L.I.-4, L.I.-11, ST-44, Du-14.
Commentary: if started early enough, acupuncture can be very effective. Daily treatments are necessary. If symptoms worsen despite acupuncture, antibiotics have to be prescribed in order to prevent abscess formation. Acupuncture can always be used in addition to conventional treatment with antibiotics to speed up the healing process.

Acupuncture points

Du-14 **Location:** below the spinous process of C7.
Notes: meeting point of all *Yang* meridians; strengthens the immune system, drains heat; for fever, use sedating needling techniques.

Ex-preaxillary breast point **Location:** on a line connecting the end of the axillary fold and the nipple, at the border of the mamillary tissue.
Notes: regulates the mammary glands; local point.

G.B.-41 **Location:** between the 4th and 5th metatarsal bones, lateral to the tendon of the extensor digitorum longus.
Notes: opening point of the *Dai Mai*, *Shu*-stream point, distal point for the thorax; promotes lactation.

L.I.-4 **Location:** on the highest point of the adductor pollicis.
Notes: *Yuan*-source point; clears Heat together with L.I.-11 and Du-14.

L.I.-11 **Location:** with the arm in maximum flexion, at the radial end of the cubital crease.
Notes: *He*-sea point, tonification point; clears Damp-Heat and Wind, stimulates the immune system, sedating effect for fever.

LIV-3 **Location:** in the depression distal to the junction of the 1st and 2nd metatarsal bones.
Notes: *Yuan*-source and *Shu*-stream point; calms the Liver *Yang*, harmonizes the flow of Liver *Qi*, spasmolytic.

P-6 **Location:** 2 cun proximal to the midpoint of the palmar aspect of the wrist crease, between the tendons of the flexor carpi radialis and palmaris longus.
Notes: opening point of the *Yin Wei Mai*; distal point of the breasts (meridian pathway!).

Ren-17 **Location:** on the midline of the sternum, level with the 4th ICS, between the nipples.
Notes: front-*Mu* point of the Pericardium; unbinds the chest, promotes lactation.

S.I.-1 **Location:** on the little finger, next to the ulnar corner of the nail.
Notes: *Jing*-well point; promotes lactation, opens and invigorates the meridian.

SP-6 **Location:** 3 cun superior to the highest prominence of the medial malleolus, on the posterior border of the tibia.
Notes: group *Luo*-connecting point for the 3 *Yin* meridians of the leg; promotes the production of Blood (*Xue*).

ST-16 **Location:** on the midclavicular line, 3rd ICS, lateral to Ren-18.
Notes: regulates the *Qi* flow in the thorax 'as if a window is opened'.

ST-18 **Location:** in the 5th ICS, on the lower border of the breast, on the midclavicular line.
Notes: regulates the functions of the breasts.

ST-36 **Location:** 1 cun lateral to the anterior crest of the tibia, 1.5 cun inferior to the lower border of the head of the fibula (G.B.-34).
Notes: *He*-sea point, master point of hormones; tonifies the Stomach and Spleen, and therefore *Qi* and Blood (*Xue*); distal point for the breasts, stabilizing and strengthening.

ST-44 **Location:** on the interdigital fold between the 2nd and 3rd toes.
Notes: drains Heat from the Stomach meridian and the breasts.

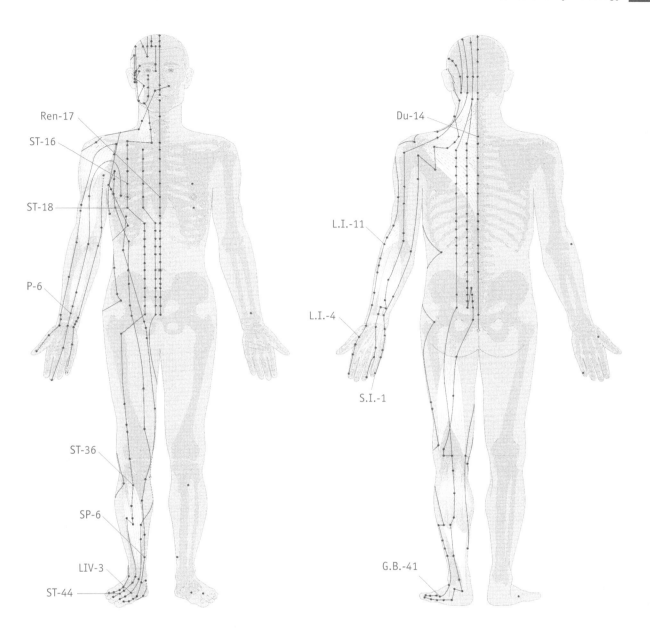

6.8 Nervous system and psychological disorders

A. Meng, G. Kubiena (6.8.1)

6.8.1 Headache and migraine

Headache and migraine respond very well to acupuncture. The point combinations described below are the quintessence of a study trip to the Beijing College for TCM in September 1994.

The classification of headache and the resulting therapy is carried out according to two criteria: location and pathogenesis.

Individual point combination

Therapy according to location of pain

Frontal – Yang Ming (L.I./ST)

L.I.-4, ST-8 [ST-1 Bi], ST-36, BL-2, G.B.-14.

Temporal – Shao Yang (T.B./G.B.)

T.B.-5, G.B.-8, (G.B.-41), Ex-HN-5 (*Tai Yang*).

Occipital – Tai Yang (S.I./BL)

S.I.-3, BL-10, BL-60, G.B.-20.

Vertex – Jue Yin (LIV/P)

LIV-3, KID-1, Du-20, Ex-HN-1 (*Si Shen Cong*).

Therapy according to pathogenesis

External factors – Wind and Cold

LU-7, L.I.-4, reducing method.

Rising Liver Yang

Tonify SP-6, reduce LIV-2.

Qi/Blood (Xue) deficiency

ST-36 and Ren-6, both tonifying methods.

Acupuncture points

BL-2 **Location:** at the junction of a vertical line through the medial end of the eyebrow/inner canthus and a horizontal line through the supraorbital foramen. **Notes:** local point.

BL-10 **Location:** at the insertion of the trapezius at the external occipital protuberance. **Notes:** eliminates Wind, locally unblocks the meridians, especially for headaches and occipital pain, benefits the brain and eyes; combined with G.B.-20 vagotonic – standard combination for the autonomic nervous system.

BL-60 **Location:** midway between the Achilles tendon and the highest prominence of the lateral malleolus. **Notes:** *Jing* river point, master point for pain along the meridian pathway; relaxes the tendons, invigorates the blood circulation.

Du-20 **Location:** on a line connecting the apices of the ears. **Notes:** meeting point of all divergent meridians, therefore effective for psychosomatic disorders, harmonizing.

Ex-HN-1 **Location:** 1 cun anterior, posterior and lateral to Du-20.

Ex-HN-5 **Location:** in the depression at the temple. **Notes:** eliminates Wind-Heat.

G.B.-8 **Location:** 1.5 cun superior to the apex of the ear. **Notes:** eliminates Wind and Heat; for headaches.

G.B.-14 **Location:** 1 cun superior to the midpoint of the eyebrow, on the pupil line. **Notes:** promotes the flow in the meridians, benefits the eyes.

G.B.-20 **Location:** posterior to the mastoid, between the trapezius and sternocleidomastoid, on the lower border of the occipital bone. **Notes:** dispels Wind from the head, subdues internal/external Wind and Liver Fire, tonifies the sympathetic nervous system – combine with BL-10 (basic combination for the autonomic nervous system), benefits the brain and eyes.

G.B.-41 **Location:** between the 4th and 5th metatarsal bones, lateral to the tendon of the extensor digitorum longus. **Notes:** opening point of the *Dai Mai*, *Shu*-stream point, distal point for the temples.

KID-1 **Location:** where the two pads of the toes meet, in the depression formed with plantar flexion. **Notes:** *Jing*-well point, shock point, sedation point; descends Liver Fire, calms the Spirit; for eye symptoms, photophobia.

L.I.-4 **Location:** on the highest point of the adductor pollicis. **Notes:** *Yuan*-source point, command point for the face, moves *Qi*, unblocks the meridians, especially with LIV-3 (4 gates); with LU-7, eliminates external pathogens.

LIV-2 **Location:** on the interdigital web between the 1st and 2nd toes, lateral to the metatarsophalangeal joint. **Notes:** *Ying*-spring point, sedation point; clears Liver Fire, calming.

LIV-3 **Location:** in the depression distal to the junction of the 1st and 2nd metatarsal bones. **Notes:** *Yuan*-source and *Shu*-stream point; calms the Liver Yang, harmonizes the flow of Liver *Qi*, spasmolytic.

LU-7 **Location:** 1.5 cun proximal to the wrist crease, at the radial artery. **Notes:** *Luo*-connecting point, opening point of the *Ren Mai*, command point for the head and throat, master point for stagnation; with L.I.-4, eliminates external pathogens.

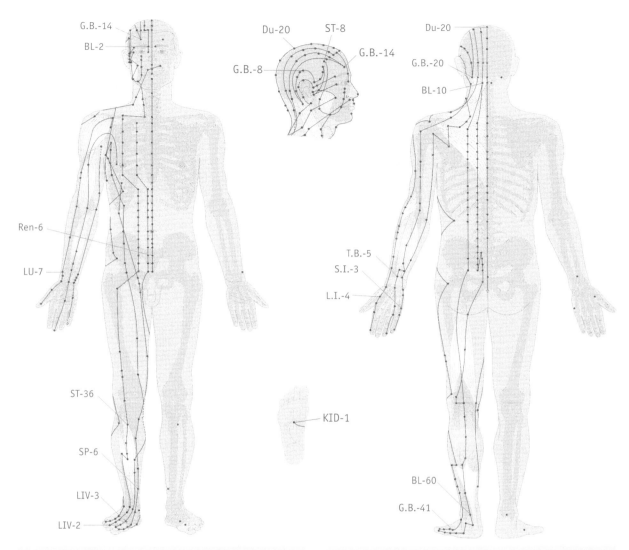

Ren-6 **Location:** 1.5 cun inferior to the umbilicus.
  Notes: 'Sea of *Qi*' – tonifies the Kidneys, original *Qi* and *Yang Qi*; pulls rising *Yang* downward.

S.I.-3 **Location:** when a fist is made, on the dorsum of the hand, in the depression at the end of the most distal palmar crease.
  Notes: opening point of the *Du Mai*, therefore able to eliminate external and internal Wind from the *Du Mai*; has an effect on the central nervous system; benefits the Spirit.

SP-6 **Location:** 3 cun superior to the highest prominence of the medial malleolus, on the posterior border of the tibia.
  Notes: as group *Luo*-connecting point, tonifies the Spleen, Kidneys and Liver; also tonifies the *Qi*, Blood (*Xue*) and *Yin*, nourishing, moves the Blood (*Xue*), eliminates Dampness.

ST-8 **Location:** at the corner of the forehead, 3 cun superior and 1 cun posterior to the frontozygomatic suture.
  Notes: alleviates headaches due to Wind-Heat (common cold) or digestive problems with dizziness (Dampness and Phlegm).

ST-36 **Location:** 1 cun lateral to the anterior crest of the tibia, 1.5 cun inferior to the lower border of the head of the fibula (G.B.-34).
  Notes: *He*-sea point, master point of hormones; tonifies the Stomach and Spleen, and therefore *Qi* and Blood (*Xue*), calming and tonifying.

T.B.-5 **Location:** 2 cun proximal to the midpoint of the dorsal wrist crease, opposite P-6.
  Notes: *Luo*-connecting point, opening point of the *Yang Wei Mai* – dominates the surface, eliminates external pathogens, especially Wind-Heat.

6.8.2 *Trigeminal neuralgia (1)*

Here the focus is on the idiopathic form of trigeminal neuralgia which tends to be the more common form in patients over 40 years of age.

TCM

Location of pain: this is considered the leading criterion.
Differentiation into four syndromes: Wind symptoms, excess of Liver *Yang*, Heat stagnation in the Stomach, Heat due to *Yin* deficiency.
Clinical application: the first treatments should take place at shorter intervals, daily or 2–3 treatments per week. After 4–5 treatments, change to weekly treatments; 10–20 treatments represent a treatment course. Select 6–10 points per treatment.

The point prescription comprises the basic point combination and additional points. The needle should reach the deeper levels of the point; depending on the constitution and the current condition of the patient, tonifying needle techniques (mainly for the local points) or reducing techniques (usually for the distal points) should be applied. Threading (reaching several points with one insertion) can be helpful in reducing the number of needles used.

Western medication should be reduced slowly and only after discussion with the prescribing physician. In most cases, a reduction in pain intensity, frequency of attacks and reduction of medication to be taken 'as needed' can be observed. A repeated course of treatment is recommended after 6–12 months.

In cases where neurosurgical palliative treatment was unsuccessful, the response to acupuncture may also be less promising.

Basic point combination

L.I.-4, ST-25, ST-44, T.B.-17, G.B.-20.

Individual point combination

Differentiation according to location of pain

First branch

BL-2, G.B.-14, Ex-HN-4 (*Yu Yao*), Ex-HN-5 (*Tai Yang*), local pressure-sensitive points.

Second branch

ST-2 [ST-5 Bi], ST-3 [ST-6 Bi], L.I.-20, ST-7 [ST-2 Bi], S.I.-18, local pain point.

Third branch

ST-4 [ST-7 Bi], ST-6 [ST-3 Bi], ST-7 [ST-2 Bi], Ren-24, local pain point.

Acupuncture points

BL-2 **Location:** at the junction of the medial end of the eyebrow and a vertical line through the inner canthus and supraorbital foramen.

Ex-HN-4 **Location:** in the centre of the eyebrow.

Ex-HN-5 **Location:** in the depression at the temple.
Notes: eliminates Wind-Heat.

G.B.-14 **Location:** 1 cun superior to the midpoint of the eyebrow, on the pupil line.
Notes: promotes the flow in the meridians, benefits the eyes.

G.B.-20 **Location:** posterior to the mastoid, between the trapezius and sternocleidomastoid, on the lower border of the occipital bone.
Notes: dispels Wind from the head, subdues internal/external Wind and Liver Fire; with BL-10 tonifies the sympathetic nervous system ('vegetative foundation'), benefits the brain and eyes, most important point for Wind disorders affecting the head.

L.I.-4 **Location:** on the dorsum of the hand, on the highest point of the muscle bulge between the 1st and 2nd metacarpal bones.
Notes: *Yuan*-source point, command point for the face, moves *Qi*, unblocks the meridians, especially with LIV-3 (4 gates); with LU-7, eliminates external pathogens.

L.I.-20 **Location:** in the nasiolabial groove, at the level of the midpoint of the lateral border of the ala nasi.

Ren-24 **Location:** in the centre of the mentolabial groove.
Notes: local point.

S.I.-18 **Location:** on the anterior border of the insertion of the masseter on the maxilla. Ask the patient to clench their teeth and/or open the mouth
Notes: master point for trismus; alleviates pain.

ST-2 **Location:** on the pupil line, in the depression at the infraorbital foramen.

ST-3 **Location:** at the junction of the pupil line with a horizontal line through the lower border of the ala nasi.

ST-4 **Location:** 1 cun lateral to the corner of the mouth; needle towards the mandibular angle.

ST-6 **Location:** 1 cun anterior and superior to the mandibular angle.

ST-7 **Location:** below the midpoint of the zygomatic arch.

ST-25 **Location:** 2 cun lateral to the anterior midline, lateral to Ren-8 and the umbilicus.
Notes: front-*Mu* point of the Large Intestine; regulates *Qi*, clears Heat.

ST-44 **Location:** on the interdigital fold between the 2nd and 3rd toes.
Notes: *Ying*-spring point; clears Wind-Heat from the face.

T.B.-17 **Location:** on the anterior border of the mastoid.
Notes: eliminates obstruction due to Wind.

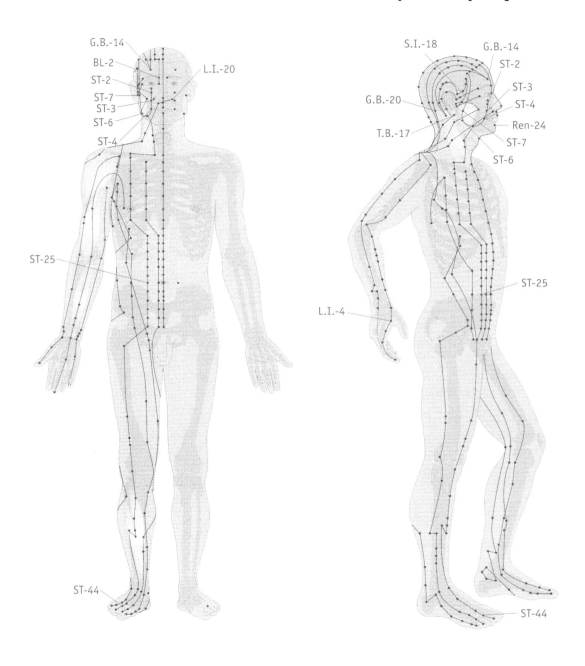

6.8.2 *Trigeminal neuralgia (2)*

Differentiation according to cause

Wind symptoms

T.B.-5, G.B.-2.
Sudden onset, generally unilateral, pulsating, like pin-pricks, possibly muscle twitching.
Tongue coating: thin, whitish.
Pulse: wiry-tight (*Xuan Jin*).

Excess of Liver Yang

LIV-3, G.B.-43.
Headaches, vertigo, bitter taste in the mouth, red eyes. Clear relationship between pain attacks and inner restlessness.
Tongue body: red.
Tongue coating: yellow.
Pulse: wiry and rapid (*Xuan Shu*).

Heat stagnation in the Stomach

L.I.-2, ST-41, ST-44.
Head and tooth aches, pain around the eyebrows; foul breath.
Tongue body: red.
Tongue coating: yellow.
Pulse: rapid and forceful.

Yin deficiency Heat

KID-3, Ren-4.
Tightness in the chest, frequent belching, reduced appetite.
Pulse: wiry – indicates Liver *Qi* stagnation (*Gan Qi Yu Jie*).

Acupuncture points

G.B.-2 **Location:** with the mouth open, in the depression anterior to the intertragic notch, posterior to the ascending ramus of the mandible.

G.B.-20 **Location:** posterior to the mastoid, between the trapezius and sternocleidomastoid, on the lower border of the occipital bone.
Notes: dispels Wind from the head, subdues internal/external Wind and Liver Fire, tonifies the sympathetic nervous system – combined with BL-10, standard combination for the autonomic nervous system, benefits the brain and eyes; most important point for wind disorders affecting the head.

G.B.-43 **Location:** on the web between the 4th and 5th toes, closer to the metatarsophalangeal joint of the 4th toe.
Notes: *Ying*-spring point, tonification point, subdues Liver *Yang*.

KID-3 **Location:** midway between the highest prominence of the medial malleolus and the Achilles tendon.
Notes: *Yuan*-source and *Shu*-stream point; with BL-23, tonifies the Kidney *Yin*.

L.I.-2 **Location:** with the hand in a fist that curls around the thumb, in the depression distal to the metacarpophalangeal joint, at the junction of the red and white skin.
Notes: eliminates Heat from the Large Intestine.

LIV-3 **Location:** in the depression distal to the junction of the 1st and 2nd metatarsal bones.
Notes: *Yuan*-source and *Shu*-stream point; calms the Liver *Yang*, harmonizes the flow of Liver *Qi*, spasmolytic.

Ren-4 **Location:** 2 cun superior to the upper border of the pubic symphysis.
Notes: meeting point of the 3 lower Yin meridians (SP, KID, LIV), front-*Mu* point of the Small Intestine; tonifying – strengthens the Essence (*Jing*), *Qi*, *Yang*, Blood and *Yin*; roots the *Hun* (ethereal soul).

ST-41 **Location:** on the ankle, between the tendons of the extensor hallucis longus and the extensor digitorum longus.
Notes: clears Stomach Heat.

T.B.-5 **Location:** 2 cun proximal to the midpoint of the dorsal wrist crease, opposite P-6.
Notes: *Luo*-connecting point, opening point of the *Yang Wei Mai* – dominates the surface, eliminates external pathogens, especially Wind-Heat; master point of the small joints.

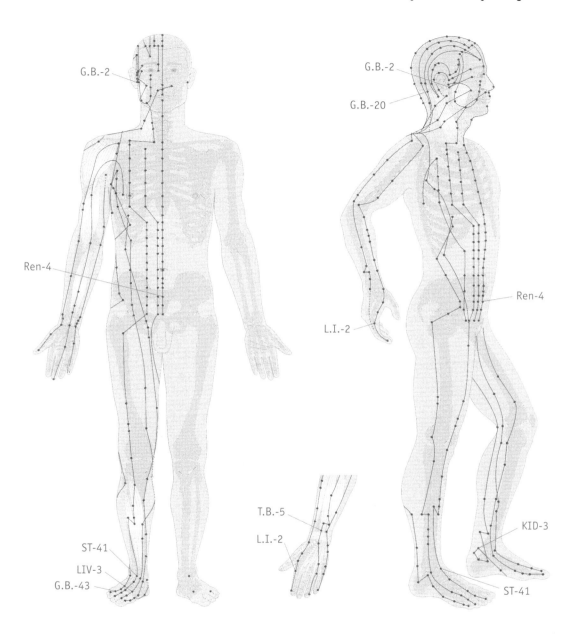

6.8.3 Intercostal neuralgia

TCM refers to this disorder as hypochondriac pain that is caused by *Qi* stagnation or by *Qi* and Blood (*Xue*) stagnation.

Basic point combination

G.B.-40, LIV-3, LIV-14, BL-18; Ex-B-2. Select appropriate points on the *Hua Tuo* line; ear acupuncture: 39 thoracic spine, 42 thorax, 26a thalamus.

Individual point combination

Excess type

Severe pain, worse with pressure.
Basic point combination: LIV-14, T.B.-6, G.B.-34.
Qi **stagnation:** distending pain that changes location, severity dependent on the emotional state, frequent sighing.
LIV-3, G.B.-40.
Blood (*Xue*) stagnation: severe, stabbing, fixed pain.
BL-17, BL-18.

Deficiency type

Dull chronic pain. **TCM:** poor diet and stagnation in the collaterals of the Liver as well as internal Heat caused by chronic stagnation.
Blood (*Xue*) deficiency: dizziness, blurred vision, thready, choppy pulse.
Yin **deficiency:** dry mouth, restlessness, hardly any tongue coating, thready and rapid pulse.
LIV-14, BL-18, BL-23, ST-36, SP-6, LIV-3.

Acupuncture points

BL-17 **Location:** 1.5 cun lateral to the spinous process of T7.
  Notes: as *Hui*-meeting point of the Blood (*Xue*), tonifies and regulates the blood; as back-*Shu* point of the diaphragm, removes diaphragmatic constriction.

BL-18 **Location:** 2 cun lateral to the spinous process of T9.
  Notes: back-*Shu* point of the Liver; moves *Qi*, together with BL-17 also moves Blood (*Xue*) for excess patterns; with BL-23, LIV-14 and LIV-3, tonifies the Blood (*Xue*) and Essence (*Jing*) for deficiency patterns; regulates the Liver, alleviates pain.

BL-23 **Location:** 1.5 cun lateral to the lower border of the spinous process of L2.
  Notes: back-*Shu* point of the Kidneys; strengthens the lumbar region, tonifies the Kidney *Yin* and *Yang*, has an effect on the hormones, strengthening for chronic disorders, corticotrophic; moxa may be beneficial.

Ex-B-2 **Location:** paravertebral points after *Hua Tuo* (*Hua Tuo* points).
  Notes: have an effect on the segments.

G.B.-34 **Location:** in a depression anterior and inferior to the head of the fibula.
  Notes: *He*-sea point; special point for hypochondriac pain; regulates the flow of Gall Bladder *Qi*.

G.B.-40 **Location:** in the depression anterior and inferior to the lateral malleolus.
  Notes: *Yuan*-source point, special point for hypochondriac pain; regulates the flow of Gall Bladder *Qi*.

LIV-3 **Location:** in the depression distal to the junction of the 1st and 2nd metatarsal bones.
  Notes: *Yuan*-source and *Shu*-stream point; calms the Liver *Yang*, harmonizes the flow of Liver *Qi*, spasmolytic.

LIV-14 **Location:** on the midclavicular line, in the 6th ICS, directly below the nipple.
  Notes: front-*Mu* point of the Liver; promotes the smooth flow of Liver *Qi*, alleviates hypochondriacal pain.

SP-6 **Location:** 3 cun superior to the highest prominence of the medial malleolus, on the posterior border of the tibia.
  Notes: as group *Luo*-connecting point, tonifies the Spleen, Kidneys and Liver; also tonifies the *Qi*, Blood (*Xue*) and *Yin*.

ST-36 **Location:** 1 cun lateral to the anterior crest of the tibia, 1.5 cun inferior to the lower border of the head of the fibula (G.B.-34).
  Notes: *He*-sea point, master point of hormones, hypertension; harmonizes the flow of *Qi* and Blood (*Xue*), especially when combined with BL-20, LIV-3, and SP-4 or SP-6, tonifies the Stomach and Spleen, stabilizing, strengthening, psychologically harmonizing.

T.B.-6 **Location:** 3 cun proximal to the midpoint of the dorsal wrist crease.
  Notes: invigorates the collaterals, disperses Blood stagnation, regulates the thorax; with G.B.-34 for hypochondriacal pain.

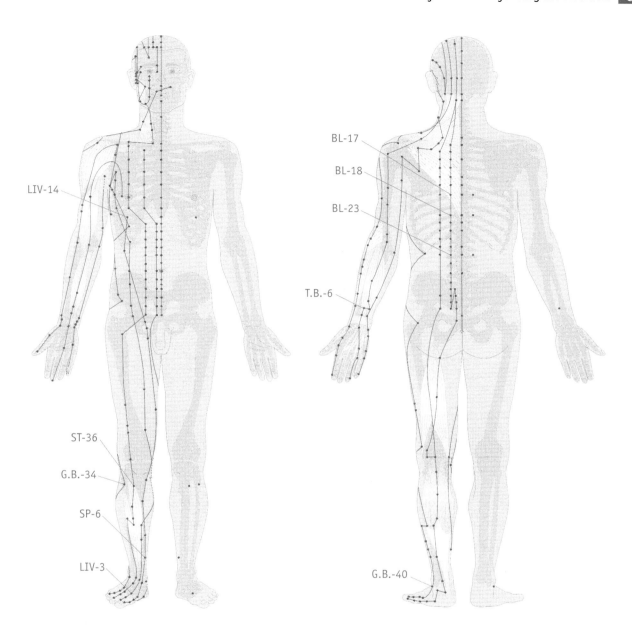

LIV-14

BL-17
BL-18
BL-23

T.B.-6

ST-36
G.B.-34
SP-6
LIV-3

G.B.-40

6.8.4 Facial paresis (1)

TCM does not distinguish between peripheral and central facial paralysis, but describes various disorders that roughly match the Western differentiation. TCM postulates a deficiency of the body's defence system (*Zheng Qi*), so that external pathogenic factors (such as draught) can disturb the circulation in the meridians of the face. This results in poor nourishment of the facial musculature, triggering the typical symptoms of facial paralysis. This form represents the idiopathic or inflammatory peripheral facial paralysis.

Internal Wind can also cause facial paralysis, corresponding more closely to central facial paralysis.

Basic point combination

L.I.-4, ST-7 [ST-2 Bi] or T.B.-5, T.B.-17 or G.B.-20, sedating method.

Individual point combination

Idiopathic or inflammatory peripheral facial paralysis

Absence of any other neurological symptoms.
TCM: external Wind leads to a sudden, unilateral facial paralysis, possibly with localized redness and swelling.
Tongue body: red; **tongue coating:** thin, white; **pulse:** superficial and rapid (*Fu Shu*) or superficial and tight (*Fu Jin*).

Point selection according to location

VIII/1: BL-2, T.B.-23, G.B.-14, G.B.-8 or Ex-HN 5 (*Tai Yang*).
VIII/2: ST-1 [ST-4 Bi] or ST-2 [ST-5 Bi], S.I.-18, BL-20.
VIII/3: ST-4 [ST-7 Bi], ST-6 [ST-3 Bi].

Accompanied by chills and fever

Du-14 [Du-13 Bi].

Accompanied by strong tearing

BL-2, Ex-HN-4 (*Yu Yao*).
Technique: gentle (tonifying) manipulation for local points, strong (sedating) manipulation for distal points.

For peripheral facial paralysis, electroacupuncture is recommended once the acute stage has subsided. Electroacupuncture should be applied for 10–15 minutes, either continuous or dense-disperse setting. There should be no pain, but slight muscle twitching may be visible. Select 1–3 point pairs per treatment.

Local points are needled only on the affected side, distal points bilaterally.

It is also possible to use transcutaneous electrical nerve stimulation (TENS) at the above points. Initially perform daily treatments; after 4–5 treatments switch to twice-weekly and then once-weekly treatments. Electrostimulation should not be too strong or too long, because it can trigger a facial spasm.

Acupuncture points

BL-2 **Location:** at the junction of the medial end of the eyebrow and a vertical line through the inner canthus and the supraorbital foramen.

BL-20 **Location:** 1.5 cun lateral to the lower border of the spinous process of T11.
Notes: back-*Shu* point of the Spleen; tonifies the Spleen and Stomach, and therefore the production of *Qi* and Blood (*Xue*).

Du-14 **Location:** below the spinous process of C7.
Notes: meeting point of all *Yang* meridians; disperses Wind, Cold, Heat or tonifies – depending on the method of stimulation.

Ex-HN-4 **Location:** in the centre of the eyebrow.

Ex-HN-5 **Location:** in the depression at the temple.

Ex-UE-11 **Location:** at the tips of the 10 fingers, approximately 0.1 cun from the fingernail.
Notes: disperse Wind-Heat.

G.B.-8 **Location:** 1.5 cun superior to the apex of the ear.
Notes: eliminates Wind-Heat and meridian obstructions.

G.B.-14 **Location:** 1 cun superior to the midpoint of the eyebrow, on the pupil line.
Notes: promotes the flow in the meridians, benefits the eyes.

G.B.-20 **Location:** posterior to the mastoid, between the trapezius and sternocleidomastoid, on the lower border of the occipital bone.
Notes: dispels Wind from the head, subdues internal/external Wind and Liver Fire, tonifies the sympathetic nervous system – combined with BL-10 standard combination for the autonomic nervous system, benefits the brain and eyes.

L.I.-4 **Location:** on the dorsum of the hand, on the highest point of the muscle bulge between the 1st and 2nd metacarpal bones.
Notes: *Yuan*-source point, command point for the face; moves *Qi*, unblocks the meridians, especially with LIV-3 (4 gates); with LU-7 eliminates external pathogens.

S.I.-18 **Location:** on the anterior border of the insertion of the masseter on the maxilla. Ask the patient to clench their teeth and/or open the mouth.
Notes: a secondary vessel connects S.I.-18 with BL-1; meeting point with the Gall Bladder meridian, master point for trismus.

ST-1 **Location:** on the pupil line, on the lower border of the orbit.

ST-4 **Location:** 1 cun lateral to the corner of the mouth. Needle towards the mandibular angle.

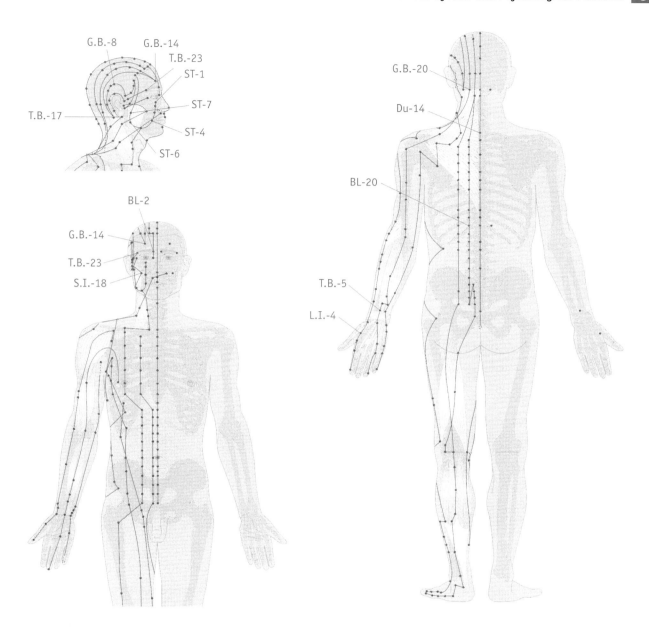

ST-6 **Location:** 1 cun anterior and superior to the mandibular angle.

ST-7 **Location:** inferior to the midpoint of the zygomatic arch.

T.B.-5 **Location:** 2 cun proximal to the midpoint of the dorsal wrist crease, opposite P-6.
Notes: *Luo*-connecting point, opening point of the *Yang Wei Mai* – dominates the surface, eliminates external pathogens, especially Wind-Heat; master point of the small joints.

T.B.-17 **Location:** on the anterior border of the mastoid.
Notes: eliminates Wind and obstruction form the meridians and collaterals.

T.B.-23 **Location:** in a depression at the lateral end of the eyebrow.
Notes: meeting point with the Gall Bladder meridian; dispels Wind, benefits the eyes, supports the ears.

6.8.4 Facial paresis (2)

Facial paralysis accompanied by further neurological symptoms

TCM: internal Wind due to Liver and Kidney deficiency.

May also have sudden onset as unilateral facial paralysis, but may be accompanied by vertigo, tinnitus, unilateral symptoms such as hemihypo-aesthesia, disturbed sense of taste, deviated tongue; **tongue body:** dark red; **tongue coating:** whitish; pulse: wiry (*Xuan*). This picture corresponds to the prodromal stage of a cerebral insult, so Western investigation is absolutely essential.

Tinnitus

S.I.-19, T.B.-3, T.B.-17, T.B.-21.

Disturbed sense of taste

Ren-24.

Points addressing the eye

L.I.-4, BL-2 (affected side only) and Ex-HN-5 (*Tai Yang*).

Points addressing the mouth and eye

ST-6 [ST-3 Bi] (affected side only), Du-26.

Facial tic

S.I.-18, Ex-HN-5 (*Tai Yang*)
Technique: needle local points ipsilaterally and gently, distal points bilaterally and with stronger stimulation. In cases of central paralysis (also facial paralysis), electroacupuncture is not recommended, as it could exacerbate the rigor.

Acupuncture points

BL-2 **Location:** at the junction of the medial end of the eyebrow and a vertical line through the inner canthus and the supraorbital foramen.

Du-26 **Location:** at the junction of the upper and middle third of the philtrum.
Notes: local point for the upper lip.

Ex-HN-5 **Location:** in the depression at the temple.

L.I.-4 **Location:** on the dorsum of the hand, on the highest point of the muscle bulge between the 1st and 2nd metacarpal bones.
Notes: *Yuan*-source point, command point for the face, moves *Qi*, unblocks the meridians, especially with LIV-3 (4 gates); with LU-7 eliminates external pathogens.

Ren-24 **Location:** in the centre of the mentolabial groove.
Notes: local point.

S.I.-18 **Location:** on the anterior border of the insertion of the masseter on the maxilla. Ask the patient to clench their teeth and/or open the mouth.
Notes: a secondary branch connects S.I.-18 with BL-1; meeting point with the Gall Bladder meridian, master point for trismus.

S.I.-19 **Location:** with the mouth open, in the depression between the tragus and mandibular angle.
Notes: local point, located close to where the facial nerve emerges.

ST-6 **Location:** 1 cun anterior and superior to the mandibular angle.

T.B.-3 **Location:** on the dorsum of the hand, between the 4th and 5th metacarpal bones, with the hand in a loose fist in the depression proximal to the metacarpophalangeal joints.
Notes: *Shu*-stream point; eliminates *Qi* stagnation, Wind and Heat, especially for disorders affecting the eyes and ears.

T.B.-17 **Location:** on the anterior border of the mastoid.
Notes: eliminates Wind and obstruction form the meridians and collaterals, benefits the ears.

T.B.-20 **Location:** directly above the apex of the ear, on the hairline.
Notes: local point; a collateral descends from here to the cheek.

T.B.-21 **Location:** at the level of the supratragic notch, with the mouth open in the depression superior to the condyloid process of the mandible.
Notes: local point; from here a branch a branch descends to the cheek.

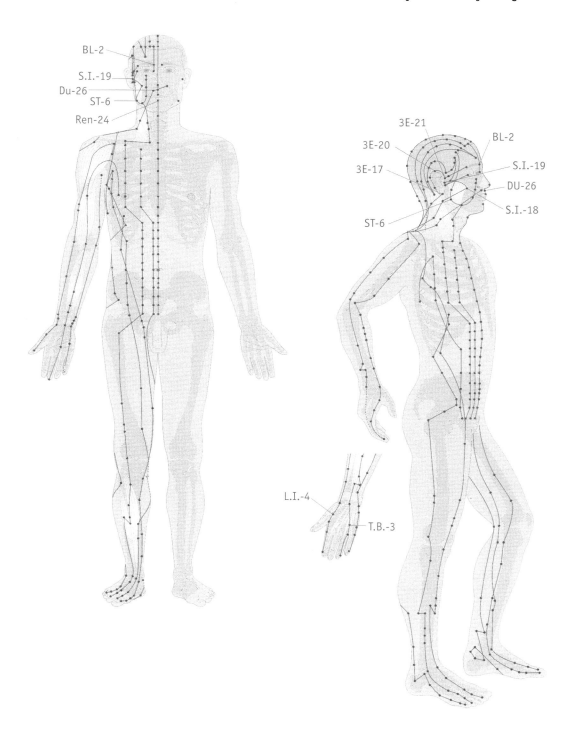

BL-2
S.I.-19
Du-26
ST-6
Ren-24

3E-21
3E-20
3E-17
ST-6
BL-2
S.I.-19
DU-26
S.I.-18

L.I.-4
T.B.-3

6.8.5 Cerebral insult, hemiparesis, post-acute therapy (1)

In China, acupuncture treatments are started during the acute stage of a cerebral insult.

> In contrast, in the West, acupuncture is considered an adjunctive therapy, administered only once the clinical picture has become stable (approximately 1 week after the stroke).

TCM

Certain triggers will lead to a stroke: overwhelming emotions, irregular daily schedule and other factors that disturb the harmony of *Yin* and *Yang* within the body. The result is a disturbed circulation of the vital energy *Qi* and Blood (*Xue*) in the meridians (which roughly correspond to the vascular system). Any obstruction, stagnation or stasis can then trigger the symptoms of a stroke.

Other aetiological factors include: poor diet and exhaustion, which compromise metabolic processes in the body. As a result the composition of the Body Fluids changes and a meridian ('vessel') can suddenly become blocked.

TCM: sudden 'Wind' stirs up 'Phlegm', which then blocks the meridians (paresis).

Transient ischaemic attack (TIA) stage

Fleeting, non-psychiatric symptoms; **TCM:** slight disturbance at the *Luo* collateral level.

Basic point combination

L.I.-11, L.I.-15, ST-36, G.B.-34, Du-20, Du-23, Ex-HN-3 (*Yin Tang*).

Individual point combination

Vertigo

ST-8 [ST-1 Bi], G.B.-20.

Disturbed sleep

HE-7 and Ex-HN-1 (*Si Shen Cong*).

Inner restlessness

L.I.-4 and LIV-3.

Cerebral infarction

TCM

Disturbance at the meridian (*Jing*) level.

Basic point combination

L.I.-11, ST-44, P-6, LIV-3, Du-26, Ren-6 (Ren-8 **M**).

Cerebral haemorrhage

P-6, Du-20, bloodletting at the fingertips (Ex-UE-11, *Shi Xuan*); Du-16.

Subarachnoid haemorrhage, massive cerebral haemorrhage, increased intracranial pressure, meningoencephalitis; **TCM:** at the level of the *Zang Fu* organs.

Select only emergency points: In China, acupuncture is also used as an adjunctive therapy for unconsciousness, dyspnoea, spasms of the extremities, constipation, high temperature, severe headaches, etc.

If the patient is comatose with anisocoria or wide pupil sizes, as well as pale, cyanotic, mucous membranes, urinary and faecal incontinence, shallow breathing and cold sweat, acupuncture is also used as a supportive measure in China.

Commonly used points include ST-11, ST-44, P-6, LIV-3, Du-26, Ren-4, Ren-6, Ren 8 **M**.

> In the West, acupuncture is to be used in this situation only if indications are absolutely clear and unequivocal.

TCM: differentiation according to affected level and severity

Location according to TCM	Clinical symptoms	Differential diagnosis according to Western medicine
Luo level (secondary vessels)	Hemihypo-aesthesia, vertigo, tinnitus	Increased blood viscosity, vascular sclerosis (TIA, prodromal stage)
Jing level (meridians)	Hemiparesis, hemihypo-aesthesia, aphasia	Blocked blood vessel, embolism
Fu level (*Yang* organs)	Loss of consciousness coupled with paresis, constipation, retention of urine	Blocked blood vessel, cerebral haemorrhage
Zang level (*Yin* organs)	Soporose, comatose, headaches, occipital stiffness, high temperature, Damp rattling breathing sounds, drooling	Increased intracranial pressure

Acupuncture points

Du-16   **Location:** 1 cun superior to the occipital hairline, in the depression inferior to the external occipital protuberance.
Notes: for disorders affecting the head and sensory organs; eliminates pathogenic Wind from the head.

Du-20   **Location:** on a line connecting the apices of the ears, 7 cun superior the posterior hairline.
Notes: meeting point of all divergent meridians, therefore effective for psychosomatic disorders, harmonizing; has an effect on the precentral gyrus and the motor zone; raises the *Qi*.

Du-23   **Location:** 1 cun within the anterior hairline.
Notes: disperses Wind.

Du-26   **Location:** at the junction of the upper and middle third of the philtrum.
Notes: restores consciousness and *Yang*, calms the Spirit.

Ex-HN-1   **Location:** 1 cun anterior, posterior and lateral to Du-20.

Ex-HN-3   **Location:** midway between the eyebrows.

G.B.-20   **Location:** posterior to the mastoid, between the trapezius and sternocleidomastoid, on the lower border of the occipital bone.
Notes: dispels Wind from the head, subdues internal/external Wind and Liver Fire, tonifies the sympathetic nervous system – combined with BL-10, standard combination for the autonomic nervous system, benefits the brain and eyes.

G.B.-34   **Location:** in a depression anterior and inferior to the head of the fibula.
Notes: *He*-sea point and *Hui*-meeting point of the tendons; subdues rebellious *Qi*; promotes the smooth flow of Liver *Qi*.

HE-7   **Location:** at the ulnar aspect of the wrist crease, on the radial side of the pisiform bone.
Notes: *Yuan*-source point, *Shu*-stream point, sedation point; calms the Spirit, pacifies the Heart.

L.I.-4   **Location:** on the dorsum of the hand, on the highest point of the muscle bulge between the 1st and 2nd metacarpal bones.
Notes: moves *Qi*, especially with LIV-3 (4 gates).

L.I.-11   **Location:** with the arm fully flexed, at the radial end of the cubital crease.
Notes: *He*-sea point, tonification point; eliminates Damp-Heat and Wind, benefits the tendons and joints.

L.I.-15   **Location:** with the arm abducted, in the anterior of the two depressions inferior to the acromioclavicular joint, between the anterior and medial third of the deltoid.
Notes: master point for pareses affecting the upper extremities.

LIV-3   **Location:** in the depression distal to the junction of the 1st and 2nd metatarsal bones.
Notes: *Yuan*-source and *Shu*-stream point; calms the Liver *Yang*, harmonizes the flow of Liver *Qi*, spasmolytic.

P-6   **Location:** 2 cun proximal to the midpoint of the palmar aspect of the wrist crease, between the tendons of the flexor carpi radialis and palmaris longus.
Notes: opening point of the *Yin Wei Mai*; master point for nausea; regulates the Triple Burner, the *Jue Yin*, Heart *Qi* and Blood (*Xue*), unbinds the chest, harmonizes the Stomach, calms the Spirit.

Ren-4   **Location:** 2 cun superior to the upper border of the pubic symphysis.
Notes: meeting point of the 3 lower Yin meridians (SP, KID, LIV), front-*Mu* point of the Small Intestine; tonifying – strengthens the Essence (*Jing*), *Qi*, *Yang*, Blood (*Xue*) and *Yin*; roots the ethereal soul (*Hun*).

Ren-6   **Location:** 1.5 cun inferior to the umbilicus.
Notes: 'Sea of *Qi*' – tonifies the Kidneys, original *Qi* and *Yang Qi*; pulls rising *Yang* downward; use moxa for cold sweat.

Ren-8   **Location:** in the centre of the umbilicus.

ST-8   **Location:** at the corner of the forehead, 3 cun superior and 1 cun posterior to the frontozygomatic suture.
Notes: alleviates headaches due to Wind-Heat (common cold) or digestive problems with dizziness (Dampness and Phlegm).

ST-11   **Location:** on the upper border of the clavicle, at the junction of the shaft and the head, between the clavicular and sternal insertions of the sternocleidomastoid.

ST-36   **Location:** 1 cun lateral to the anterior crest of the tibia, 1.5 cun inferior to the lower border of the head of the fibula (G.B.-34).
Notes: *He*-sea point, master point of hormones; tonifies the Stomach and Spleen, and therefore *Qi* and Blood (*Xue*), calming and tonifying.

ST-44   **Location:** on the interdigital fold between the 2nd and 3rd toes.
Notes: descends counterflow Stomach *Qi*, eliminates Stomach Heat.

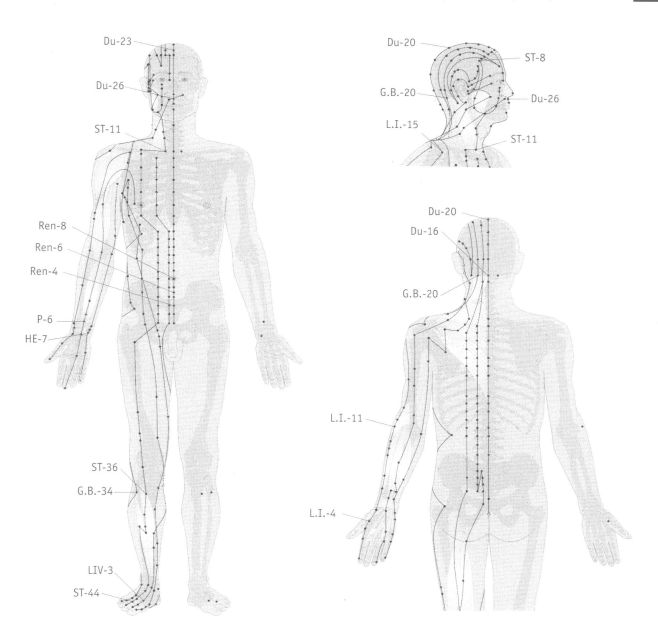

6.8.5 Cerebral insult, hemiparesis, rehabilitation following insult (2)

After approximately 3 months, all patients with hemiparesis can be rehabilitated, following a standard protocol. Point selection is based on the location of the symptoms.

Individual point combination

Aphasia

HE-5, BL-10, G.B.-20, Du-23 needled towards Du-20.

Hemianopsia

BL-10, G.B.-20.

Pseudobulbar symptoms

P-6, G.B.-20, Du-26, Ren-23.

Hemiparesis of the upper extremity

LU-5, L.I.-4, L.I.-11, L.I.-15, HE-1, P-3, P-7, T.B.-5, G.B.-20, Ex-UE-9 (*Ba xie*).

Acupuncture points

BL-10 **Location:** at the insertion of the trapezius at the external occipital protuberance.
Notes: eliminates Wind, locally unblocks the meridians, especially for headaches and occipital pain, benefits the brain and eyes; combined with G.B.-20 vagotonic – standard combination for the autonomic nervous system.

Du-23 **Location:** on the midline, 1 cun within the anterior hairline.
Notes: disperses Wind.

Du-26 **Location:** at the junction of the upper and middle third of the philtrum.
Notes: restores consciousness and *Yang*, calms the Spirit.

Ex-UE-9 **Location:** when a loose fist is made, 4 points on the dorsal aspect of each hand, on the interdigital webs between the heads of the 1st to 5th metacarpal bones.
Notes: relax the tendons, dispel Wind-Cold, invigorate the Blood (*Xue*).

G.B.-20 **Location:** posterior to the mastoid, between the trapezius and sternocleidomastoid, on the lower border of the occipital bone.
Notes: dispels Wind from the head, subdues internal/external Wind and Liver Fire, tonifies the sympathetic nervous system – combined with BL-10, standard combination for the autonomic nervous system, benefits the brain and eyes.

HE-1 **Location:** in the centre of the axilla, medial to the axillary artery.
Notes: special point for posterior apoplectic paresis of the upper extremity.

HE-5 **Location:** 1 cun proximal to HE-7.
Notes: *Luo*-connecting point; tonifies and regulates Heart *Qi*, distal point for the tongue (aphasia).

LU-5 **Location:** on the cubital crease, radial to the tendon of the biceps.
Notes: *He*-sea point, sedation point; distal point for the face; clears Lung-Heat and Phlegm.

P-3 **Location:** on the cubital crease, ulnar to the tendon of the biceps (LU-5 is located radial to the tendon).
Notes: *He*-sea point; has a local spasmolytic effect, activates the channel, calms the Spirit.

P-6 **Location:** 2 cun proximal to the midpoint of the palmar aspect of the wrist crease, between the tendons of the flexor carpi radialis and palmaris longus.
Notes: opening point of the *Yin Wei Mai*; master point for nausea; regulates the Triple Burner, the *Jue Yin*, Heart *Qi* and Blood (*Xue*), unbinds the chest, harmonizes the Stomach, calms the Spirit.

P-7 **Location:** on the anterior aspect of the wrist joint, between the tendons of the flexor carpi radialis and palmaris longus.
Notes: *Yuan*-source point, *Shu*-stream point, sedation point; calms the Heart and Spirit; local point for contractures.

Ren-23 **Location:** superior to the larynx, above the hyoid bone, at the junction of the neck and the chin.
Notes: extinguishes internal Wind, promotes speech due to its direct effect on the tongue (for aphasia), clears Heat, resolves Phlegm.

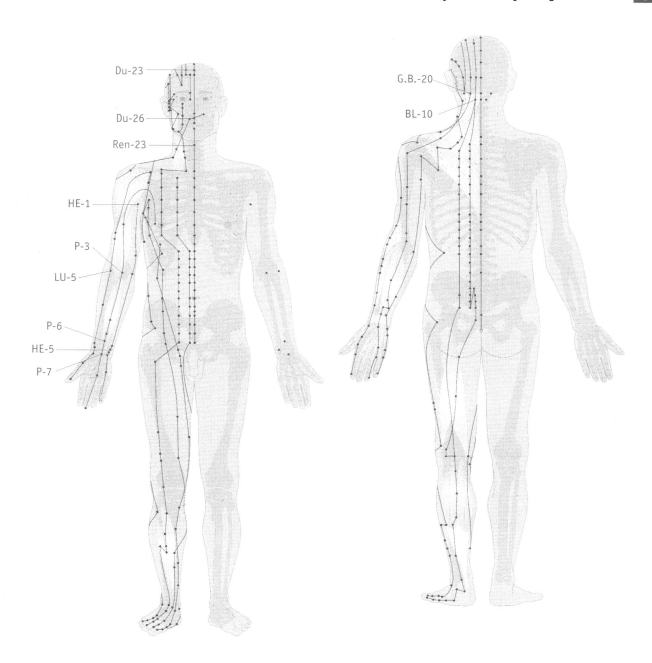

Du-23
Du-26
Ren-23
HE-1
P-3
LU-5
P-6
HE-5
P-7

G.B.-20
BL-10

6.8.5 *Cerebral insult, hemiparesis, rehabilitation following insult (3)*

Pain in the shoulder joint

Bloodletting at local pressure-sensitive points: L.I.-15, ST-38, S.I.-9, S.I.-14.

Hemiparesis of the lower extremity

SP-6, BL-40 [BL-54 Bi], BL-60, KID-3, G.B.-30, G.B.-34, Ex-LE-10.

Talipes equinus

ST-41, BL-60, KID-9, G.B.-40 needled towards KID-6.
Method: medium-strength stimulation, less strong for chronic cases. Initially treat ipsilaterally, later bilaterally.

Electrostimulation

L.I.-4, L.I.-11, L.I.-15, T.B.-5, G.B.-30, G.B.-31, G.B.-34, G.B.-39.

Select 2–3 point pairs per treatment, according to the location of the complaint (pain, paresis, swelling). When a needle sensation (*De Qi*) is obtained, commence electrostimulation; 15–30 minutes daily, with a break on Saturday/Sunday. Continue with all other therapies, medication, physiotherapy, speech therapy, etc.

Details of electrostimulation: 0–35 V, wave width 0.05 ms, 2–4 Hz, continuous impulses. This will trigger slight, rhythmic muscle contractions. If the treatment increases the rigor, electrostimulation should not be continued. Electrostimulation is contraindicated during the acute stage of a cerebral haemorrhage and haemorrhagic insult.

Acupuncture points

BL-40 **Location:** in the centre of the popliteal crease, between the tendons of the semitendinosus and the biceps.
Notes: *He*-sea point; eliminates stagnation of *Qi* and Blood (*Xue*), relaxes the tendons, activates the collaterals.

BL-60 **Location:** midway between the Achilles tendon and the highest prominence of the lateral malleolus.
Notes: *Jing*-river point, master point for pain along the meridian pathway; relaxes the tendons, invigorates the circulation of blood.

Ex-LE-10 **Location:** 4 points on the dorsum of the foot, 0.5 cun proximal to the interdigital folds.
Notes: relax the tendons, dispel Wind-Cold, invigorate the Blood (*Xue*).

G.B.-30 **Location:** on a line connecting the greater trochanter and the sacral hiatus, at the junction of the lateral and medial third.
Notes: master point for sciatica and paresis of the lower extremity.

G.B.-31 **Location:** on the lateral aspect of the thigh where the trouser seam would be. With the arms hanging down, the middle finger will indicate this point.
Notes: eliminates Wind, unblocks the collaterals, relaxes the tendons.

G.B.-34 **Location:** in a depression anterior and inferior to the head of the fibula.
Notes: *He*-sea point, *Hui*-meeting point of the tendons; subdues rebellious *Qi*; smoothes the flow of Liver *Qi*.

G.B.-39 **Location:** 3 cun superior to the lateral malleolus, on the anterior border of the fibula (Zeitler, Kö/Wa: on the posterior border).
Notes: *Hui*-meeting point of the marrow (brain substance = marrow), group *Luo*-connecting point of the 3 *Yang* of the leg (ST, G.B., BL).

G.B.-40 **Location:** in the depression anterior and inferior to the lateral malleolus.
Notes: *Yuan*-source point; harmonizes the flow of Liver *Qi*, special point for hypochondriacal pain; local point for the ankle.

KID-3 **Location:** midway between the highest prominence of the medial malleolus and the Achilles tendon.
Notes: *Yuan*-source and *Shu*-stream point; tonifies the Kidney *Yin* and *Yang*, strengthens the knees, benefits the Essence (*Jing*) and therefore the brain.

KID-9 **Location:** 6 cun superior to the medial malleolus, 1.5 cun posterior to the medial crest of the tibia, on the tibial border of the medial belly of the gastrocnemius.
Notes: *Xi*-cleft point of the *Yin Wei Mai*; calms the Spirit, tonifies Kidney *Yin*.

L.I.-4 **Location:** on the highest point of the adductor pollicis.
Notes: *Yuan*-source point, command point for the face; moves *Qi*, unblocks the meridians, especially with LIV-3 (4 gates); with LU-7 eliminates external pathogens.

L.I.-11 **Location:** with the arm fully flexed, at the radial end of the cubital crease.
Notes: *He*-sea point, tonification point; eliminates Damp-Heat and Wind, benefits the tendons and joints.

L.I.-15 **Location:** with the arm abducted, in the anterior of the two depressions inferior to the acromioclavicular joint, between the anterior and medial third of the deltoid.
Notes: master point for paresis of the upper extremities.

S.I.-9 **Location:** with the arm hanging down, 1 cun superior to the end of the posterior axillary fold.
Notes: strengthens the collaterals, eliminates Wind; local point for disorders of the shoulder.

S.I.-14 **Location:** on the upper part of the scapula; 3 cun lateral to the lower border of the spinous process of T1.
Notes: outer back-*Shu* point of the shoulder.

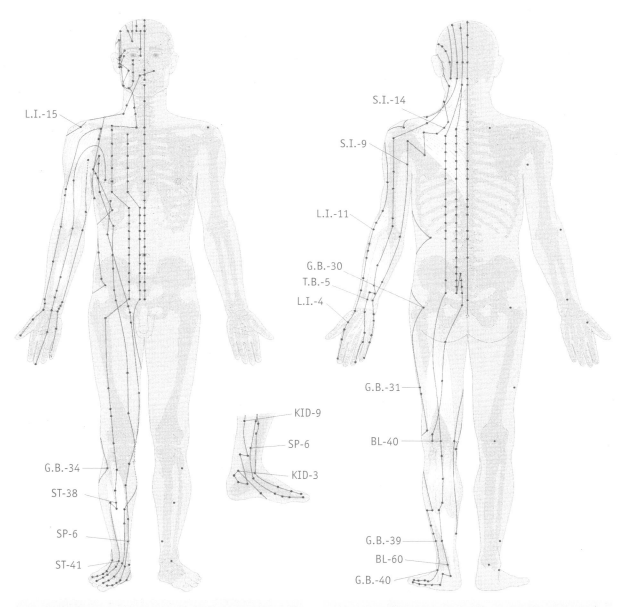

SP-6 **Location:** 3 cun superior to the highest prominence of the medial malleolus, on the posterior border of the tibia.
Notes: as group *Luo*-connecting point, tonifies the Spleen, Kidneys and Liver; also tonifies the *Qi*, Blood (*Xue*) and *Yin*, nourishing, moves the Blood (*Xue*), eliminates Dampness.

ST-38 **Location:** 0.5 cun lateral to the anterior crest of the tibia, 7 cun inferior to the lower border of the head of the fibula, midway between the highest prominence of the medial malleolus and the knee joint space.
Notes: important distal point for the shoulder.

ST-41 **Location:** on the anterior aspect of the ankle, between the tendons of the extensor hallucis longus and extensor digitorum longus.
Notes: *Jing*-river point and tonification point; resolves *Qi* stagnation in the leg.

T.B.-5 **Location:** 2 cun proximal to the midpoint of the dorsal wrist crease, opposite P-6.
Notes: *Luo*-connecting point, opening point of the *Yang Wei Mai* – dominates the surface, eliminates external pathogens, especially Wind-Heat; master point of the small joints.

6.8.6 *Motion sickness*

TCM considers a general weakness of the body as a primary factor, particularly *Qi* and Blood (*Xue*) deficiency.

Basic point combination

P-6.
Acupuncture or acupressure at P-6, both during acute stages or as a preventive measure: alternating pressing of the right/left P-6 for 2–5 minutes with intermittent pressure until *De Qi* (→ 3.2) is obtained.

Individual point combination

Hypotension

ST-36, BL-17, BL-20, Du-20, Ren-6.
Gentle stimulation; retain the needles for approximately 30 minutes. Possibly moxa at ST-36, Ren-6.
TCM: *Qi* and Blood (*Xue*) deficiency (hypotension, weak constitution): just before or at the end of a trip, symptoms such as dizziness, floaters, nausea, gag reflex, pale complexion, palpitations, etc. will occur – in other words, cardiovascular symptoms accompanied by general weakness. Prophylactic treatment of the gastrointestinal tract is recommended.

Hypertension

LIV-3, LIV-2, G.B.-20, G.B.-43, Ex-HN-3 (*Yin Tang*), Ex-HN-5 (*Tai Yang*).
TCM: choleric type, excess of Liver *Yang*: Shortly before start of trip or towards the end, onset of symptoms such as dizziness, lightheadedness, tension headache; reddish cheeks, fullness in the chest, impatient, irascible, tiredness; symptoms worse with stress; **tongue body:** reddish; **tongue coating:** yellow; **pulse:** wiry. The major aspect is a Liver disharmony, as is often seen with arterial hypertension, neurasthenia and hyperthyroidism.

Pyknic[1] constitution

ST-8 [ST-1 Bi], ST-40, SP-4, P-6, Ren-12.
Medium-strength stimulation; needle retention 20–30 minutes.
TCM: pasty type, stagnation of Phlegm and Dampness in the gastrointestinal tract (Middle Burner): symptoms as above, no appetite; **tongue body:** pale; **tongue coating:** slippery (rather more Stomach-related symptoms).

[1]Pyknic: a person of medium height, stockily built, with a tendency to become overweight and a stolid temperament. One of three constitutional types (asthenic, athletic and pyknic) posited by the German psychiatrist Ernst Kretschmer.

Acupuncture points

BL-17 **Location:** 1.5 cun lateral to the spinous process of T7.
Notes: as *Hui*-meeting point of the Blood (*Xue*), tonifies and regulates the Blood; as back-*Shu* point of the diaphragm, removes diaphragmatic constriction.

BL-20 **Location:** 1.5 cun lateral to the lower border of the spinous process of T11.
Notes: back-*Shu* point of the Spleen; tonifies the Spleen and Stomach, and therefore the production of *Qi* and Blood (*Xue*); eliminates Dampness.

Du-20 **Location:** on a line connecting the apices of the ears, 7 cun superior the posterior hairline.
Notes: meeting point of all divergent meridians, therefore effective for psychosomatic disorders; harmonizing.

Ex-HN-3 **Location:** midway between the eyebrows.
Notes: miracle point for headaches.

Ex-HN-5 **Location:** in the depression at the temple.
Notes: important point for temporal headaches.

G.B.-20 **Location:** posterior to the mastoid, between the trapezius and sternocleidomastoid, on the lower border of the occipital bone.
Notes: dispels Wind from the head, subdues internal/external Wind and Liver Fire, tonifies the sympathetic nervous system – combined with BL-10, standard combination for the autonomic nervous system, benefits the brain and eyes.

G.B.-43 **Location:** between the 4th and 5th toes, proximal to the margin of the web, closer to the metatarsophalangeal joint of the 4th toe.
Notes: subdues Liver *Yang*.

LIV-2 **Location:** on the interdigital web between the 1st and 2nd toes, lateral to the metatarsophalangeal joint.
Notes: *Ying*-spring point, sedation point; clears Liver Fire, calming.

LIV-3 **Location:** in the depression distal to the junction of the 1st and 2nd metatarsal bones.
Notes: *Yuan*-source and *Shu*-stream point; calms the Liver *Yang*, harmonizes the flow of Liver *Qi*, spasmolytic.

P-6 **Location:** 2 cun proximal to the midpoint of the palmar aspect of the wrist crease, between the tendons of the flexor carpi radialis and palmaris longus.
Notes: opening point of the *Yin Wei Mai*; master point for nausea; regulates the Triple Burner, the *Jue Yin*, Heart *Qi* and Blood (*Xue*), unbinds the chest, harmonizes the Stomach, calms the Spirit; most important point for motion sickness.

Ren-6 **Location:** 1.5 cun inferior to the umbilicus.
Notes: 'Sea of *Qi*' – tonifies the Kidneys, original *Qi* and *Yang Qi*; pulls rising *Yang* downwards.

Ren-12 **Location:** midway between the umbilicus and the xiphoid process.
Notes: *Hui*-meeting point of the hollow organs (*Fu*), front-*Mu* point of the Stomach; tonifies the Stomach and Spleen, regulates Stomach *Qi*, eliminates Dampness.

SP-4 **Location:** in the depression at the junction of the base and shaft of the 1st metatarsal bone, at the junction of the red and white skin.
Notes: *Luo*-connecting point, opening point of the *Chong Mai*; tonifies the Spleen and calms the Stomach.

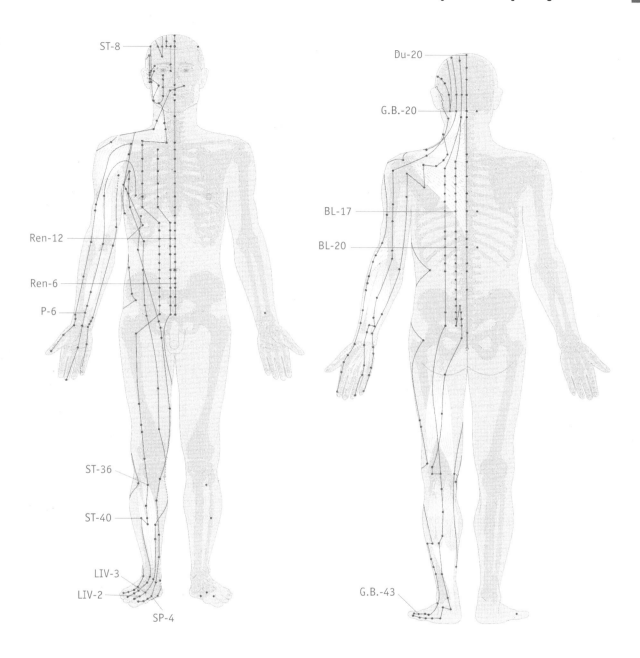

ST-8 **Location:** at the corner of the forehead, 3 cun superior and 1 cun posterior to the frontozygomatic suture.
Notes: alleviates headaches due to Wind-Heat (common cold) or to digestive problems with dizziness (Dampness and Phlegm).
ST-36 **Location:** 1 cun lateral to the anterior crest of the tibia, 1.5 cun inferior to the lower border of the head of the fibula (G.B.-34).

Notes: *He*-sea point, master point of hormones; tonifies the Stomach and the Spleen, and therefore *Qi* and Blood (*Xue*), calming and strengthening.
ST-40 **Location:** at the midpoint of the lower leg, 2 cun lateral to the anterior crest of the tibia.
Notes: *Luo*-connecting point (connects with the Spleen), therefore specifically for Dampness and Phlegm.

241

6.8.7 Insomnia (1)

The following section refers to chronic insomnia: sleep is too short, there is frequent wakening or inability to get back to sleep after wakening.

Insomnia due to heat, cold, consumption of tea, coffee or other stimulants, or due to psychological or physical stress, is not considered as a disorder by TCM. If the cause of the insomnia is known (e.g. pain, asthma, pruritus), this will be treated as the primary root.

Basic point combination

KID-6, BL-62, HE-7, SP-6.

Individual point combination

TCM differentiates four main patterns of insomnia.

Key symptom: disturbed sleep

BL-15, BL-20, P-6.
TCM: Heart *Yin* deficiency: difficulty falling asleep, inner restlessness, much dreaming, forgetfulness, frequent sweating, heat sensation in the palms and soles of the feet, dry mouth and throat; **tongue body:** dry, reddish; **pulse:** thin and rapid (*Xi Shu*). This is the most common type.

Key symptom: difficulty falling and staying asleep

BL-15, BL-23, KID-3.
TCM: hyperactivity accompanied by physical weakness. Heat symptoms due to Kidney and Heart *Yin* deficiency (*Yin Xu Hou Wang*). Difficulty falling and staying asleep, vertigo, tinnitus, night sweating, inner restlessness, forgetfulness, much dreaming, weak extremities, may have nocturnal emissions; **tongue body:** reddish, little coating; **pulse:** thin and rapid (*Xi Shu*).

Acupuncture points

BL-15 **Location:** 1.5 cun lateral to the lower border of the spinous process of T5.
Notes: back-*Shu* point of the Heart; combine with HE-7 for insomnia.

BL-18 **Location:** 2 cun lateral to the spinous process of T9.
Notes: back-*Shu* point of the Liver; resolves *Qi* stagnation, for hypochondriacal distension.

BL-20 **Location:** 1.5 cun lateral to the lower border of the spinous process of T11.
Notes: back-*Shu* point of the Spleen; tonifies the Spleen and Stomach, and therefore the production of *Qi* and Blood (*Xue*).

BL-21 **Location:** 1.5 cun lateral to the lower border of the spinous process of T12.
Notes: back-*Shu* point of the Stomach, master point of the Stomach.

BL-23 **Location:** 1.5 cun lateral to the lower border of the spinous process of L2.
Notes: back-*Shu* point of the Kidneys; tonifies the *Qi*, *Yang*, *Yin* and Essence (*Jing*) of the Kidneys.

BL-62 **Location:** below the tip of the lateral malleolus.
Notes: opening point of the *Yang Qiao Mai*, which carries *Yang* energy to the eye and controls the opening of the eyelids; together with KID-6, master point of insomnia.

HE-7 **Location:** at the ulnar aspect of the wrist crease, on the radial side of the pisiform bone.
Notes: *Yuan*-source point, *Shu*-stream point, sedation point; tonifies the Heart Blood, cools Heat and Fire, clears Heat at the *Ying* level, calms the Spirit, pacifies the Heart, opens the orifices of the Heart, resolves *Qi* stagnation in the Heart and chest, improves memory and alleviates insomnia.

KID-3 **Location:** midway between the highest prominence of the medial malleolus and the Achilles tendon.
Notes: *Yuan*-source and *Shu*-stream point; tonifies the Kidney *Yin* and *Yang*, benefits the Essence (*Jing*).

KID-6 **Location:** directly below the medial malleolus, often in a small cleft.
Notes: specifically tonifies *Yin*, calms the Spirit; opening point of the *Yin Qiao Mai* which carries *Yin* energy to the eyes and controls the closing of the eyelids; with BL-62, master point for insomnia.

P-6 **Location:** 2 cun proximal to the midpoint of the palmar aspect of the wrist crease, between the tendons of the flexor carpi radialis and palmaris longus.
Notes: opening point of the *Yin Wei Mai*; regulates Heart *Qi* and Blood, calms the Spirit.

SP-6 **Location:** 3 cun superior to the highest prominence of the medial malleolus, on the posterior border of the tibia.
Notes: as group *Luo*-connecting point tonifies the Spleen, Kidneys and Liver; also tonifies the *Qi*, Blood (*Xue*) and *Yin*, nourishing, moves the Blood (*Xue*).

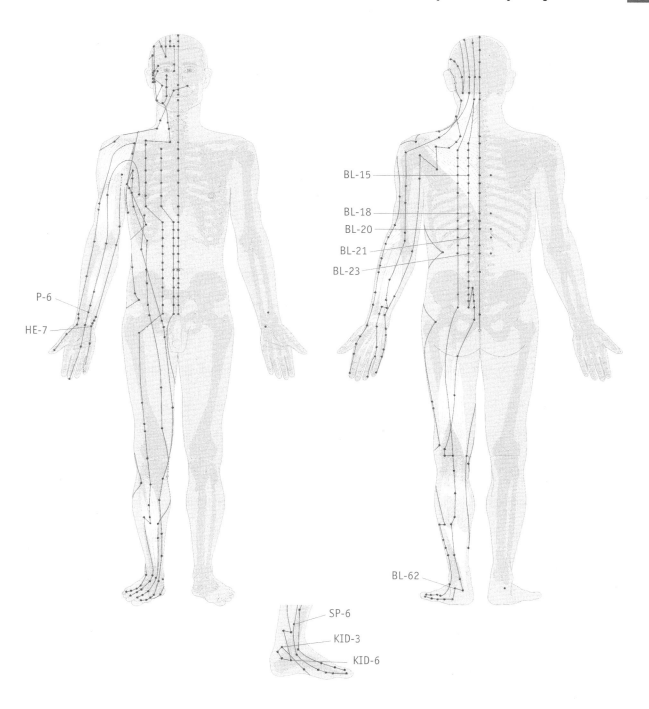

P-6

HE-7

BL-15

BL-18

BL-20

BL-21

BL-23

BL-62

SP-6

KID-3

KID-6

6.8.7 Insomnia (2)

Key symptom: digestive problems

ST-36, ST-40, BL-21, Ren-12.
TCM: disharmony in the gastrointestinal tract: fullness, often with belching; difficult bowel movements; **pulse:** wiry and slippery (*Shu Hua*).

Key symptom: depressive mood

BL-18, LIV-2 or LIV-3, Du-20.
TCM: Fire symptoms in the Liver and Gall Bladder organs: depressive or irascible, vertigo, headache, hypochondriac distension; **tongue coating:** yellow; **pulse:** wiry (*Xuan*).

Acupuncture points

BL-18 **Location:** 2 cun lateral to the spinous process of T9.
Notes: back-*Shu* point of the Liver; resolves *Qi* stagnation and distension in the hypochondrium.

BL-21 **Location:** 1.5 cun lateral to the lower border of the spinous process of T12.
Notes: back-*Shu* point of the Stomach, master point of the Stomach.

Du-20 **Location:** on a line connecting the apices of the ears, 7 cun superior the posterior hairline.
Notes: meeting point of all divergent meridians, therefore effective for psychosomatic disorders; an internal branch of the Liver meridian terminates here; harmonizing.

LIV-2 **Location:** on the interdigital web between the 1st and 2nd toes, lateral to the metatarsophalangeal joint.
Notes: *Ying*-spring point, sedation point; clears Liver Fire, calming.

LIV-3 **Location:** in the depression distal to the junction of the 1st and 2nd metatarsal bones.
Notes: *Yuan*-source and *Shu*-stream point; calms the Liver Yang, harmonizes the flow of Liver *Qi*, spasmolytic.

Ren-12 **Location:** midway between the umbilicus and the xiphoid process.
Notes: front-*Mu* point of the Stomach; tonifies the Stomach and Spleen, regulates Stomach *Qi*.

ST-36 **Location:** 1 cun lateral to the anterior crest of the tibia, 1.5 cun inferior to the lower border of the head of the fibula (G.B.-34).
Notes: *He*-sea point; harmonizes the Stomach and Spleen, promotes the digestion of undigested food.

ST-40 **Location:** at the midpoint of the lower leg, 2 cun lateral to the anterior crest of the tibia.
Notes: *Luo*-connecting point (connects with the Spleen); promotes digestion and the transformation of Phlegm.

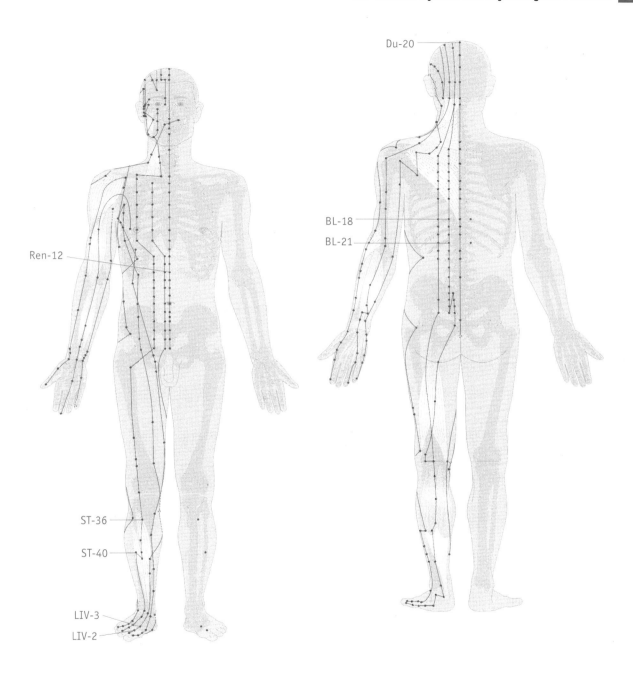

Du-20

BL-18
BL-21

Ren-12

ST-36

ST-40

LIV-3
LIV-2

6.8.8 Tremor

In TCM, tremors of the head as well as tremors of the hand and feet can be due to either *Feng Yang* (Wind *Yang*) or *Xu Feng* (empty Wind).

Basic point combination

L.I.-4, SP-6, G.B.-20, LIV-3, Du-20.
Additional points depending on the location of the tremor:
Hand: T.B.-4.
Foot: P-6 or G.B.-34.
Head: L.I.-11, S.I.-3, BL-62.

Individual point combination

Excess type (*Feng Yang*) (*Feng* = Wind)

G.B.-34, KID-7.
Technique: L.I.-4, G.B.-20, G.B.-34, Du-20 with even method; SP-6, KID-7 with tonifying method; LIV-3 with sedating method. Needle retention: approximately 20 minutes.

Mostly caused by psychovegetative imbalances: Liver *Qi* stagnation due to a depressive disorder can lead to Liver Fire. Wind develops as a result of the Fire, with typical Wind symptoms such as tremors of the head, hands or feet. The overall picture is one of *Yang* and excess. Tremor, vertigo, headaches, restlessness, sleep disturbances; **tongue body:** red; **tongue coating:** slightly yellow; **pulse:** wiry and rapid (*Xuan Shu*).

Deficiency type: *Xu Feng* (*Xu* = deficiency, *Feng* = Wind)

ST-36, P-6.
Method: Du-20, G.B.-20 with even method; P-6, L.I.-4 and LIV-3 with reducing method; ST-36 and SP-6 with tonifying method. Needle retention: approximately 20 minutes.

More common in elderly patients after a febrile disease that strongly depleted Kidney and Liver *Yin*. The deficient (*Xu*) character of this pattern leads to so-called endogenous Wind with cervical dystonia as well as tremors of the hands and feet. The overall picture is one of *Yin* and deficiency. Tremors, emotional exhaustion, palpitations, dryness of the mouth and throat; **tongue body:** red to dark red; **tongue coating:** little or no coating; **pulse:** thin and rapid (*Xi Shu*).

Acupuncture points

BL-62 **Location:** below the tip of the lateral malleolus.
Notes: opening point of the *Yang Qiao Mai*, which strengthens the effect of S.I.-3 (opening point of the *Du Mai*).

Du-20 **Location:** on a line connecting the apices of the ears, 7 cun superior the posterior hairline.
Notes: meeting point of all divergent meridians; an internal branch of the Liver meridian terminates here.

G.B.-20 **Location:** posterior to the mastoid, between the trapezius and sternocleidomastoid, on the lower border of the occipital bone.
Notes: dispels Wind from the head, subdues internal/external Wind and Liver Fire.

G.B.-34 **Location:** in a depression anterior and inferior to the head of the fibula.
Notes: *He*-sea point and *Hui*-meeting point of the tendons; relaxes the tendons; smoothes the flow of Liver *Qi*.

KID-7 **Location:** 2 cun superior to KID-3 (KID-3: midway between the highest prominence of the medial malleolus and the Achilles tendon).
Notes: *Jing*-river point, tonification point; tonifies the Kidneys, especially Kidney *Yang*.

L.I.-4 **Location:** on the highest point of the adductor pollicis.
Notes: *Yuan*-source point, command point for the face; moves *Qi*, unblocks the meridians, especially with LIV-3 (4 gates).

L.I.-11 **Location:** with the arm fully flexed, at the radial end of the cubital crease.
Notes: *He*-sea point, tonification point; eliminates Damp-Heat and Wind, benefits the tendons and joints.

LIV-3 **Location:** in the depression distal to the junction of the 1st and 2nd metatarsal bones.
Notes: *Yuan*-source and *Shu*-stream point; calms the Liver *Yang* and the 'Wind' following it, spasmolytic.

P-6 **Location:** 2 cun proximal to the midpoint of the palmar aspect of the wrist crease, between the tendons of the flexor carpi radialis and palmaris longus.
Notes: opening point of the *Yin Wei Mai*; master point for nausea; regulates the Triple Burner, the *Jue Yin*, Heart *Qi* and Blood (*Xue*), calms the Spirit.

S.I.-3 **Location:** when a fist is made, on the dorsum of the hand, in the depression at the end of the most distal palmar crease.
Notes: opening point of the *Du Mai*, therefore able to eliminate external and internal Wind from the *Du Mai*; has an effect on the central nervous system, benefits the Spirit.

SP-6 **Location:** 3 cun superior to the highest prominence of the medial malleolus, on the posterior border of the tibia.
Notes: as group *Luo*-connecting point, tonifies the Spleen, Kidneys and Liver; also tonifies the *Qi*, Blood (*Xue*) and *Yin*, nourishing, moves the Blood (*Xue*).

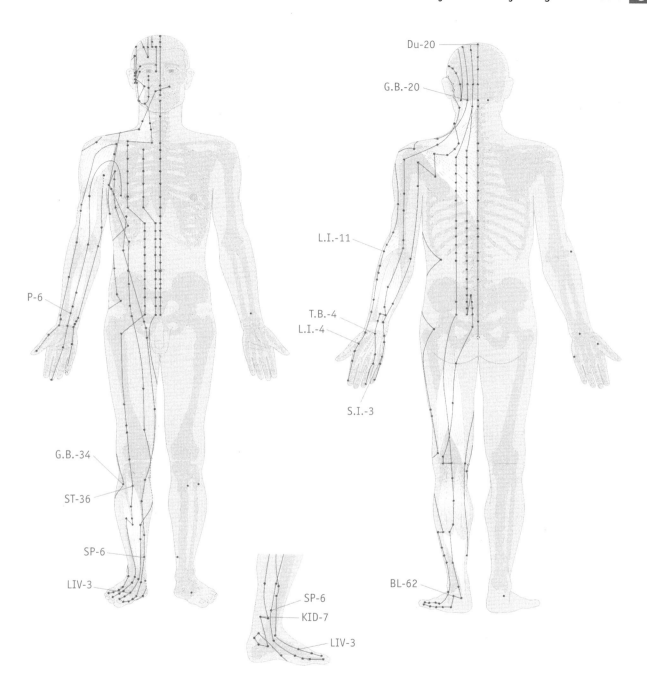

ST-36 **Location:** 1 cun lateral to the anterior crest of the tibia, 1.5 cun inferior to the lower border of the head of the fibula (G.B.-34).
Notes: *He*-sea point, master point of hormones; tonifies the Stomach and the Spleen, and therefore *Qi* and Blood (*Xue*), calming and strengthening.

T.B.-4 **Location:** on the wrist crease, in the depression lateral to the tendon of the extensor digitorum longus.
Notes: *Yuan*-source point; here used as a local point to relax the tendons.

6.8.9 Parkinson's disease

As for tremors, TCM recognizes two patterns for Parkinson's disease. Depending on the pattern, the basic point combination can be modified accordingly.

Basic point combination

BL-18, BL-23, G.B.-20, G.B.-34, Du-14 [Du-13 Bi] Du-20.
Scalp acupuncture: Parkinson zone.
Method (scalp acupuncture): several needles are inserted at a distance of 1 cm from one another.

Individual point combination

With much Phlegm

ST-40.

Spleen deficiency symptoms (digestive imbalance)

ST-36, BL-20.

Dorsalgia

BL-40 [BL-54 Bi] and local pressure-sensitive points on the back.

More severe rigor

L.I.-4, P-3.
Scalp acupuncture: anti-Parkinson zone: parallel to and 1.5 cm anterior to the motor zone, which is used as a line of reference with the following reference points:

Point A: 0.5 cm posterior to the midpoint of the line connecting Ex-HN-3 (*Yin Tang*, 'point de Merveille') and the external occipital protuberance – this will be a point very close to DU-20.

Point B: at the junction of a line connecting the highest point of the eyebrow and the external occipital protuberance and a vertical line through the midpoint of the zygomatic arch (approximately 0.5 cm superior to the zygomatic arch).

Acupuncture points

BL-18 **Location:** 2 cun lateral to the spinous process of T9.
Notes: back-*Shu* point of the Liver; tonifies and regulates Liver *Qi* and Blood (*Xue*).

BL-20 **Location:** 1.5 cun lateral to the lower border of the spinous process of T11.
Notes: back-*Shu* point of the Spleen; tonifies the Spleen and Stomach, and therefore the production of *Qi* and Blood (*Xue*).

BL-23 **Location:** 1.5 cun lateral to the lower border of the spinous process of L2.
Notes: back-*Shu* point of the Kidneys; tonifies the *Qi*, *Yang*, *Yin* and Essence (*Jing*) of the Kidneys.

BL-40 **Location:** in the centre of the popliteal crease, between the tendons of the semitendinosus and the biceps.
Notes: *He*-sea point; eliminates stagnation of *Qi* and Blood (*Xue*), relaxes the tendons, activates the collaterals.

Du-14 **Location:** below the spinous process of C7.
Notes: meeting point of all *Yang* meridians.

Du-20 **Location:** on a line connecting the apices of the ears, 7 cun superior the posterior hairline.
Notes: meeting point of all divergent meridians, also terminal point of an internal branch of the Liver meridian; in scalp acupuncture, local point for the motor/Parkinson zone.

G.B.-20 **Location:** posterior to the mastoid, between the trapezius and sternocleidomastoid, on the lower border of the occipital bone.
Notes: dispels Wind from the head, subdues internal/external Wind.

G.B.-34 **Location:** in a depression anterior and inferior to the head of the fibula.
Notes: *He*-sea point and *Hui*-meeting point of the tendons, relaxing point; smoothes the flow of Liver *Qi*.

L.I.-4 **Location:** on the highest point of the adductor pollicis.
Notes: *Yuan*-source point, command point for the face; moves *Qi*, unblocks the meridians, especially with LIV-3 (4 gates).

P-3 **Location:** on the cubital crease, ulnar to the tendon of the biceps (LU-5 is located radial to the tendon).
Notes: *He*-sea point; local spasmolytic effect, for tremors affecting the upper extremity.

ST-36 **Location:** 1 cun lateral to the anterior crest of the tibia, 1.5 cun inferior to the lower border of the head of the fibula (G.B.-34).
Notes: *He*-sea point, master point of hormones; tonifies the Stomach and the Spleen, and therefore *Qi* and Blood (*Xue*), stabilizing.

ST-40 **Location:** at the midpoint of the lower leg, 2 cun lateral to the anterior crest of the tibia.
Notes: *Luo*-connecting point (connects with the Spleen); therefore specifically for Dampness and Phlegm.

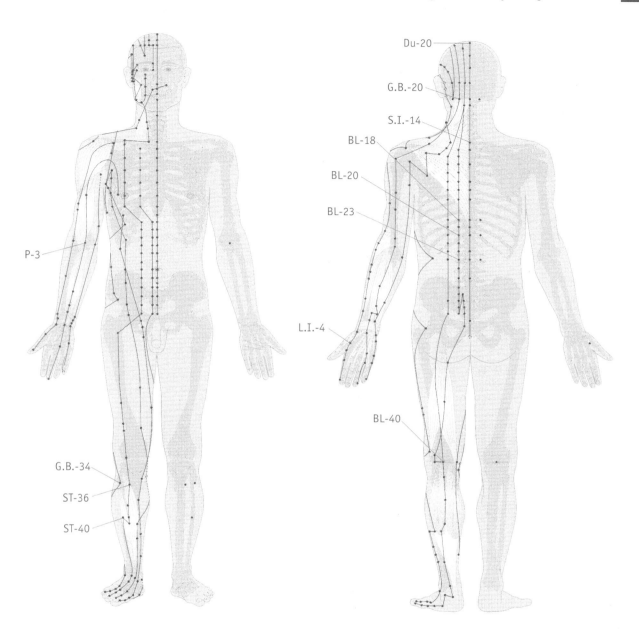

6.8.10 Lack of concentration, poor memory (1)

TCM differentiates five patterns of concentration and memory disorders, which may be congenital, dependent or non-dependent on age. It is of interest that TCM does not use the term 'lack of concentration'. The Heart stores the substantial aspect *Shen*, which represents the material foundation of the Spirit. Thus, points on the Heart meridian will always be used in the treatment of this type of disorder.

Basic point combination

ST-36, SP-6, HE-7, BL-15 or P-6, Ex-HN-1 (*Si Shen Cong*) or Du-20.

Individual point combinations

Pre-senile forgetfulness

KID-3, BL-23, G.B.-39, Du-4 **M**, Ren-4 **M** or Ren-6, BL-11. **TCM:** Kidney Essence (*Jing*) deficiency: helpless, despairing, forgetful, listless, premature hair loss, brittle and greying hair, loose teeth, weak joints; slow gait; **tongue body:** pale; **tongue coating:** white; **pulse:** empty (*Xu*). **Aetiology:** major causes are stress, extreme tiredness and the patient's constitution. **Commentary:** in TCM, Essence (*Jing*) represents the material substrate of a person's constitution. Essence (*Jing*) is responsible for development, ageing and fertility (*Shen Jing Kui Xu*).

Acupuncture points

BL-11 **Location:** 1.5 cun lateral to the lower border of the spinous process of T1.
Notes: *Hui*-meeting point of the bones; secondary action on the Essence (*Jing*) and therefore the brain.
BL-15 **Location:** 1.5 cun lateral to the lower border of the spinous process of T5.
Notes: back-*Shu* point of the Heart; combined with HE-7 tonifies the Heart *Qi* and *Yin*.
BL-23 **Location:** 1.5 cun lateral to the lower border of the spinous process of L2.
Notes: back-*Shu* point of the Kidneys; tonifies the *Qi, Yang, Yin* and Essence (*Jing*) of the Kidneys; counterbalances rising Liver *Yang*.
Du-4 **Location:** on the posterior midline, below the spinous process of L2.
Notes: *Ming Men* (Gate of Vitality); tonifies Kidney *Yang* in particular, but also Kidney *Yin*, firms the Essence (*Jing*), strengthening.

Du-20 **Location:** on a line connecting the apices of the ears, 7 cun superior the posterior hairline.
Notes: meeting point of all divergent meridians; strengthens the brain.
Ex-HN-1 **Location:** 1 cun anterior, posterior and lateral to Du-20.
Notes: subdues internal Wind, strengthens the brain.
G.B.-39 **Location:** 3 cun superior to the lateral malleolus, on the anterior border of the fibula (Zeitler, Kö/Wa: on the posterior border).
Notes: *Hui*-meeting point of the marrow (brain substance = marrow).
HE-3 **Location:** with the elbow fully flexed, between the medial end of the cubital crease and the medial epicondyle.
Notes: *He*-sea point, master point for depression.
HE-7 **Location:** at the ulnar aspect of the wrist crease, on the radial side of the pisiform bone.
Notes: *Yuan*-source point, *Shu*-stream point, sedation point; tonifies the Heart Blood, where the Spirit (*Shen*) is anchored, calms the Spirit, improves memory and alleviates insomnia.
KID-3 **Location:** midway between the highest prominence of the medial malleolus and the Achilles tendon.
Notes: *Yuan*-source and *Shu*-stream point; tonifies the Kidney *Yin* and *Yang*, strengthens the knees, benefits the Essence (*Jing*) and therefore the brain.
P-6 **Location:** 2 cun proximal to the midpoint of the palmar aspect of the wrist crease, between the tendons of the flexor carpi radialis and palmaris longus.
Notes: opening point of the *Yin Wei Mai*; regulates Heart *Qi* and Blood, calms the Spirit.
Ren-4 **Location:** 2 cun superior to the upper border of the pubic symphysis.
Notes: meeting point of the 3 lower *Yin* meridians (SP, KID, LIV), front-*Mu* point of the Small Intestine (which is paired with the Heart); tonifying – strengthens the Essence (*Jing*), *Qi, Yang*, Blood and *Yin*; roots the ethereal soul (*Hun*).
Ren-6 **Location:** 1.5 cun inferior to the umbilicus.
Notes: 'sea of *Qi*' – tonifies the Kidneys, original *Qi* and *Yang Qi*; holds the *Qi* together.
SP-6 **Location:** 3 cun superior to the highest prominence of the medial malleolus, on the posterior border of the tibia.
Notes: as group *Luo*-connecting point, tonifies the Spleen, Kidneys and Liver; also tonifies the *Qi*, Blood (*Xue*) and *Yin*, nourishing, moves the Blood (*Xue*).
ST-36 **Location:** 1 cun lateral to the anterior crest of the tibia, 1.5 cun inferior to the lower border of the head of the fibula (G.B.-34).
Notes: *He*-sea point, master point of hormones; tonifies the Stomach and Spleen, and therefore *Qi* and Blood (*Xue*), stabilizing and strengthening.

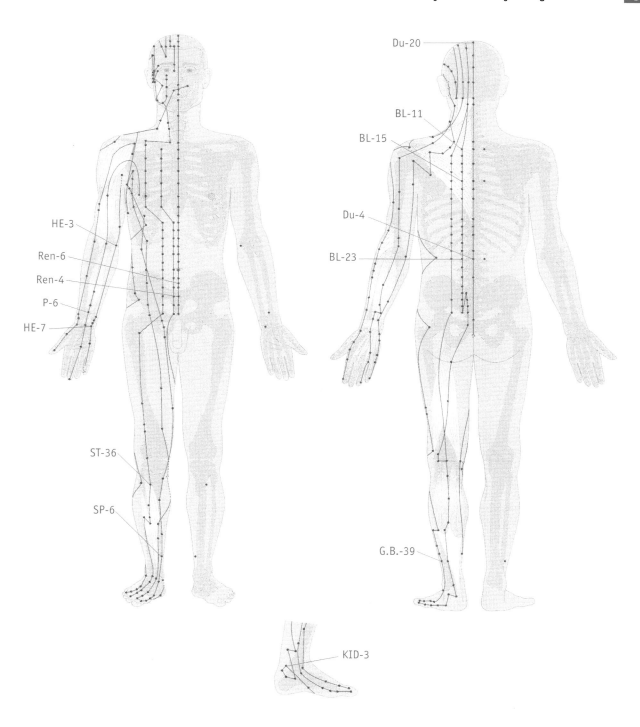

6.8.10 Lack of concentration, poor memory (2)

Lack of concentration accompanied by high stress levels and hectic environment

BL-23, KID-3.
TCM: disharmony between the Heart and the Kidneys (*Xin Shen Bu Jiao*): very often forgetful, inner restlessness and emptiness, insomnia, palpitations and nervous agitation, vertigo, tinnitus, lower back pain and weakness of the knees, vivid dreams with seminal emissions (men), much sweating, nocturia; **tongue body:** red; **tongue coating:** little; **pulse:** thin and rapid (*Xi Shu*).

Senile forgetfulness

BL-20 M, Ren-12 M.
TCM: *Qi/Yang* deficiency of the Heart and Spleen: pale complexion, forgetfulness with nervous agitation, less sleep, much dreaming, shortness of breath, anxious, little appetite, tiredness, bloating, loose stools, menstrual difficulties; **tongue body:** pale; **tongue coating:** white; **pulse:** thin and frail (*Xi Ruo*).

Pre-psychotic stage caused by emotional stress

BL-20, Ren-12 M.
TCM: 'turbid Phlegm disturbing the Heart (*Tan Zhu Rao Xin*): forgetfulness, desire to lie down, feeling despair, dizziness, blurry vision, palpitations, insomnia, chest tightness, much mucus in the throat; **tongue coating:** white, slippery; **pulse:** wiry, slippery (*Xuan Hua*).

With cardiovascular disease

Acupuncture is contraindicated.
TCM: 'stagnated Blood severely obstructs the Heart' (*Yu Xue Gong Xin*): sudden forgetfulness, dysarthria, difficulty swallowing, abdominal pain with muscular defence, cyanosis of the lips and fingertips, clear urine, dark stools; **pulse:** knotted (*Jie Dai*). These symptoms indicate acute, severe cardiovascular disease.

Acupuncture points

BL-20 **Location:** 1.5 cun lateral to the lower border of the spinous process of T11.
Notes: back-*Shu* point of the Spleen; tonifies the Spleen and Stomach, and therefore the production of *Qi* and Blood (*Xue*).

BL-23 **Location:** 1.5 cun lateral to the lower border of the spinous process of L2.
Notes: back-*Shu* point of the Kidneys; tonifies the *Qi, Yang, Yin* and Essence (*Jing*) of the Kidneys, counterbalances rising Liver *Yang*.

KID-3 **Location:** midway between the highest prominence of the medial malleolus and the Achilles tendon.
Notes: *Yuan*-source and *Shu*-stream point; tonifies the Kidney *Yin* and *Yang*, strengthens the knees, benefits the Essence (*Jing*) and therefore the brain.

Ren-12 **Location:** midway between the umbilicus and the xiphoid process.
Notes: front-*Mu* point of the Stomach; tonifies the Stomach and Spleen, and therefore *Qi* and Blood (*Xue*).

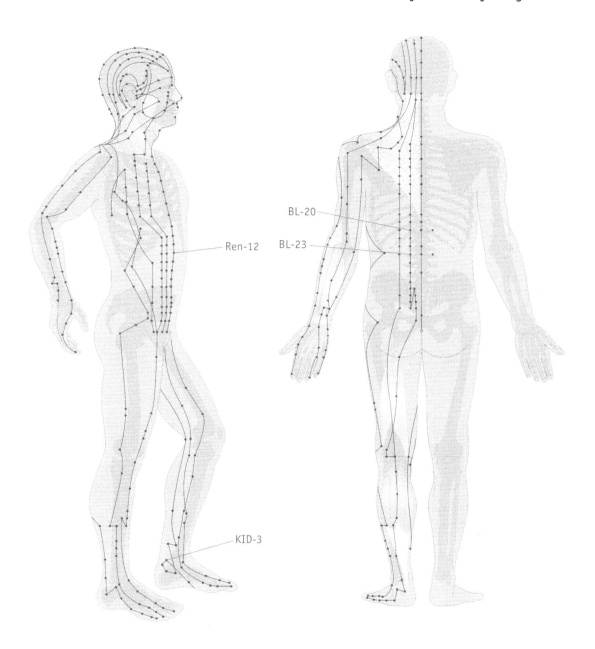

Ren-12

BL-20

BL-23

KID-3

6.8.11 Depressive disorder (1)

TCM considers depression as Liver *Qi* stagnation, causing digestive difficulties (Spleen) and also involving the Heart.

Clinical symptoms: despondence, listlessness, hypochondriacal distension, easily irritated, weepy, globus hystericus, disturbed sleep.

TCM: Liver *Qi* stagnation and Spleen deficiency (*Gan Yu Pi Xu*): common in women around the age of 7 × 7 years, when, biologically speaking, emptiness and deficiency of the *Ren Mai* and *Chong Mai* (extraordinary meridians) occur. Other underlying stress-related diseases may also play a role as causative factors.

Symptoms: inner restlessness, difficulty falling asleep, mistrust, unfocused, possibly compulsive behaviour, vertigo, reduced appetite, loose stools, tightness in the chest, bloating; **tongue body:** dull, pale; **tongue coating:** thick, white; **pulse:** wiry and thin (*Xuan Xi*). These symptoms are often seen with endogenous or reactive depression, depression in the elderly, menopausal syndrome, neurasthenia and paranoia.

Current antidepressant medication should not be discontinued abruptly, but should be changed only after consulting with the treating physician.

In addition: both *Tai Qi Quan* as well as *Qi Gong* (Chinese breathing and concentration exercises) have proven to be very helpful for depressive disorders.

Key symptoms: depression and emotional instability

TCM

Inner restlessness, emotionally unstable, insomnia.

Basic point combination

G.B.-34, LIV-3.

Individual point combination

Headaches

Ex-HN-5 (*Tai Yang*), needle towards G.B.-8 and Du-20.

Insomnia

SP-6.

Key symptoms: depression and impatience

TCM

Depression, impatience, restlessness, mistrust.

Basic point combination

T.B.-6, LIV-14, BL-20.

Individual point combination

Bloating

ST-36, ST-40.

Globus hystericus

KID-6, Ren-22 [Ren-21 Bi].

Diarrhoea

ST-36 and Ren-12.

Acupuncture points

BL-20 Location: 1.5 cun lateral to the lower border of the spinous process of T11.
Notes: back-*Shu* point of the Spleen; tonifies the Spleen/Stomach and therefore the production of *Qi* and Blood (*Xue*).

Du-20 Location: on a line connecting the apices of the ears, 7 cun superior the posterior hairline.
Notes: meeting point of all divergent meridians; strengthens the brain.

Ex-HN-5 Location: in the depression at the temple.

G.B.-8 Location: 1.5 cun superior to the apex of the ear.

G.B.-34 Location: in a depression anterior and inferior to the head of the fibula.
Notes: *He*-sea point; subdues rebellious *Qi*; promotes the smooth flow of Liver *Qi*.

KID-6 Location: directly below the medial malleolus, often in a small cleft.
Notes: tonifies *Yin*; opening point of the *Yin Qiao Mai* – due to the meridian pathway effective for globus sensation; calms the Spirit.

LIV-3 Location: in the depression distal to the junction of the 1st and 2nd metatarsal bones.
Notes: *Yuan*-source and *Shu*-stream point; subdues rising Liver *Yang*, harmonizes the flow of Liver *Qi*.

LIV-14 Location: on the midclavicular line, in the 6th ICS, directly below the nipple.
Notes: front-*Mu* point of the Liver; promotes the smooth flow of Liver *Qi*, harmonizes the Liver and Stomach.

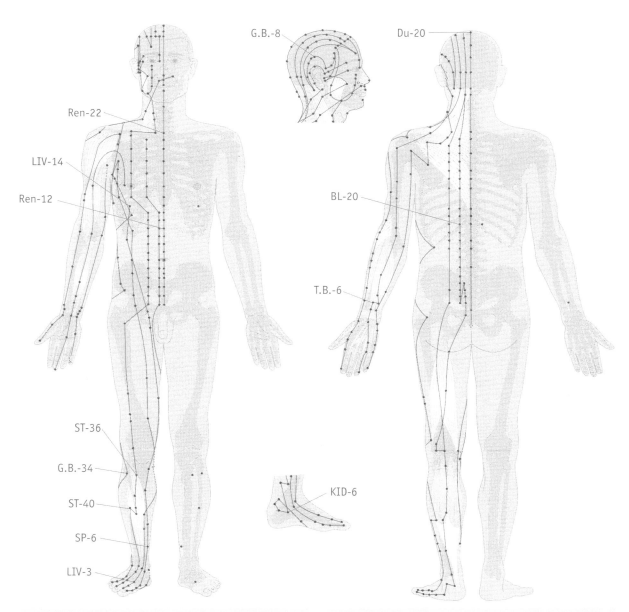

G.B.-8

Du-20

Ren-22

LIV-14

Ren-12

BL-20

T.B.-6

ST-36

G.B.-34

ST-40

SP-6

LIV-3

KID-6

Ren-12 **Location:** midway between the umbilicus and xiphoid process.
Notes: front-*Mu* point of the Stomach; tonifies the Stomach and Spleen, regulates Stomach *Qi*.

Ren-22 **Location:** in the centre of the jugulum.
Notes: resolves Phlegm; local point for globus sensation.

SP-6 **Location:** 3 cun superior to the highest prominence of the medial malleolus, on the posterior border of the tibia.
Notes: as group *Luo*-connecting point tonifies the Spleen, Kidneys and Liver; also tonifies the *Qi*, Blood (*Xue*) and *Yin*; calms the Spirit.

ST-36 **Location:** 1 cun lateral to the anterior crest of the tibia, 1.5 cun inferior to the lower border of the head of the fibula (G.B.-34).
Notes: *He*-sea point; tonifies the Stomach and Spleen.

ST-40 **Location:** at the midpoint of the lower leg, 2 cun lateral to the anterior crest of the tibia.
Notes: *Luo*-connecting point (connects with the Spleen), therefore specifically for Dampness and Phlegm.

T.B.-6 **Location:** 3 cun proximal to the centre of the dorsal wrist crease.
Notes: regulates the *Qi* in the chest, mobilizes *Qi* stagnation in the 3 Burners.

6.8.11 Depressive disorder (2)

Key symptoms: depression and inner restlessness, irascibility

TCM

Inner restlessness, irascibility, easily startled, much crying.

Basic point combination

HE-7, BL-15.

Individual point combination

Nocturnal emissions

BL-23, KID-3, SP-6.

Menstrual disorder

SP-10, P-6.

Tinnitus

G.B.-2, Ren-4.

Acupuncture points

BL-15 **Location:** 1.5 cun lateral to the lower border of the spinous process of T5.
Notes: back-*Shu* point of the Heart; combined with HE-7, tonifies the Heart *Qi* and *Yin*.

BL-23 **Location:** 1.5 cun lateral to the lower border of the spinous process of L2.
Notes: back-*Shu* point of the Kidneys; tonifies the *Qi*, *Yang*, *Yin* and Essence (*Jing*) of the Kidneys; counterbalances rising Liver *Yang*.

G.B.-2 **Location:** with the mouth open, in the depression anterior to the intertragic notch, posterior to the ascending ramus of the mandible.
Notes: raises the clear *Qi* to the ear and descends the turbid *Qi* from the ear.

HE-7 **Location:** at the ulnar aspect of the wrist crease, on the radial side of the pisiform bone.
Notes: *Yuan*-source point, *Shu*-stream point, sedation point; tonifies the Heart Blood, clears Heat, calms the Spirit and the Heart, opens the orifices of the Heart, resolves *Qi* stagnation in the Heart and chest, improves memory and alleviates insomnia.

KID-3 **Location:** midway between the highest prominence of the medial malleolus and the Achilles tendon.
Notes: *Yuan*-source and *Shu*-stream point; tonifies the Kidney *Yin* and *Yang*, benefits the Essence (*Jing*), stabilizes the Spirit and emotions (anxiety, psychological instability).

P-6 **Location:** 2 cun proximal to the midpoint of the palmar aspect of the wrist crease, between the tendons of the flexor carpi radialis and palmaris longus.
Notes: opening point of the *Yin Wei Mai*, has an effect on the Heart, Heart *Qi* and Blood (*Xue*), harmonizes the Stomach, calms the Spirit, especially with HE-7.

Ren-4 **Location:** 2 cun superior to the upper border of the pubic symphysis.
Notes: meeting point of the 3 lower *Yin* meridians (SP, KID, LIV), front-*Mu* point of the Small Intestine; tonifying – strengthens the Essence (*Jing*), *Qi*, *Yang*, Blood (*Xue*) and *Yin*, roots the ethereal soul (*Hun*).

SP-6 **Location:** 3 cun superior to the highest prominence of the medial malleolus, on the posterior border of the tibia.
Notes: as group *Luo*-connecting point, tonifies the Spleen, Kidneys and Liver; also tonifies the *Qi*, Blood (*Xue*) and *Yin*, calms the Spirit.

SP-10 **Location:** 2 cun superior to the upper medial patellar border.
Notes: 'Sea of Blood'; nourishes, cools and invigorates the Blood (*Xue*).

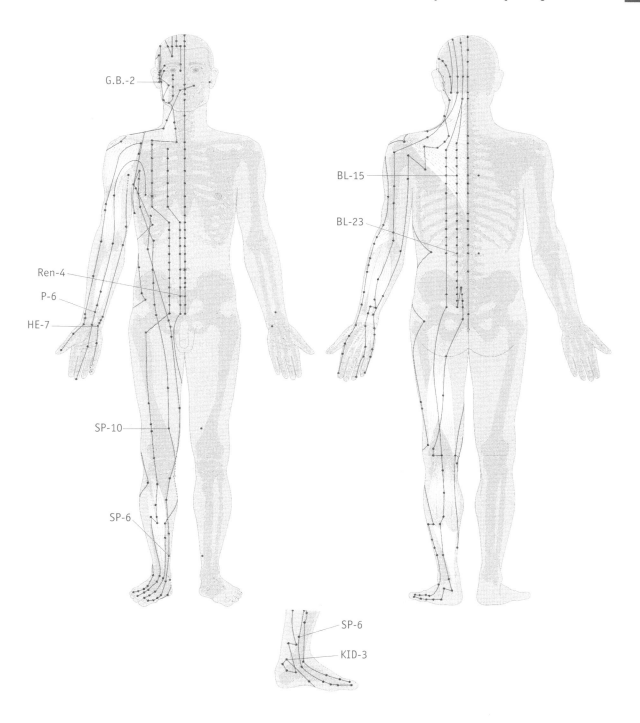

G.B.-2

BL-15

BL-23

Ren-4

P-6

HE-7

SP-10

SP-6

SP-6

KID-3

6.8.11 Depressive disorder (3)

Key symptoms: depression and anxiety

TCM

Depression, worrying, anxiety.

Basic point combination

P-6, HE-7.

Individual point combination

Reduced appetite

Ren-6, Ren-12.

Palpitations

BL-15, BL-18.

Key symptoms: depression and apathy

TCM

Dominant symptoms: apathy, lack of motivation, no enthusiasm.

Basic point combination

BL-23, Du-4.

Individual point combination

Impotence

Ren-2, Ren-4.

Loss of appetite

ST-36, BL-20 and Ren-4 **M**.

Anxiety

BL-15, BL-18.

Acupuncture points

BL-15 **Location:** 1.5 cun lateral to the lower border of the spinous process of T5.
Notes: back-*Shu* point of the Heart; combined with HE-7, tonifies the Heart *Qi* and *Yin*.

BL-18 **Location:** 2 cun lateral to the spinous process of T9.
Notes: back-*Shu* point of the Liver; tonifies and moves Liver *Qi* and Blood (*Xue*).

BL-20 **Location:** 1.5 cun lateral to the lower border of the spinous process of T11.
Notes: back-*Shu* point of the Spleen; tonifies the Spleen and Stomach, and therefore the production of *Qi* and Blood (*Xue*).

BL-23 **Location:** 1.5 cun lateral to the lower border of the spinous process of L2.
Notes: back-*Shu* point of the Kidneys; tonifies the *Qi*, *Yang*, *Yin* and Essence (*Jing*) of the Kidneys; counterbalances rising Liver *Yang*.

Du-4 **Location:** on the posterior midline, below the spinous process of L2, at the same level as BL-23 and BL-47.

HE-7 **Location:** at the ulnar aspect of the wrist crease, on the radial side of the pisiform bone.
Notes: *Yuan*-source point, *Shu*-stream point, sedation point; tonifies the Heart Blood, cools Heat, calms the Spirit and the Heart, opens the orifices of the Heart, improves memory and alleviates insomnia.

P-6 **Location:** 2 cun proximal to the midpoint of the palmar aspect of the wrist crease, between the tendons of the flexor carpi radialis and palmaris longus.
Notes: opening point of the *Yin Wei Mai*; has an effect on the Heart, Heart *Qi* and Blood (*Xue*), harmonizes the Stomach, calms the Spirit, especially with HE-7.

Ren-2 **Location:** on the upper border of the pubic symphysis, in the crease that forms when bending forward; level with KID-11, SP-12, ST-30.
Notes: together with Ren-3, forms the energetic centre of reproduction.

Ren-4 **Location:** 2 cun superior to the upper border of the pubic symphysis.
Notes: meeting point of the 3 lower *Yin* (SP, KID, LIV), front-*Mu* point of the Small Intestine; tonifying – strengthens the Essence (*Jing*), *Qi*, *Yang*, Blood (*Xue*) and *Yin*, roots the ethereal soul (*Hun*).

Ren-6 **Location:** 1.5 cun inferior to the umbilicus.
Notes: 'Sea of *Qi*' – tonifies the Kidneys, original *Qi* and *Yang Qi*; holds the *Qi* together.

Ren-12 **Location:** midway between the umbilicus and the xiphoid process.
Notes: front-*Mu* point of the Stomach; tonifies the Stomach and Spleen, regulates Stomach *Qi*.

ST-36 **Location:** 1 cun lateral to the anterior crest of the tibia, 1.5 cun inferior to the lower border of the head of the fibula (G.B.-34).
Notes: *He*-sea point, epithet 'Divine Serenity'; tonifies the Stomach and Spleen.

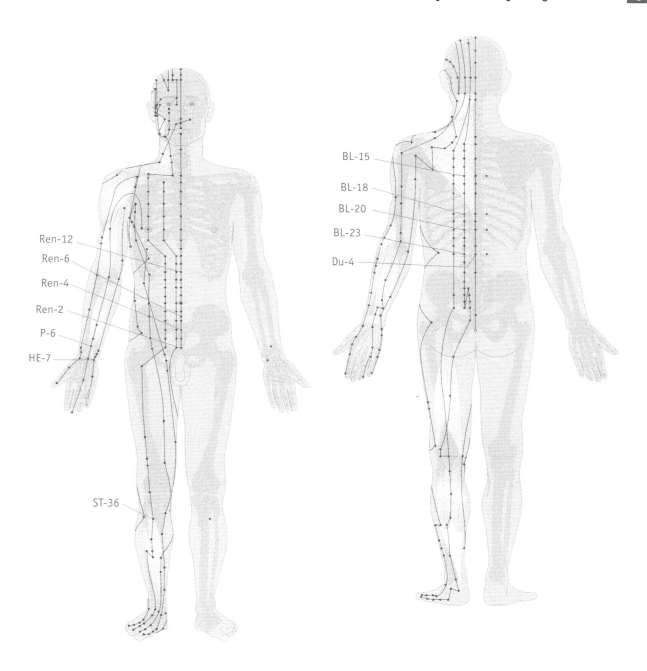

Ren-12
Ren-6
Ren-4
Ren-2
P-6
HE-7

ST-36

BL-15
BL-18
BL-20
BL-23
Du-4

6.9 Skin disorders

B. Sommer

Skin disorders can be caused either by any of the external pathogens, or by pathological substances generated within the body (e.g. Damp-Heat, Fire toxins). They may also be caused by deficiency conditions (e.g. Blood Dryness).

In TCM, the skin is seen as part of the Lungs and Large Intestine, so that skin disorders are often treated with points on these meridians. The Lungs house the corporeal soul (*Po*), which is responsible for the autonomic nervous system. As the most sensitive of all souls, the corporeal soul responds to any psychological upset. Weeping or vesicular dermatoses are an expression of Spleen and Stomach imbalances, and have to be treated accordingly. Itching is considered as a symptom of Wind, so that points on the Liver meridian are often selected for treatment.

The stresses of life today are often an exacerbating factor in many skin disorders. Therefore, a calming point prescription that will often have a positive 'side-effect' on the skin is recommended as the first treatment:

- Relaxing point prescription: L.I.-4, LIV-3, ST-36.

The choice of distal and local points is determined mainly by the location of the disorder; it is equally important to identify the underlying pattern accurately, in order to add the appropriate points and choose the correct needling technique. Pathogenic factors and pathological substances have to be eliminated, requiring a reducing needling technique, whereas deficiency patterns call for tonifying methods.

In general, needling directly into any affected areas should be avoided. An exception is efflorescences covering larger areas with signs of chronic Blood stagnation (dark bluish-red discoloration, lichenification, for example with chronic inverse psoriasis).

6.9.1 Acne vulgaris

The location of the affected areas will point to the site of the disharmony within the body, whereas the type of efflorescence tends to be indicative of the underlying pattern. Perioral acne with purulent pustules is a sign of Damp-Heat or Fire toxins (pus) in the *Yang Ming* (L.I. and ST meridians, perioral zone). Chronic acne with bluish-red knots indicates Blood stagnation, whereas hardened acne scars represent Phlegm.

Basic point combination

LU-5, L.I.-4, Ren-9.
Ear acupuncture: points on the reflex zones representing areas affected by acne. The addition of 101 Lung, 22 endocrine system and 13 adrenal gland has proven beneficial.

Individual point combination

Select appropriate metabolic points (after Bischko)

L.I.-4, BL-40 [BL-54 Bi], BL-58, KID-6, LIV-13.

Facial acne

S.I.-3, LU-5.

Acne near the lips

ST-45.

Acne around the nose

Ex-HN-3 (*Yin Tang*).

Acne on the back

S.I.-3, BL-62, Du-14 [Du-13 Bi].

Inverse acne, in the axilla

G.B.-38, G.B.40, P-1; if treatments are not successful, inverse acne (axilla, inguinal region) might require surgery.

Acne with pruritus

BL-13, BL-42, L.I.-11, LIV-5.

Severely purulent acne

T.B.-5, S.I.-16, L.I.-11, SP-9.

Acupuncture points

BL-13 **Location:** 1.5 cun lateral to the spinous process of T3.
Notes: back-*Shu* point of the Lungs.

BL-40 **Location:** in the centre of the popliteal crease, between the tendons of the semitendinosus and the biceps femoris.
Notes: *He*-sea point; eliminates Blood-Heat, *Qi* and Blood (*Xue*) stagnation (e.g. for acne with bluish-red nodes); Bi: master point for skin diseases.

BL-42 **Location:** 3 cun lateral to the spinous process of T3, lateral to BL-13 (back-*Shu* point of the LU), at the medial border of the scapula.
Notes: the name 'Gate of the Corporeal Soul *Po*' explains the action of this point: stops pruritus; also for psychosomatic disorders.

BL-58 **Location:** 1 cun distal and lateral to BL-57, on the lateral border of the gastrocnemius, on the soleus.
Notes: *Luo*-connecting point (connects to KID-3), metabolic point, clears Heat and resolves stagnation.

BL-62 **Location:** below the prominence of the lateral malleolus.
Notes: opening point of the *Yang Wei Mai*.

Du-14 **Location:** below the spinous process of C7.
Notes: meeting point of all *Yang* meridians.

Ex-HN-3 **Location:** at the midpoint between the eyebrows.
Notes: clears Heat; local point.

G.B.-38 **Location:** 4 cun superior to the lateral malleolus, on the anterior border of the fibula.
Notes: clears Damp-Heat.

G.B.-40 **Location:** on the junction of a horizontal line through the prominence of the lateral malleolus and a vertical line through the greatest circumference of the lateral malleolus, over the calcaneocuboidal joint.
Notes: distal point for the hypochondrium.

KID-6 **Location:** below the prominence of the medial malleolus.
Notes: metabolic point, opening point of the *Yin Qiao Mai*; tonifies *Yin* – Phlegm is the substitute for deficient *Yin*! Cools Blood (*Xue*), calms the Spirit.

L.I.-4 **Location:** on the dorsum of the hand, at the highest point of the muscle bulge between the 1st and 2nd metacarpal bones.
Notes: *Yuan*-source point, metabolic point, command point of the face, combined with L.I.-3 (master point for acne); important point for all skin disorders.

L.I.-11 **Location:** with the arm fully flexed at the radial end of the cubital crease.
Notes: *He*-sea point, tonification point; eliminates Damp-Heat and Wind.

LIV-5 **Location:** on the medial border of the tibia, 5 cun superior to the medial malleolus.
Notes: *Luo*-connecting point; specific effect on pruritus; clears Damp-Heat, firms the Essence (*Jing*); effective for related to the genital organs, sexual intercourse or puberty.

LIV-13 **Location:** on the lower border of the free end of the 11th rib.
Notes: metabolic point, front-*Mu* point of the Spleen; invigorates the Blood circulation, resolves congealed Blood (*Xue*).

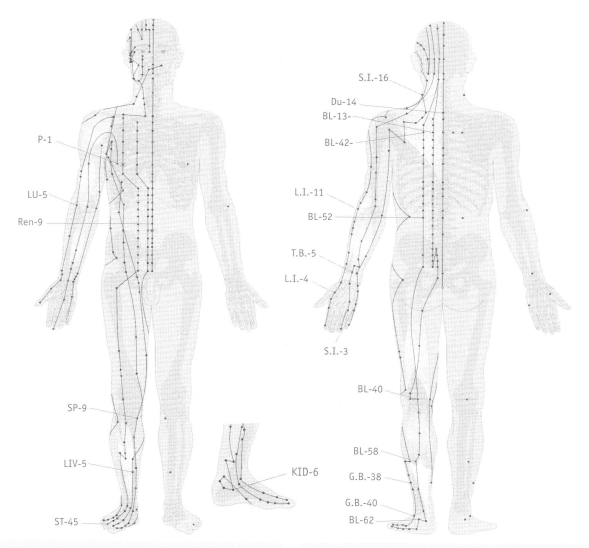

LU-5 **Location:** on the cubital crease, radial to the tendon of the biceps.
 Notes: *He*-sea point, sedation point, distal point for the face; clears Lung Heat and resolves Phlegm.
P-1 **Location:** in the 4th ICS, 1 cun lateral to the midclavicular line or the nipple.
 Notes: local point.
Ren-9 **Location:** 1 cun superior to the umbilicus.
 Notes: promotes the transformation of Fluids and Dampness.
S.I.-3 **Location:** when a fist is made, on the dorsum of the hand, in the depression at the end of the most distal palmar crease.
 Notes: opening point of the *Du Mai* with an effect on the central nervous system; eliminates Wind, Heat and Dampness.
S.I.-16 **Location:** on the posterior border of the sternocleidomastoid, at the level of the upper border of the thyroid cartilage.

 Notes: eliminates Heat toxins; local point for severe dermatoses affecting the upper back and occiput.
SP-9 **Location:** with the knee flexed in the depression inferior to the medial condyle of the tibia, at the same level as G.B.-34.
 Notes: *He*-sea point; eliminates Dampness and Heat.
ST-45 **Location:** on the 2nd toe, near the lateral corner of the nail.
 Notes: *Jing*-well point; clears Fire from the Stomach, face and skin.
T.B.-5 **Location:** 2 cun proximal to the midpoint of the dorsal wrist crease, opposite P-6.
 Notes: *Luo*-connecting point, opening point of the *Yang Wei Mai* – dominates the surface, eliminates external pathogens, especially Wind-Heat; specific action for hot or purulent dermatoses.

6.9.2 Neurodermatitis and other forms of eczema (1)

Synonym: atopic eczema, endogenous eczema.

> Eczemas are often wrongly interpreted as an expression of hyperfunction.

TCM interprets eczema as a deficiency or *Yin* disorder. Therefore, as few needles as possible should be used and only tonifying needling techniques should be applied.

Neurodermatitis can be treated with the same points as eczema, but the psychological aspect has to be considered to a greater extent.

'Curing' the atopic predisposition with acupuncture is, by its very definition, not possible, but the period of remission between flare-ups can be extended and the condition of the skin can also be stabilized for a longer period of time without the use of steroids. Some authors (e.g. Stiefvater) suggest acupuncture should not be administered for at least 2 months after the application of steroids, but in clinical practice this is hardly feasible and, based on our experience, it is not necessary to be so strict. However, the patient should be informed that steroids will reduce the effect of acupuncture.

Both moxibustion and laser provide good results. Laser is recommended particularly in the treatment of children. In addition to the treatment of indicated points, laser can be applied to particularly affected skin areas.

> Any episode of neurodermatitis or even herpetic eczema should be treated with conventional medicine. Consulting a dermatologist is strictly recommended.

Basic point combination

L.I.-4, L.I.-11, ST-36, SP-6, HE-3, BL-40 [BL-54 Bi].
Ear acupuncture: points on the reflex zones representing affected areas; also beneficial: 101 Lung, 29 occiput, 22 endocrine system, 13 adrenal gland.

In TCM the skin is associated with the Lungs and the Large Intestine. For longstanding eczema it is therefore recommended to combine the *Yuan*-source point of the affected *Yin* meridian (LU-9) and the back-*Shu* point of the Lung on the Bladder meridian (BL-13).
In addition, blood-letting at BL-40 [BL-54 Bi] is thought to have an antihistaminic effect.
TCM: the treatment goal is to clear Blood Heat, which is considered the cause of red exanthemas.

Individual point combination

Acute eczema

T.B.-5, BL-52 [BL-47 Bi].

Acupuncture points

BL-13 **Location:** 1.5 cun lateral to the spinous process of T3.
Notes: back-*Shu* point of the Lungs.

BL-40 **Location:** in the centre of the popliteal crease, between the tendons of the semitendinosus and the biceps femoris.
Notes: *He*-sea point; eliminates Blood-Heat, *Qi* and Blood (*Xue*) stagnation (e.g. for acne with bluish-red nodes); Bischko: master point for skin diseases.

BL-52 **Location:** 3 cun lateral to the spinous process of L2, lateral to BL-23 (back-*Shu* point of the KID).
Notes: has a connection to the soul of the Kidneys (*Zhi*, willpower); corticotrophic point.

HE-3 **Location:** with the elbow fully flexed, between the medial end of the cubital crease and the medial epicondyle.
Notes: *He*-sea point, master point for depression; clears Heat, lifts the emotions.

L.I.-4 **Location:** on the dorsum of the hand, at the highest point of the muscle bulge between the 1st and 2nd metacarpal bones.
Notes: *Yuan*-source point, metabolic point, command point of the face, combine with L.I.-3 (master point for acne); important point for all skin disorders.

L.I.-11 **Location:** with the arm fully flexed at the radial end of the cubital crease.
Notes: *He*-sea point, tonification point; eliminates Damp-Heat and Wind.

LU-9 **Location:** on the wrist crease, radial to the radial artery.
Notes: *Shu*-stream point, *Yuan*-source point; tonifies Lung *Qi* and *Yin*; combine with BL-13 for chronic Lung deficiency patterns.

SP-6 **Location:** 3 cun superior to the highest prominence of the medial malleolus, on the posterior border of the tibia.
Notes: regulates the skin – Dampness, Dryness, Heat; group *Luo*-connecting point (SP, LIV, KID), tonifies *Qi*, Blood (*Xue*) and *Yin*, nourishes and moves the Blood (*Xue*).

ST-36 **Location:** 1 cun lateral to the anterior crest of the tibia, 1.5 cun inferior to the lower border of the head of the fibula (G.B.-34).
Notes: *He*-sea point of the Stomach, master point for hormones; tonifies the Stomach and the Spleen, and therefore *Qi* and Blood (*Xue*); calming and strengthening.

T.B.-5 **Location:** 2 cun proximal to the midpoint of the dorsal wrist crease, opposite P-6.
Notes: *Luo*-connecting point, opening point of the *Yang Wei Mai* – dominates the surface, eliminates external pathogens, especially Wind-Heat; specific action for hot or purulent dermatoses.

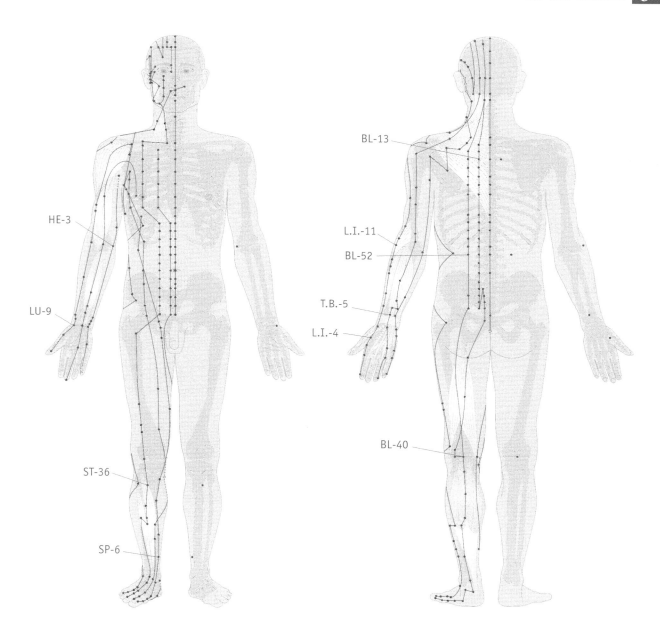

HE-3

LU-9

ST-36

SP-6

BL-13

L.I.-11

BL-52

T.B.-5

L.I.-4

BL-40

6.9.2 Neurodermatitis and other forms of eczema (2)

Individual point combination

Hand and foot eczema

S.I.-3, S.I.-5, KID-3, P-7, BL-58, T.B.-5.

Weeping eczema

SP-9, BL-52 [BL-47 Bi], Ren-9.

Chronic eczema

LU-9, BL-13.

Acupuncture points

BL-13 Location: 1.5 cun lateral to the spinous process of T3.
Notes: back-*Shu* point of the Lungs.

BL-52 Location: 3 cun lateral to the spinous process of L2, lateral to BL-23 (back *Shu* point of the KID).
Notes: has a connection to the soul of the Kidneys (*Zhi*, willpower).

BL-58 Location: 1 cun distal and lateral to BL-57, on the lateral border of the gastrocnemius, on the soleus.
Notes: *Luo*-connecting point (connects to KID-3), metabolic point; clears Heat and resolves stagnation (according to TCM, impaired circulation is caused by the stagnation of *Qi* and Blood).

KID-3 Location: between the highest prominence of the medial malleolus and the Achilles tendon.

Notes: *Yuan*-source point, *Shu*-stream point; tonifies Kidney *Yin*, *Yang* and Essence (*Jing*), stabilizes the Spirit and emotions.

LU-9 Location: on the wrist crease, radial to the radial artery.
Notes: *Shu*-stream point, *Yuan*-source point; tonifies Lung *Qi* and *Yin*.

P-7 Location: on the anterior aspect of the wrist joint, between the tendons of the flexor carpi radialis and palmaris longus.
Notes: *Yuan*-source point, *Shu*-stream point, sedation point; clears Heat; also as local point for dermatoses; calms the Heart and the Spirit.

Ren-9 Location: 1 cun superior to the umbilicus.
Notes: promotes the transformation of Fluids and Dampness.

S.I.-3 Location: when a fist is made, on the dorsum of the hand, in the depression at the end of the most distal palmar crease.
Notes: opening point of the *Du Mai* with an effect on the central nervous system; eliminates Wind, Heat and Dampness.

S.I.-5 Location: on the ulnar aspect of the wrist crease, distal to the styloid process of the ulna and proximal to the triquetrum bone.
Notes: *Jing*-river point, Fire point; dispels Damp-Heat.

SP-9 Location: with the knee flexed in the depression inferior to the medial condyle of the tibia, at the same level as G.B.-34.
Notes: *He*-sea point; eliminates Dampness and Heat.

T.B.-5 Location: 2 cun proximal to the midpoint of the dorsal wrist crease, opposite P-6.
Notes: *Luo*-connecting point, opening point of the *Yang Wei Mai* – dominates the surface, eliminates external pathogens, especially Wind-Heat; specific action for hot or purulent dermatoses.

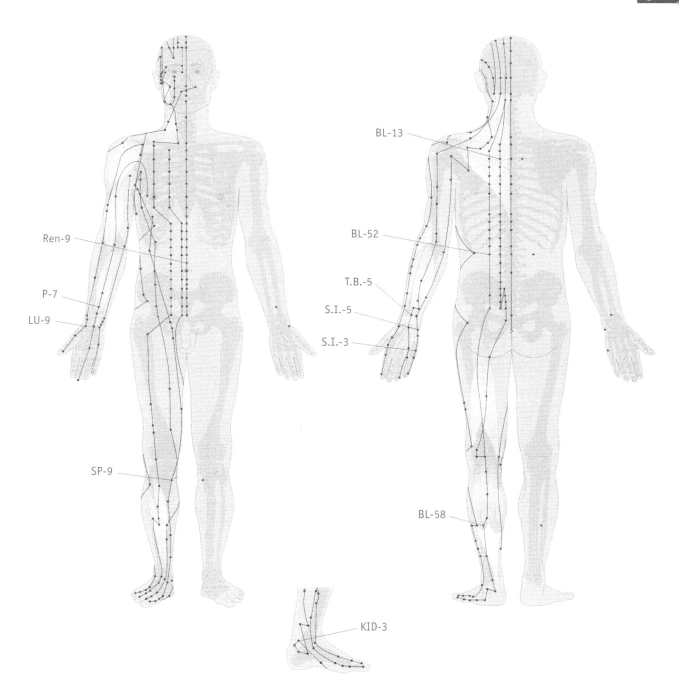

Ren-9

P-7

LU-9

SP-9

BL-13

BL-52

T.B.-5

S.I.-5

S.I.-3

BL-58

KID-3

6.9.2 Neurodermatitis and other forms of eczema (3)

Individual point combination

Severe pruritus

LU-7, SP-10, LIV-5, BL-13.

Accompanied by oedema

SP-9.

Facial eczema

LU-5, L.I.-4.

Select appropriate points from the following metabolic points after Bischko

L.I.-4, BL-40 [BL-54 Bi], BL-58, KID-6, LIV-13.
Extra point: Ex-LE-4 (*Nei Xi Yan*)

Acupuncture points

BL-13   Location: 1.5 cun lateral to the spinous process of T3.
Notes: back-*Shu* point of the Lungs.

BL-40   Location: in the centre of the popliteal crease, between the tendons of the semitendinosus and the biceps femoris.
Notes: *He*-sea point; eliminates Blood-Heat, *Qi* and Blood (*Xue*) stagnation (e.g. for acne with bluish-red nodes); Bi: master point for skin diseases.

BL-58   Location: 1 cun distal and lateral to BL-57, on the lateral border of the gastrocnemius, on the soleus.
Notes: *Luo*-connecting point (connects to KID-3), metabolic point; clears Heat and resolves stagnation.

Ex-LE-4   Location: with the knee flexed, the inner eye of the knee is in a depression medial to the patellar ligament (lateral to the tendon is the outer eye of the knee, which is also identical with ST-35).
Notes: local point.

KID-6   Location: below the prominence of the medial malleolus.
Notes: metabolic point, opening point of the *Yin Qiao Mai*; tonifies *Yin* – Phlegm is the substitute for deficient *Yin*! Cools Blood (*Xue*), calms the Spirit.

L.I.-4   Location: on the dorsum of the hand, at the highest point of the muscle bulge between the 1st and 2nd metacarpal bones.
Notes: *Yuan*-source point, metabolic point, command point of the face, combine with L.I.-3 (master point for acne); important point for all skin disorders.

LIV-5   Location: on the medial border of the tibia, 5 cun superior to the medial malleolus.
Notes: *Luo*-connecting point; specific effect on pruritus; clears Damp-Heat, firms the Essence (*Jing*); effective for dermatoses related to the genital organs, sexual intercourse or puberty.

LIV-13   Location: on the lower border of the free end of the 11th rib.
Notes: metabolic point, front-*Mu* point of the Spleen; invigorates the Blood circulation, resolves congealed Blood (*Xue*).

LU-5   Location: on the cubital crease, radial to the tendon of the biceps.
Notes: *He*-sea point, sedation point; distal point for the face, clears Lung Heat and resolves Phlegm.

LU-7   Location: 1.5 cun proximal to the wrist crease, superior to the radial artery.
Notes: *Luo*-connecting point, opening point for the *Ren Mai*, master point for stagnation; sedating effect for headaches in conjunction with the onset of a cold, tonifies Lung and Kidney *Yin*, dispels external pathogenic factors.

SP-9   Location: with the knee flexed in the depression inferior to the medial condyle of the tibia, at the same level as G.B.-34.
Notes: *He*-sea point; eliminates Dampness and Heat.

SP-10   Location: with the knee flexed, 2 cun superior to the upper patellar border, medial to the vastus medialis.
Notes: 'Sea of Blood' – cools, tonifies, invigorates the Blood (*Xue*).

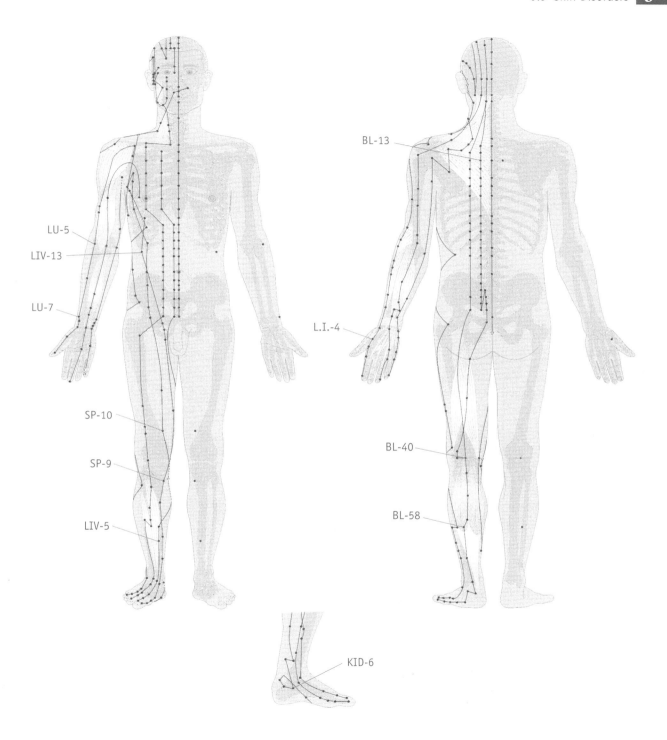

BL-13

LU-5

LIV-13

LU-7

L.I.-4

SP-10

BL-40

SP-9

LIV-5

BL-58

KID-6

6.9.3 Herpes zoster and post-herpetic neuralgia (1)

The prognosis for acute herpes zoster is generally better than for post-herpetic neuralgia. The sooner acupuncture is administered, the better the results regarding both shortening and alleviating post-herpetic pain.

TCM

Herpes zoster is associated with the Liver and Gall Bladder, and is therefore treated by using points on their pertaining meridians.

The acute stage of the disease is interpreted as Wind-Heat; as soon as purulent blisters occur it is considered as Damp-Heat. Fever, severe pain and aggressive efflorescences are a sign of toxic Heat; post-herpetic neuralgia is a manifestation of residual Heat with Wind; recurring herpes zoster is interpreted as a *Wen Bing*: the virus is a form of Damp-Heat lurking in the *Qi* level. Eliminating the pathogen is a crucial aspect of the treatment.

Method: distal points are always strongly stimulated in a reducing manner. Freshly affected areas of skin are surrounded by 4–5 needles. In addition, the front-*Mu* and the back-*Shu* points of the affected segments should be needled.

Ear acupuncture can further support the treatment: normal or intradermal needles are inserted at pressure-sensitive points on the helix, in the 'vegetative' groove anterior to it, and also at the thalamus point.

Laser treatment of the affected skin areas also contributes to the healing process.

Complications (zoster ophthalmicus, zoster oticus, danger of cerebral involvement) require intravenous virus-static therapy and preferably a multidisciplinary approach. This does not exclude concurrent or subsequent acupuncture therapy.

Basic point combination

BL-60, LIV-3, P-7, local points surrounding the skin lesion, especially at the beginning and end of the elongated efflorescences.

Ear acupuncture: points on the helix between the points 72–78 (Chinese) or 25–30 (Nogier); alternatively, pressure-sensitive points representing the affected locations of the efflorescences as well as the thalamus point.

Individual point combination

Herpes zoster affecting the head

 Caution: involvement of the optical or brain nerves (accompanying treatment by specialists, may require hospitalization).

Herpes zoster affecting the mastoid and ear

T.B.-3, T.B.-17, G.B.-20, G.B.-34, LIV-5.
During the early stages: G.B.-41, T.B.-5.

Cervical herpes zoster

T.B.-16 or G.B.-21, S.I.-16.

Thoracic herpes zoster

G.B.-40, G.B.-41. Micromassage on hand point 3; front-*Mu* points and back-*Shu* points of the affected segments.

Acupuncture points

BL-60 **Location:** midway between the Achilles tendon and the highest prominence of the lateral malleolus.
  Notes: *Jing*-river point, master point for pain along the meridian pathway.
G.B.-20 **Location:** posterior to the mastoid, between the trapezius and sternocleidomastoid muscles, on the lower border of the occiput.
  Notes: eliminates Wind from the head.
G.B.-21 **Location:** on the highest point of the shoulder, midway between the acromion and the spinous process of C7.
  Notes: clears Heat; contraindicated during pregnancy.
G.B.-34 **Location:** with the knee flexed, in the depression anterior and inferior to the head of the fibula.
  Notes: *He*-sea point, *Hui*-meeting point of the tendons, master point of the musculature; relaxes the tendons, promotes the smooth flow of Liver *Qi*.
G.B.-40 **Location:** on the junction of a horizontal line through the prominence of the lateral malleolus and a vertical line through the greatest circumference of the lateral malleolus, over the calcaneocuboidal joint.
  Notes: distal point for the hypochondrium.
G.B.-41 **Location:** in the depression distal to the junction of the 4th and 5th metatarsal bones.
  Notes: *Shu*-stream point, opening point of the *Dai Mai*; eliminates Damp-Heat and Fire, promotes the harmonious flow of Liver *Qi*, alleviates pain.
Hand point 3 **Location:** on the thumb, at the radial end of the palmar crease at the distal phalangeal joint.

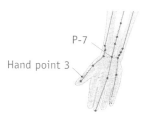

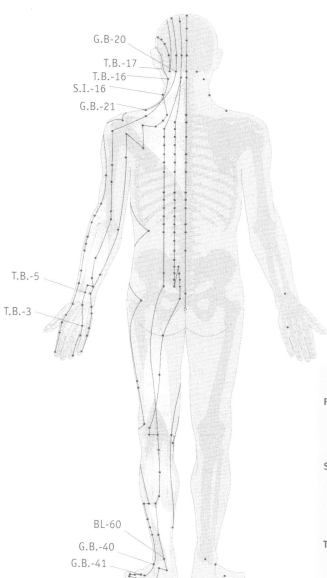

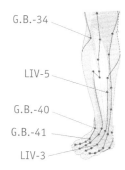

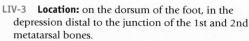

Notes: *Luo*-connecting point; effective for pruritus; clears Damp-Heat.

P-7 **Location:** on the anterior aspect of the wrist joint, between the tendons of the flexor carpi radialis and palmaris longus.
Notes: *Yuan*-source point and *Shu*-stream point, sedation point; clears Heat, local point for dermatoses; calms the Heart and Spirit.

S.I.-16 **Location:** on the posterior border of the sternocleidomastoid, at the level of the upper border of the thyroid cartilage.
Notes: eliminates Heat toxins; local point for severe dermatosis related to the genital organs, sexual intercourse or puberty.

T.B.-3 **Location:** when a loose fist is made on the dorsum of the hand, between the 4th and 5th metacarpal bones, in the depression proximal to the metacarpophalangeal joints.
Notes: eliminates Wind-Heat for disorders of the eyes and ears, resolves *Qi* stagnation.

T.B.-5 **Location:** 2 cun proximal to the midpoint of the dorsal wrist crease, opposite P-6.
Notes: *Luo*-connecting point, opening point of the *Yang Wei Mai* – dominates the surface, eliminates all external pathogens.

T.B.-16 **Location:** on the posterior border of the sternocleidomastoid, at the level of the mandibular angle, inferior to T.B.-17.
Notes: local point.

T.B.-17 **Location:** on the anterior border of the mastoid.
Notes: eliminates Wind; local point.

LIV-3 **Location:** on the dorsum of the foot, in the depression distal to the junction of the 1st and 2nd metatarsal bones.
Notes: *Yuan*-source point and *Shu*-stream point; subdues Liver *Yang*, eliminates Liver Wind, harmonizes the flow of Liver *Qi*, regulates the flow of *Qi* and thus also the Blood (*Xue*) flow, eliminates Damp-Heat from the Liver and Gall Bladder.

LIV-5 **Location:** on the medial border of the tibia, 5 cun superior to the medial malleolus.

6.9.3 Herpes zoster and post-herpetic neuralgia (2)

For general weakness

L.I.-10, SP-6, ST-36, HE-3, KID-10, BL-60.

Post-herpetic neuralgia

Basic point combination as with acute herpes zoster. Also sedating method for distal points.
Laser: treat affected skin areas as well as distal points. Daily treatments for 5–6 days, then slowly reduce to 1 weekly treatment.

> Bilateral needling of only G.B.-40 towards KID-6 (*Zhao Hai*). Initially gentle, then stronger stimulation. The extra point *Long Yan* (Dragon's Eye) may be added: on the little finger; when a loose fist is made, the point is on the radial aspect of the crease of the metacarpophalangeal joint (after *He* and *Meng*).

Acupuncture points

BL-60   Location: midway between the Achilles tendon and the highest prominence of the lateral malleolus.
Notes: *Jing*-river point, master point for pain along the meridian pathway.

G.B.-40   Location: on the junction of a horizontal line through the prominence of the lateral malleolus and a vertical line through the greatest circumference of the lateral malleolus, over the calcaneocuboidal joint.
Notes: distal point for the hypochondrium.

HE-3   Location: with the elbow fully flexed, between the medial end of the cubital crease and the medial epicondyle.
Notes: *He*-sea point, master point for depression; lifts the emotions.

KID-6   Location: below the prominence of the medial malleolus.
Notes: metabolic point, opening point of the *Yin Qiao Mai*; tonifies *Yin* – Phlegm is the substitute for deficient *Yin*! Cools Blood (*Xue*), calms the Spirit.

KID-10   Location: with the knee flexed, at the medial end of the popliteal crease, between the tendons of the semitendinosus and semimembranosus.
Notes: *He*-sea point; cools Fire.

L.I.-10   Location: on the radial aspect of the forearm, 3 cun distal to L.I.-11, on the belly of the extensor muscles.
Notes: resolves swellings.

SP-6   Location: 3 cun superior to the highest prominence of the medial malleolus, on the posterior border of the tibia.
Notes: regulates the skin – Dampness, Dryness, Heat; group *Luo*-connecting point (SP, LIV, KID), tonifies *Qi*, Blood (*Xue*) and *Yin*, nourishes and moves the Blood (*Xue*).

ST-36   Location: 1 cun lateral to the anterior crest of the tibia, 1.5 cun inferior to the lower border of the head of the fibula (G.B.-34).
Notes: *He*-sea point of the Stomach, master point for hormones; tonifies the Stomach and the Spleen, and therefore *Qi* and Blood (*Xue*); calming and strengthening.

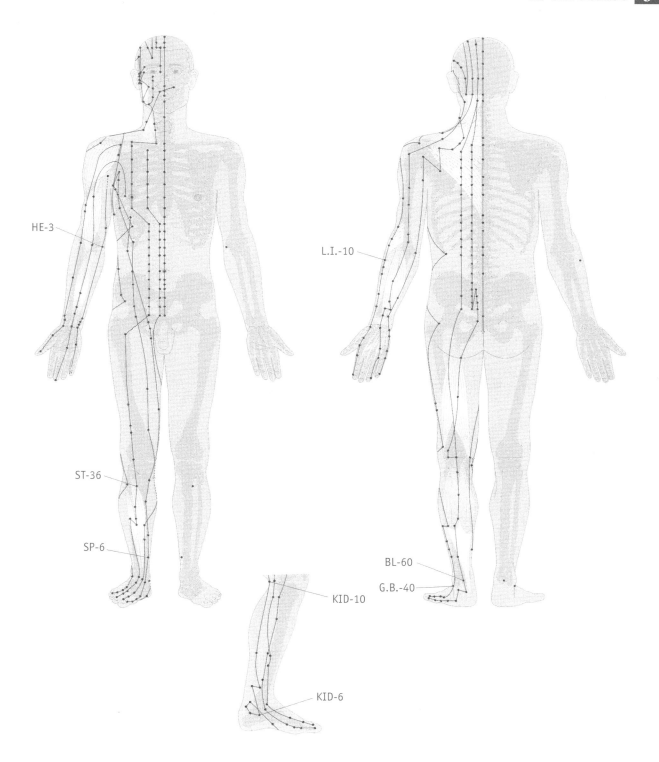

HE-3

L.I.-10

ST-36

SP-6

BL-60

G.B.-40

KID-10

KID-6

6.9.4 Pruritus

Generalized itching always presents a great strain for the patient and often does not respond well to either conventional treatment or acupuncture. As the causes, especially for chronic pruritus, can vary considerably, specialists of both internal medicine and dermatology should also be consulted.

▌ Acupuncture should be given only once diagnostic tests for fungal or parasitic infections have been carried out.

Taking a detailed medical history allows the therapist to determine the affected meridians, which can then be treated. Although rigid point prescriptions generally do not work well here, some basic point combinations that have proven beneficial are described below.

In contrast, localized itching, as well as anal and vulvar itching, tends to respond better to acupuncture.

TCM

Pruritus is considered as Wind or Wind-Heat. Idiopathic pruritus may be due to the wanderings of the soul that cannot be anchored because of Blood deficiency or anxiety.

Basic point combination

L.I.-11, SP-6, LIV-5, Ex-LE-3 (*Bai Chong Wo*).
Ear acupuncture: 22 endocrine system, 71 urticaria, 101 Lungs.

Individual point combination

Vulvar, scrotal, perianal pruritus

LIV-5, SP-10, BL-57. Du-1 as local point, Du-2, Ren-1, SP-9. Despite being very effective, the local points are, unfortunately, rarely used because of their inconvenient location.

Pruritus around the eyes and eyelids

G.B.-1, LIV-3.

Pruritus of the ears

G.B.-2, G.B.-12, T.B.-17.

Facial pruritus

LU-5.

Acupuncture points

BL-57 **Location:** 1.5 cun lateral to the spinous process of T7.
  Notes: eliminates Damp-Heat from the Lower Burner.
Du-1 **Location:** between the coccyx and the anus.
  Notes: drains Damp-Heat.
Du-2 **Location:** in the sacral hiatus.
  Notes: may be used instead of Du-1 (location!); eliminates Damp-Heat.
Ex-LE-3 **Location:** 1 cun superior to SP-10 (SP-10: with the knee flexed 2 cun superior to the upper medial border of the patella, in a depression on the quadriceps femoris).
  Notes: 'Nest of the 100 worms' – important point for pruritus, especially if due to parasites.
G.B.-1 **Location:** 0.5 cun lateral to the outer canthus of the eye, in the depression lateral to the orbit.
  Notes: dispels Wind-Heat, eliminates Fire, benefits the eyes.
G.B.-2 **Location:** with the mouth open, in the depression anterior to the antitragic notch, posterior to the condyloid process of the mandible.
  Notes: local point for itching of the ears.
G.B.-12 **Location:** posterior and inferior to the mastoid, insertion of the sternocleidomastoid; ask the patient to rotate the head contralaterally.
  Notes: eliminates Wind.
L.I.-11 **Location:** with the arm fully flexed at the radial end of the cubital crease.
  Notes: *He*-sea point, tonification point; eliminates Damp-Heat and Wind.
LIV-3 **Location:** on the dorsum of the foot, in the depression distal to the junction of the 1st and 2nd metatarsal bones.
  Notes: *Yuan*-source point and *Shu*-stream point; subdues Liver *Yang*, eliminates Liver Wind, harmonizes the flow of Liver *Qi*.
LIV-5 **Location:** on the medial border of the tibia, 5 cun superior to the medial malleolus.
  Notes: *Luo*-connecting point; specific effect on pruritus; clears Damp-Heat, firms the Essence (*Jing*); effective for dermatosis related to the genital organs, sexual intercourse or puberty.
LU-5 **Location:** on the cubital crease, radial to the tendon of the biceps.
  Notes: *He*-sea point, sedation point; distal point for the face, as water point cooling for heat, tonifies *Yin*, moistens Dryness.
Ren-1 **Location:** at the perineum, between the anus and the scrotum and posterior labial commissure respectively.
  Notes: tonifies the *Yin*, drains Damp-Heat.
SP-6 **Location:** 3 cun superior to the highest prominence of the medial malleolus, on the posterior border of the tibia.
  Notes: regulates the skin – Dampness, Dryness, Heat; group *Luo*-connecting point (SP, LIV, KID); tonifies *Qi*, Blood (*Xue*) and *Yin*, nourishes and moves the Blood (*Xue*).

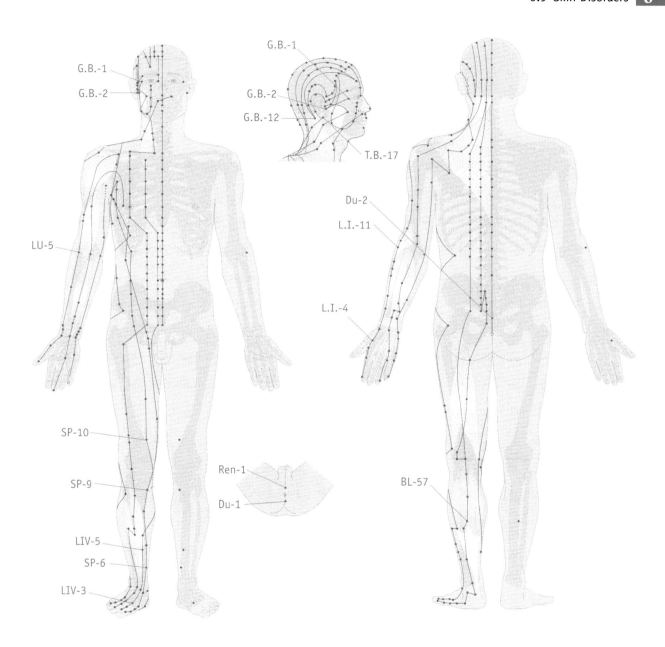

SP-9   **Location:** with the knee flexed in the depression inferior to the medial condyle of the tibia, at the same level as G.B.-34.

    Notes: *He*-sea point; eliminates Dampness and Heat.

SP-10   **Location:** with the knee flexed, 2 cun superior to the upper patellar border, medial to the vastus medialis.

Notes: 'Sea of Blood' – cools, tonifies, invigorates the Blood (*Xue*).

T.B.-17   **Location:** on the anterior border of the mastoid.

    Notes: eliminates Wind; local point.

6.9.5 Urticaria and allergies

Urticaria is also described as a common disorder in China.

TCM

TCM describes the cause of urticaria as pathogenic *Qi* attacking and injuring the meridians. In addition, enteral triggers can lead to a disharmony of the Spleen and Stomach.
Helpful advice: compared with other allergies, success rates in the treatment of urticaria are not promising. Although treatment progress can be frustrating at times, acupuncture is still recommended, especially for the more chronic forms of urticaria. In these cases, acupuncture may well provide sufficient relief to reduce medication.

Basic point combination

L.I.-4 and L.I.-11, ST-36, SP-6, BL-40 [BL-54 Bi], Du-14 [Du-13 Bi].
Ear acupuncture: 78 allergy.

Individual point combination

Allergies

LIV-3, Du-20, Ex-HN-6 (*Er Jian*, allergy point).
Ear acupuncture: 78 allergy.

Urticaria

T.B.-6, L.I.-4, L.I.-11, SP-6, SP-10 sedating.

Urticaria due to cold

KID-6, BL-23 or BL-52 [BL-47 Bi], T.B.-5.

Acupuncture points

BL-23 **Location:** 1.5 cun lateral to the spinous process of L2, lateral to Du-4.
Notes: back-*Shu* point of the Kidneys; tonifies the *Qi*, *Yang*, *Yin* and Essence (*Jing*) of the Kidneys.

BL-40 **Location:** in the centre of the popliteal crease, between the tendons of the semitendinosus and the biceps femoris.
Notes: *He*-sea point; eliminates Summer-Heat, Blood-Heat as well as Damp-Heat and Heat toxins for dermatoses; also regulates *Qi* and Blood (*Xue*) stagnation; Bi: master point for skin diseases.

BL-52 **Location:** 3 cun lateral to the spinous process of L2, lateral to BL-23 (back *Shu* point of the KID).
Notes: has a relationship with the soul of the Kidneys (*Zhi*, willpower); corticotrophic.

Du-14 **Location:** below the spinous process of C7.
Notes: meeting point of all *Yang* meridians; disperses Wind, Cold, Heat or tonifies – depending on the stimulation.

Du-20 **Location:** on a line connecting the apices of the ears, 7 cun superior the posterior hairline.
Notes: meeting point of all divergent meridians; an internal branch of the Liver terminates here.

Ex-HN-6 **Location:** at the highest point of the apex of the ear.
Notes: 'allergy point'.

KID-6 **Location:** below the prominence of the medial malleolus.
Notes: metabolic point, opening point of the *Yin Qiao Mai*; tonifies *Yin* – Phlegm is the substitute for deficient *Yin*! Cools Blood (*Xue*), calms the Spirit.

L.I.-4 **Location:** on the dorsum of the hand, at the highest point of the muscle bulge between the 1st and 2nd metacarpal bones.
Notes: *Yuan*-source point, metabolic point; eliminates Wind-Cold and Wind-Heat; combined with ST-36 tonifies *Qi* and Blood (*Xue*).

L.I.-11 **Location:** with the arm fully flexed at the radial end of the cubital crease.
Notes: *He*-sea point, tonification point; eliminates Damp-Heat and Wind.

LIV-3 **Location:** on the dorsum of the foot, in the depression distal to the junction of the 1st and 2nd metatarsal bones.
Notes: *Yuan*-source point and *Shu*-stream point; subdues Liver *Yang*, eliminates Liver Wind, harmonizes the flow of Liver *Qi*, regulates the *Qi* flow, eliminates Damp-Heat from the Liver and Gall Bladder.

SP-6 **Location:** 3 cun superior to the highest prominence of the medial malleolus, on the posterior border of the tibia.
Notes: regulates the skin – Dampness, Dryness, Heat; group *Luo*-connecting point (SP, LIV, KID); tonifies *Qi*, Blood (*Xue*) and *Yin*; nourishes and moves the Blood (*Xue*).

SP-10 **Location:** with the knee flexed, 2 cun superior to the upper patellar border, medial to the vastus medialis.
Notes: 'Sea of Blood' – cools, tonifies, invigorates the Blood (*Xue*).

ST-36 **Location:** 1 cun lateral to the anterior crest of the tibia, 1.5 cun inferior to the lower border of the head of the fibula (G.B.-34).
Notes: *He*-sea point of the Stomach, master point for hormones; tonifies the Stomach and Spleen, and therefore *Qi* and Blood (*Xue*); calming and strengthening.

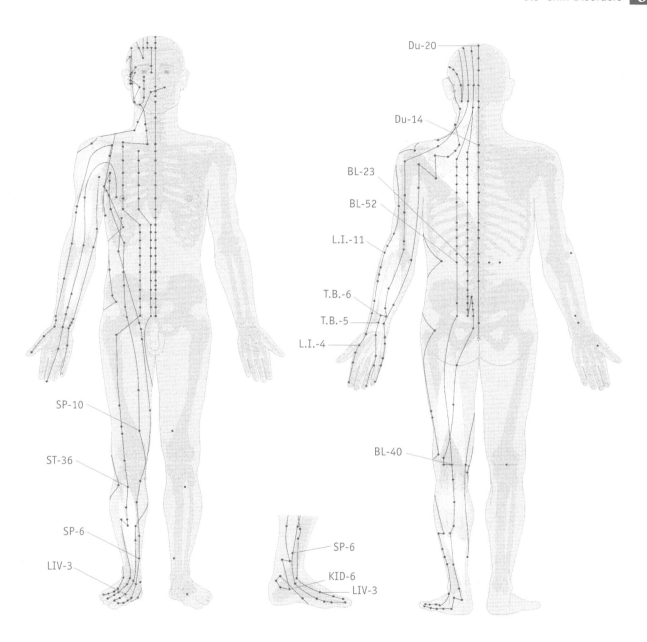

T.B.-5 Location: 2 cun proximal to the midpoint of the
dorsal wrist crease, opposite P-6.
Notes: *Luo*-connecting point, opening point of the *Yang
Wei Mai* – dominates the surface, eliminates external
pathogens, especially Wind-Heat; specific action for hot
or purulent dermatoses.

T.B.-6 Location: 3 cun proximal to the midpoint of the
dorsal wrist crease.
Notes: as Fire point eliminates Wind-Heat and Blood
(*Xue*) Heat.

6.10 Ear, nose and throat disorders

G. Kubiena

6.10.1 Rhinitis (1)

Acupuncture can help quickly and efficiently here. Particularly beneficial is the combination with phytotherapy and homoeopathy. As always, it is necessary to distinguish excess pathogenic factors and deficiency of a physiological substrate.

Basic point combination

L.I.-4. L.I.-20, BL-13.

Individual point combination

Clear the nasal passages instantly

T.B.-17, L.I.-20 or Ex-HN-8 (*Shang Yin Xiang = Bi Tong*), Ex-HN-3 (*Yin Tang*, 'point de merveille'), Du-23. Ear acupuncture: rhinopharynx (very effective).

Acute cold, no fever (excess Wind-Cold)

L.I.-4 (ginger and moxa), L.I.-20, LU-7, BL-12, BL-13 with cupping.

Acute cold, with fever (excess Wind-Heat)

L.I.-4, L.I.-20, L.I.-11, T.B.-5, BL-12, BL-13 cupping, Du-14 [Du-13 Bi]; no moxa.

Chronic rhinitis (Lung and Spleen *Qi* deficiency)

LU-9, ST-36, SP-3 or SP-6, BL-13, BL-20, Du-12, Ren-6.

Basic prophylactic treatment for colds

BL-43 [BL-38 Bi], BL-17, ST-36.

Acupuncture points

BL-12 **Location:** 1.5 cun lateral to the spinous process of T2.
   Notes: eliminates external Wind, releases the surface; promotes the descending and dispersing of Lung *Qi*.

BL-13 **Location:** 1.5 cun lateral to the spinous process of T3.
   Notes: back-*Shu* point of the Lungs; promotes the descending and dispersing of Lung *Qi*.

BL-17 **Location:** 1.5 cun lateral to the spinous process of T7.
   Notes: back-*Shu* point of the diaphragm, *Hui*-meeting point of the Blood (*Xue*); stimulates the immune system.

BL-20 **Location:** 1.5 cun lateral to the spinous process of T11.
   Notes: back-*Shu* point of the Spleen; together with ST-36 and Ren-12, tonifies the Spleen.

BL-43 **Location:** 3 cun lateral to the spinous process of T4, lateral to BL-14 (back-*Shu* point of the P), at the medial border of the scapula.
   Notes: stimulates prenatal and postnatal Essence (*Jing*), stimulates the immune system.

Du-12 **Location:** below the spinous process of T3, level with BL-13.
   Notes: tonifies the defensive *Qi* (*Wei Qi*).

Du-14 **Location:** below the spinous process of C7.
   Notes: meeting point of all *Yang* meridians; the effect depends on the technique used: reducing method to disperse Wind, Cold, Heat; tonifying method for overall strengthening.

Du-23 **Location:** on the anterior midline, 1 cun within the anterior hairline.
   Notes: dispels Wind from the nasal passages, strengthens the *Du Mai*, stops nasal discharge.

Ex-HN-3 **Location:** at the midpoint between the eyebrows.
   Notes: dispels Wind from the nasal passages; very effective for frontal headaches (hence its nickname 'point de merveille' – 'miracle point').

Ex-HN-8 **Location:** at the superior end of the nasolabial groove.
   Notes: dispels Wind from the nasal passages; use as an alternative to L.I.-20.

L.I.-4 **Location:** on the dorsum of the hand, at the highest point of the muscle bulge between the 1st and 2nd metacarpal bones.
   Notes: *Yuan*-source point, command point of the face; eliminates external Wind (with LU-7), Cold, Heat; with KID-7 induces sweating; important distal point for ENT disorders; standard point prescription for fever: L.I.-4, L.I.-11, Du-14.

L.I.-11 **Location:** with the arm fully flexed at the radial end of the cubital crease.
   Notes: *He*-sea point, tonification point; eliminates external Wind, Heat, Dampness; with L.I.-4 and Du-14 for fever.

L.I.-20 **Location:** in the nasolabial groove, at the level of the midpoint of the lateral border of the ala nasi.
   Notes: dispels external Wind, opens the nasal passages.

LU-7 **Location:** 1.5 cun proximal to the wrist crease, superior to the radial artery.
   Notes: *Luo*-connecting point, opening point for the *Ren Mai*, which, especially in women, supports the *Du Mai*; restores the Lung's dispersing and descending function.

LU-9 **Location:** on the wrist crease, radial to the radial artery.
   Notes: *Shu*-stream point, *Yuan*-source point, *Hui*-meeting point of the vessels; combined with BL-13 effect on the Lung organ, strengthens the defensive *Qi* (*Wei Qi*).

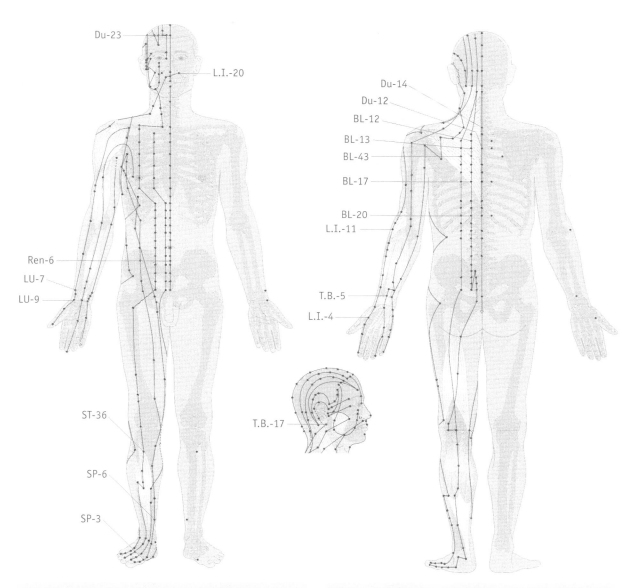

Du-23

L.I.-20

Du-14
Du-12
BL-12
BL-13
BL-43
BL-17
BL-20
L.I.-11

Ren-6
LU-7
LU-9

T.B.-5
L.I.-4

ST-36

T.B.-17

SP-6

SP-3

Ren-6 **Location:** 1.5 cun inferior to the umbilicus.
Notes: tonifies and generally invigorates *Qi*.

SP-3 **Location:** just proximal to the metatarsophalangeal joint of the big toe, over the tendon of the abductor hallucis longus.
Notes: *Shu*-stream point, *Yuan*-source point; harmonizing effect on the Stomach and Spleen, has an effect on Heart function.

SP-6 **Location:** 3 cun superior to the highest prominence of the medial malleolus, on the posterior border of the tibia.
Notes: as group *Luo*-connecting point (SP, LIV, KID), tonifies *Qi*, Blood (*Xue*) and *Yin*, nourishes and moves the Blood (*Xue*), eliminates Dampness.

ST-36 **Location:** 1 cun lateral to the anterior crest of the tibia, 1.5 cun inferior to the lower border of the head of the fibula (G.B.-34).
Notes: *He*-sea point; combined with Ren-12 and BL-20 tonifies the Spleen – the main producer of postnatal *Qi*.

T.B.-5 **Location:** 2 cun proximal to the midpoint of the dorsal wrist crease, opposite P-6.
Notes: *Luo*-connecting point, opening point of the *Yang Wei Mai* – dominates the surface, eliminates external pathogens, especially Wind-Heat.

T.B.-17 **Location:** on the anterior border of the mastoid.
Notes: meeting point with the Gall Bladder meridian; instantly unblocks the nose.

6.10.1 Rhinitis (2)

Allergic rhinitis, hay fever, pollinosis

Acute cases: treat as acute rhinitis, add G.B.-20 and ear acupuncture: 78 allergy point, 13 adrenal glands, 23 endocrine system, 55 *Shen Men*.

TCM: allergens are often distributed by the air; therefore allergic rhinitis often manifests with Wind symptoms. Depending on the symptoms, we can distinguish:

- Wind-Cold: only blocked nose, clear discharge, sneezing attacks; treat as acute cold without fever; add G.B.-20 and ear points as above.
- Wind-Heat: accompanied by fever, red eyes, sore throat; treat as acute cold with fever; add G.B.-20 and ear acupuncture as above.
- Chronic rhinitis – vasomotor rhinitis: deficiency of the Lungs, Kidneys, Spleen and *Du Mai*:
  - **Symptomatic treatment:** basic point combination plus 'clear nose' points plus G.B.-20 and ear acupuncture as above
  - **Root:** *Du Mai*: S.I.-3 and BL-62, especially in women add LU-7 and KID-6 for the *Ren Mai*; **Lung Qi:** BL-13, LU-9, Du-12; **Kidney deficiency:** BL-23 and KID-3; **Spleen Qi:** Ren-12, ST-36, BL-20; **Qi in general:** Du-4, Ren-4.

Prophylactic treatment during remission

S.I.-3, BL-62 (in women LU-7, KID-6); Du-4, Du-12, Du-14 [Du-13 Bi], Du-23, Du-24, Ren-4, BL-23, KID-3, G.B.-20, begin treatments at least 4 weeks before the expected onset of allergic rhinitis (symptoms: susceptible to colds, recurring rhinitis, weak back; tongue and complexion: pale; pulse: weak and deep; cause: weakened defence systems of the *Du Mai*, Lungs, Spleen and Kidneys).

As there are no symptoms during remission: no symptomatic points.

Acupuncture points

BL-13 **Location:** 1.5 cun lateral to the spinous process of T3.
Notes: back-*Shu* point of the Lungs; promotes the dispersing and descending of Lung *Qi*.

BL-20 **Location:** 1.5 cun lateral to the spinous process of T11.
Notes: back-*Shu* point of the Spleen; combined with ST-36 and Ren-12 tonifies the Spleen.

BL-23 **Location:** 1.5 cun lateral to the spinous process of L2.
Notes: back-*Shu* point of the Kidneys; together with KID-3/SP-6 stimulates the immune system.

BL-62 **Location:** below the prominence of the lateral malleolus.
Notes: opening point of the *Yang Qiao Mai*, supporting partner of the *Du Mai*.

Du-4 **Location:** below the spinous process of L2, at the same level as BL-23 and BL-52.
Notes: combined with Ren-4 tonifies the *Yin* and *Yang* of the *Du Mai*.

Du-12 **Location:** below the spinous process of T3, level with BL-13.
Notes: tonifies the defensive *Qi* (*Wei Qi*).

Du-14 **Location:** below the spinous process of C7.
Notes: meeting point of all *Yang* meridians; the effect depends on the technique used: reducing method to disperse Wind, Cold, Heat; tonifying method for overall strengthening; combine with L.I.-4 and L.I.-11 for fever.

Du-23 **Location:** on the anterior midline, 1 cun within the anterior hairline.
Notes: dispels Wind from the nasal passages, strengthens the *Du Mai*, stops nasal discharge.

Du-24 **Location:** on the anterior midline, 0.5 cun within the anterior hairline.
Notes: see Du-23.

G.B.-20 **Location:** posterior to the mastoid, between the trapezius and sternocleidomastoid muscles, on the lower border of the occiput.
Notes: dispels Wind, important symptomatic point for headaches.

KID-3 **Location:** between the highest prominence of the medial malleolus and the Achilles tendon.
Notes: *Yuan*-source point; combined with BL-23 tonifies the Kidneys.

KID-6 **Location:** below the prominence of the medial malleolus.
Notes: opening point of the *Yin Qiao Mai* (the partner of the *Ren Mai*).

LU-7 **Location:** 1.5 cun proximal to the wrist crease, superior to the radial artery.
Notes: opening point of the *Ren Mai*, which, particularly in women, supports the *Du Mai*; restores the dispersing and descending function of the Lung *Qi*.

LU-9 **Location:** on the wrist crease, radial to the radial artery.
Notes: *Shu*-stream point, *Yuan*-source point; tonifies Lung *Qi* and *Yin*. Combine with BL-13 for chronic Lung deficiency patterns.

Ren-4 **Location:** 2 cun superior to the upper border of the pubic symphysis (2/5 of the distance between the pubic symphysis and the umbilicus).
Notes: combined with Du-4 strengthens the *Du Mai*.

Ren-12 **Location:** midway between the umbilicus and the xiphoid process.
Notes: front-*Mu* point of the Stomach and the Middle Burner; combined with ST-36 and BL-20 supports the Spleen.

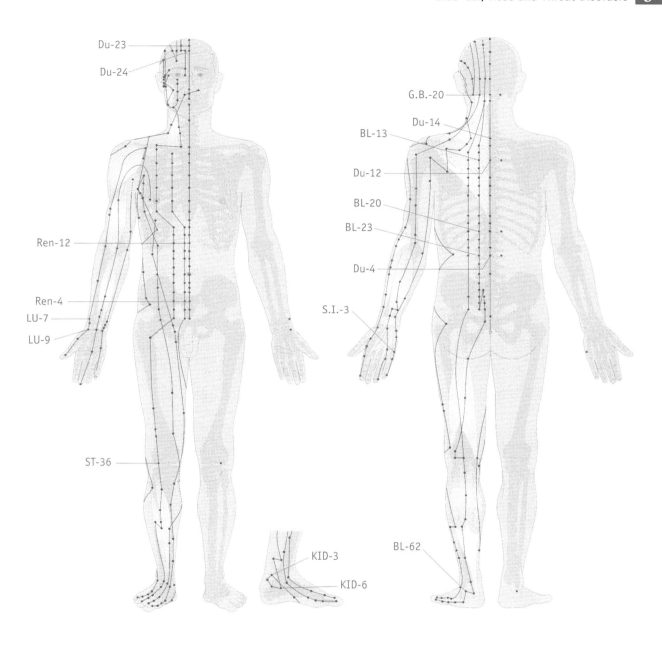

S.I.-3   Location: when a fist is made, on the dorsum of the hand, in the depression at the end of the most distal palmar crease.
Notes: opening point of the *Du Mai*; most effective if combined with BL-62.

ST-36   Location: 1 cun lateral to the anterior crest of the tibia, 1.5 cun inferior to the lower border of the head of the fibula (G.B.-34).
Notes: *He*-sea point; combined with Ren-12 and BL-20 tonifies the Spleen – the main producer of postnatal *Qi*.

6.10.2 Sinusitis

Basic point combination

L.I.-4, L.I.-20 or Ex-HN-8 (*Shang Ying Xiang = Bi Tong*).
Ear acupuncture: rhinopharynx.

Local points:

Frontal sinusitis: G.B.-14, BL-2, Ex-HN-3 (*Yin Tang*).
Maxillary sinusitis: ST-2 [ST-5 Bi], S.I.-18.
Ethmoidal and sphenoidal sinusitis: Du-16, Du-20.

Individual point combination

Acute catarrhal sinusitis (Wind-Cold)

L.I.-4 (moxa), local points.

Acute purulent sinusitis (Wind-Heat)

L.I.-4, L.I.-11, L.I.-20, T.B.-5, Du-23, BL-12 cupping.

Recurring purulent sinusitis

L.I.-4, L.I.-11, L.I.-20, LU-7, Du-14 [Du-13 Bi].

Chronic purulent sinusitis (Damp-Heat in the Stomach/Spleen)

L.I.-4, L.I.-11, L.I.-20, ST-8 [ST-1 Bi], SP-9, Ren-13, Ren-9– all with even method; Ren-12, BL-12+.

Phlegm

ST-40.

Heavy head

ST-8 [ST-1 Bi].

Swollen mucous membranes

L.I.-20, T.B.-17, ear acupuncture: rhinopharynx.

Headaches

G.B.-20, Ex-HN-3 (*Yin Tang*).

Chronic, without heat signs

Insert needles, cover with headlight box.

Fever

L.I.-4, L.I.-11, Du-14 [Du-13 Bi].

Acupuncture points

BL-2 **Location:** at the junction of a vertical line through the medial end of the eyebrow (inner canthus) and the supraorbital foramen.

BL-12 **Location:** 1.5 cun lateral to the spinous process of T2.
Notes: eliminates external Wind, releases the surface; promotes the descending and dispersing of Lung *Qi*.

BL-20 **Location:** 1.5 cun lateral to the spinous process of T11.
Notes: back-*Shu* point of the Spleen; tonifies the Stomach and Spleen, and therefore the *Qi* and Blood (*Xue*) production; eliminates Dampness.

Du-14 **Location:** below the spinous process of C7.
Notes: meeting point of all *Yang* meridians; the effect of this point depends on the technique used: reducing method to disperse Wind, Cold, Heat; tonifying method for overall strengthening; combine with L.I.-4 and L.I.-11 for fever.

Du-16 **Location:** 1 cun within the posterior hairline, in the depression inferior to the external occipital protuberance.
Notes: for disorders involving the head and sensory organs; eliminates pathogenic Wind from the head.

Du-20 **Location:** on a line connecting the apices of the ears, 7 cun superior the posterior hairline.
Notes: meeting point of all divergent meridians.

Du-23 **Location:** on the midline, 1 cun within the anterior midline.
Notes: dispels Wind from the nasal passages, strengthens the *Du Mai*, stops nasal discharge.

Ex-HN-3 **Location:** at the midpoint between the eyebrows.
Notes: dispels Wind from the nasal passages; very effective for frontal headaches (hence its nickname 'point de merveille' – 'miracle point').

Ex-HN-8 **Location:** at the superior end of the nasolabial groove.
Notes: opens the nasal passages.

G.B.-14 **Location:** 1 cun superior to the midpoint of the eyebrow, on the pupil line.
Notes: local point.

G.B.-20 **Location:** posterior to the mastoid, between the trapezius and sternocleidomastoid on the lower border of the occiput.
Notes: dispels Wind; important symptomatic point for headaches.

L.I.-4 **Location:** on the dorsum of the hand, at the highest point of the muscle bulge between the 1st and 2nd metacarpal bones.
Notes: *Yuan*-source point, command point of the face; eliminates external Wind (with LU-7), Cold, Heat; with KID-7 induces sweating; important distal point for ENT disorders; standard point prescription for fever: L.I.-4, L.I.-11, Du-14.

L.I.-11 **Location:** with the arm fully flexed, at the radial end of the cubital crease.
Notes: *He*-sea point, tonification point; eliminates external Wind, Heat and Dampness; for fever, combine with L.I.-4 and Du-14.

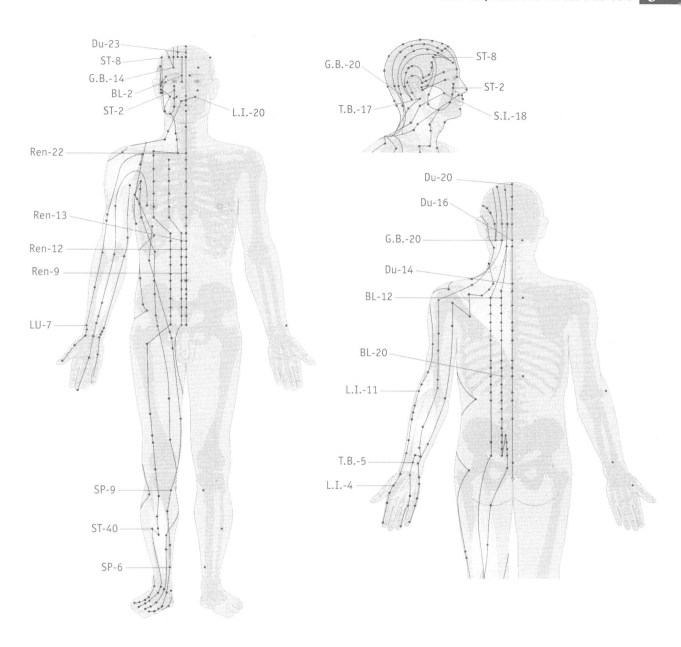

Du-23
ST-8
G.B.-14
BL-2
ST-2
L.I.-20
Ren-22
Ren-13
Ren-12
Ren-9
LU-7
SP-9
ST-40
SP-6

G.B.-20
ST-8
T.B.-17
ST-2
S.I.-18

Du-20
Du-16
G.B.-20
Du-14
BL-12
BL-20
L.I.-11
T.B.-5
L.I.-4

L.I.-20   **Location:** in the nasolabial groove, at the level of the midpoint of the lateral border of the ala nasi.
Notes: dispels external Wind, opens the nasal passages.

S.I.-18   **Location:** on the anterior border of the insertion of the masseter on the maxilla. Ask the patient to clench their teeth and/or open the mouth.
Notes: local point.

LU-7   **Location:** 1.5 cun proximal to the wrist crease, superior to the radial artery.
Notes: *Luo*-connecting point, opening point for the *Ren Mai*, master point for stagnation; combined with L.I.-4 dispels external pathogens.

Ren-9   **Location:** 1 cun superior to the umbilicus.
Notes: resolves Dampness.

Ren-12   **Location:** midway between the umbilicus and the xiphoid process.
Notes: front-*Mu* point of the Stomach and the Middle Burner; combined with ST-36 and BL-20 supports the Spleen.

Ren-13   **Location:** 5 cun superior to the umbilicus or 5/8 of the distance between the umbilicus and the xiphoid process.
Notes: for excess conditions of the Stomach.

Ren-22   **Location:** in the centre of the jugulum.
Notes: resolves Phlegm.

SP-9   **Location:** with the knee flexed in the depression inferior to the medial condyle of the tibia, at the same level as G.B.-34.
Notes: resolves Dampness.

ST-2   **Location:** on the pupil line, in the depression above the infraorbital foramen.
Notes: local point; dispels Wind, benefits the eyes.

ST-8   **Location:** at the corner of the forehead, 3 cun superior and 1 cun posterior to the frontozygomatic suture.
Notes: alleviates dull headaches and dizziness due to Dampness and Phlegm.

ST-40   **Location:** at the midpoint of the distance between the highest prominence of the medial malleolus and the knee joint space, 2 cun lateral to the anterior crest of the tibia.
Notes: *Luo*-connecting point; Phlegm!

T.B.-5   **Location:** 2 cun proximal to the midpoint of the dorsal wrist crease, opposite P-6.
Notes: *Luo*-connecting point, opening point of the *Yang Wei Mai* – dominates the surface, eliminates external pathogens, especially Wind-Heat.

T.B.-17   **Location:** on the anterior border of the mastoid.
Notes: instantly unblocks the nasal passages.

6.10.3 Otitis and tubal catarrh

▬ Good results with acupuncture and laser!

Basic point combination

T.B.-21, G.B.-20.
Ear acupuncture: rhinopharynx.

Individual point combination

Otitis externa

TCM: excess type.
T.B.-5; local treatment with laser.

Acute otitis media

TCM: excess type.
Acupuncture and laser at L.I.-4, LU-7, T.B.-5, T.B.-17, T.B.-21.
With fever: L.I.-11, Du-14 [Du-13 Bi].
With headaches: G.B.-20, Ex-HN-5 (*Tai Yang*).
Local treatment with laser – ear drum.

Recurring tubal catarrh

TCM: Spleen *Qi* deficiency (children), *Yin* deficiency (elderly patients) and Phlegm.
For children: use laser locally at T.B.-17 (opens the nasal passages and tubes), then select points from T.B.-21, S.I.-19, G.B.-2; distal points: L.I.-4, ST-36.
Boost the immune system: laser at BL-43 [BL-38 Bi], BL-17, L.I.-4, ST-36.
Tonify the Spleen: ST-36, SP-6, BL-20.
Tonify the *Yin*: KID-3, BL-23.
Phlegm: ST-40.

Acupuncture points

BL-17 **Location:** 1.5 cun lateral to the spinous process of T7.
  Notes: back-*Shu* point of the diaphragm, *Hui* meeting point of the Blood (*Xue*); strengthens the immune system.
BL-20 **Location:** 1.5 cun lateral to the spinous process of T11.
  Notes: back-*Shu* point of the Spleen; tonifies the Spleen and Stomach, eliminates Dampness.
BL-23 **Location:** 1.5 cun lateral to the spinous process of L2.
  Notes: back-*Shu* point of the Kidneys; tonifies the *Qi*, *Yang*, *Yin* and Essence (*Jing*) of the Kidneys.
BL-43 **Location:** 3 cun lateral to the spinous process of T4, lateral to BL-14 (back *Shu* point of the Pericardium), at the medial border of the scapula.
  Notes: back-*Shu* point of the Vital Region; tonifies *Qi*, deficiency, Essence (*Jing*), Lung *Yin*.
Du-14 **Location:** below the spinous process of C7.
  Notes: meeting point of all *Yang* meridians; the effect depends on the technique used: reducing method to disperse Wind, Cold, Heat; tonifying method for overall strengthening; for fever combine with L.I.-4 and L.I.-11.
Ex-HN-5 **Location:** on the temple, in a depression approximately 1 cun lateral to the midpoint of a line connecting the lateral extremity of the eyebrow and the outer canthus of the eye.
  Notes: important point for headaches.
G.B.-2 **Location:** with the mouth open, in the depression anterior to the antitragic notch, posterior to the condyloid process of the mandible.
G.B.-20 **Location:** posterior to the mastoid, between the trapezius and sternocleidomastoid muscles, on the lower border of the occiput.
  Notes: dispels Wind from the head; important point for headaches.
KID-3 **Location:** between the highest prominence of the medial malleolus and the Achilles tendon.
  Notes: *Yuan*-source point, *Shu*-stream point; tonifies Kidney *Yin, Yang* and Essence (*Jing*), especially with BL-23.
L.I.-4 **Location:** on the dorsum of the hand, at the highest point of the muscle bulge between the 1st and 2nd metacarpal bones.
  Notes: *Yuan*-source point; eliminates external Wind (with LU-7), Cold, Heat; most important distal point for ENT disorders; standard point prescription for fever: L.I.-4, L.I.-11, Du-14.
L.I.-11 **Location:** with the arm fully flexed, at the radial end of the cubital crease.
  Notes: *He*-sea point, tonification point; eliminates Damp-Heat and Wind; combine with L.I.-4 and Du-14 for fever.
LU-7 **Location:** 1.5 cun proximal to the wrist crease, superior to the radial artery.
  Notes: opening point for the *Ren Mai*; restores the dispersing and descending function of the Lung *Qi*.
S.I.-19 **Location:** with the mouth open, in the depression between the tragus and the temporomandibular joint; T.B.-21 is located superior to and G.B.-21 inferior to S.I.-19.
  Notes: local point; eliminates Heat and Wind-Heat.
SP-6 **Location:** 3 cun superior to the highest prominence of the medial malleolus, on the posterior border of the tibia.

Notes: as group *Luo*-connecting point (SP, LIV, KID) tonifies *Qi*, Blood (*Xue*) and *Yin*, nourishes and moves the Blood (*Xue*), eliminates Dampness.

ST-36 **Location:** 1 cun lateral to the anterior crest of the tibia, 1.5 cun inferior to the lower border of the head of the fibula (G.B.-34).
Notes: *He*-sea point; tonifies the Stomach and the Spleen; calming and tonifying point.

ST-40 **Location:** at the midpoint of the distance between the highest prominence of the medial malleolus and the knee joint space, 2 cun lateral to the anterior crest of the tibia.
Notes: *Luo*-connecting point; Phlegm!

T.B.-5 **Location:** 2 cun proximal to the midpoint of the dorsal wrist crease, opposite P-6.
Notes: *Luo*-connecting point, opening point of the *Yang Wei Mai* – dominates the surface, eliminates external pathogens, especially Wind-Heat.

T.B.-17 **Location:** on the anterior border of the mastoid.
Notes: opens the nasal passages and tubes, eliminates external Wind.

T.B.-21 **Location:** at the level of the supratragic incisure, with the mouth open in the depression superior to the condyloid process of the mandible.
Notes: particularly for disorders of the ears due to hyperactive Liver *Yang*; Bi: master point of the ears.

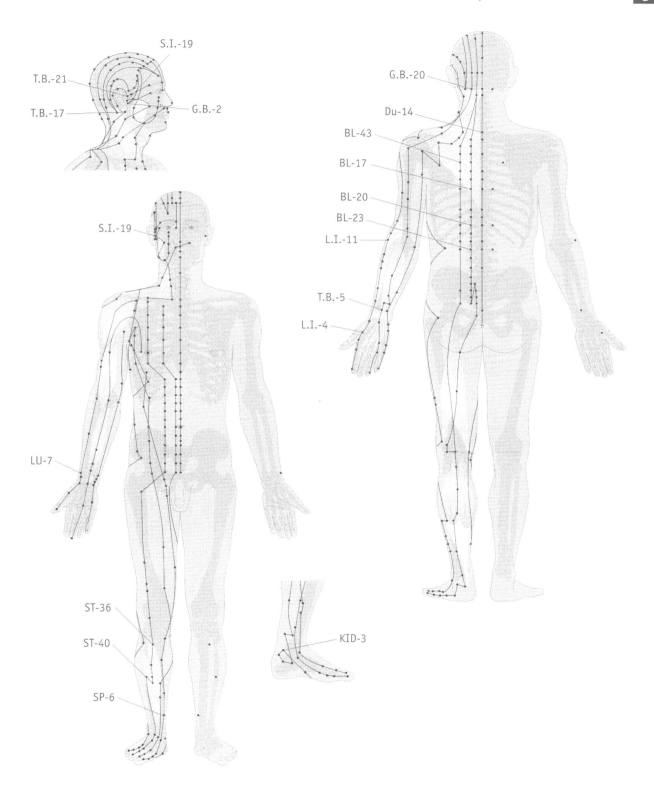

S.I.-19

T.B.-21

T.B.-17

G.B.-2

G.B.-20

Du-14

BL-43

BL-17

BL-20

BL-23

L.I.-11

T.B.-5

L.I.-4

S.I.-19

LU-7

ST-36

ST-40

SP-6

KID-3

6.10.4 Common cold and sore throat

Basic point combination

LU-10, LU-11, L.I.-4, L.I.-11, T.B.-5, Du-14 [Du-13 Bi].

Individual point combination

Onset of cold

TCM: Wind-Cold type.
Symptoms: aversion to cold, chills, fever, sore joints, blocked nose, hoarse voice, sneezing and cough with expectoration of clear runny mucus, sore throat, headaches, no sweating and no thirst. **Tongue coating:** thin, white; **pulse:** superficial, tight.
TCM: *Qi* blockage due to pathogenic factors.
Acupuncture points: L.I.-4, LU-7, Du-16, BL-12, cupping.

Highly acute infection with high temperature

TCM: Wind-Heat type, fight between the defensive *Qi* (*Wei Qi*) and Wind-Heat.
Symptoms: fever, sweating, headaches, aversion to wind, purulent discharge, sore throat, thirst. **Tongue coating:** thin, white to yellow; **pulse:** superficial, rapid.
Acupuncture points: L.I.-4, T.B.-5; LU-10 or LU-11 with bloodletting.

Headache

Du-16, G.B.-20, Ex-HN-3 (*Yin Tang*).

Severe sore throat (excess type), acute pharyngitis, tonsillitis

Bloodletting at LU-10 or LU-11, S.I.-17.

Mild sore throat (deficiency type – *Yin* deficiency) – chronic pharyngitis

KID-3+, BL-23+, LU-10-; or opening points LU-7 and KID-6, and LU-10.

Fever

L.I.-4, L.I.-11, Du-14 [Du-13 Bi].

Acupuncture points

BL-12 **Location:** 1.5 cun lateral to the spinous process of T2.
   Notes: eliminates external Wind-Cold from the *Tai Yang* (BL/S.I.), regulates the circulation of *Qi*.
BL-23 **Location:** 1.5 cun lateral to the spinous process of L2.
   Notes: back-*Shu* point of the Kidneys; for chronic pharyngitis due to *Yin* deficiency.
Du-14 **Location:** below the spinous process of C7.
   Notes: meeting point of all *Yang* meridians; the effect depends on the technique used: reducing method to disperse Wind, Cold, Heat; tonifying method for overall strengthening; combine with L.I.-4 and L.I.-11 for fever.
Du-16 **Location:** 1 cun within the posterior hairline, in the depression inferior to the external occipital protuberance.
   Notes: eliminates Wind, alleviates headaches.
Ex-HN-3 **Location:** at the midpoint between the eyebrows.
   Notes: dispels Wind from the nasal passages; very effective for frontal headaches (hence its epithet 'point de merveille' – 'miracle point').
G.B.-20 **Location:** posterior to the mastoid, between the trapezius and sternocleidomastoid muscles, on the lower border of the occiput.
   Notes: major point for headaches! Eliminates external and internal Wind and Heat.
KID-3 **Location:** between the highest prominence of the medial malleolus and the Achilles tendon.
   Notes: *Yuan*-source point; tonifies the Kidneys; for chronic pharyngitis due to *Yin* deficiency.
KID-6 **Location:** below the prominence of the medial malleolus.
   Notes: opening point of the *Yin Qiao Mai*; combine with LU-7 for sore throat due to *Yin* deficiency.
L.I.-4 **Location:** on the dorsum of the hand, at the highest point of the muscle bulge between the 1st and 2nd metacarpal bones.
   Notes: *Yuan*-source point; clears Lung Heat with L.I.-11 and eliminates Heat with L.I.-11 and Du-14 (= standard point prescription for fever), has an effect on the mucous membranes, with Cold use moxibustion.
L.I.-11 **Location:** with the arm fully flexed, at the radial end of the cubital crease.
   Notes: *He*-sea point; see also L.I.-4.
LU-7 **Location:** 1.5 cun proximal to the wrist crease, superior to the radial artery.
   Notes: *Luo*-connecting point, opening point of the *Ren Mai*, one of the 4 command points (for the face and throat).
LU-10 **Location:** at the midpoint of the 1st metacarpal bone, at the junction of the red and white skin.
   Notes: Fire point of the Lung meridian; clears Lung Heat, benefits the throat.
LU-11 **Location:** on the thumb, next to the radial corner of the nail.
   Notes: master point for throat disorders; eliminates external and internal Wind, descends and disperses the Lung *Qi*.

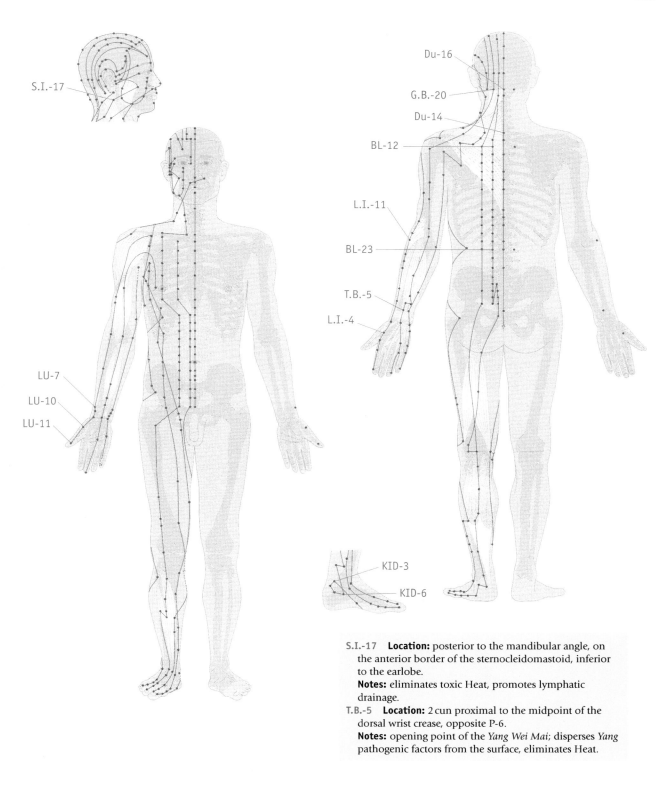

S.I.-17
Du-16
G.B.-20
Du-14
BL-12
L.I.-11
BL-23
T.B.-5
L.I.-4
LU-7
LU-10
LU-11
KID-3
KID-6

S.I.-17 **Location:** posterior to the mandibular angle, on the anterior border of the sternocleidomastoid, inferior to the earlobe.
Notes: eliminates toxic Heat, promotes lymphatic drainage.

T.B.-5 **Location:** 2 cun proximal to the midpoint of the dorsal wrist crease, opposite P-6.
Notes: opening point of the *Yang Wei Mai*; disperses *Yang* pathogenic factors from the surface, eliminates Heat.

6.10.5 Epistaxis

Acupuncture can help here very quickly. For recurring nosebleeds the cause of the bleeding (infectious disease, hypertension, coagulation disorder, malignant systemic disease) must be established.

TCM

Heat in the *Yang Ming* (Large Intestine, Stomach meridians).

Basic point combination

L.I.-4, L.I.-20, G.B.-20, Du-23.

Individual point combination

Acute infection

TCM: Excess Lung-Heat.
LU-11.

With thirst and restlessness

TCM: Stomach-Heat.
ST-44.

Premenstrual epistaxis

ST-36, BL-40 [BL-54 Bi].

Overall weak condition

TCM: *Yin* deficiency.
KID-3 or KID-6.

Acupuncture points

BL-40 **Location:** in the centre of the popliteal crease, between the tendons of the semitendinosus and the biceps femoris.
Notes: *He*-sea point; eliminates *Qi* and Blood (*Xue*) stagnation.

Du-23 **Location:** on the midline, 1 cun within the anterior hairline.
Notes: stops nosebleeds.

G.B.-20 **Location:** posterior to the mastoid, between the trapezius and sternocleidomastoid on the lower border of the occiput.
Notes: eliminates Wind and Heat.

KID-3 **Location:** between the highest prominence of the medial malleolus and the Achilles tendon.
Notes: *Yuan*-source point, *Shu*-stream point; tonifies Kidney *Yin*, *Yang* and Essence (*Jing*).

KID-6 **Location:** below the prominence of the medial malleolus.
Notes: opening point of the *Yin Qiao Mai*; tonifies *Yin*, calms the Spirit.

L.I.-4 **Location:** on the dorsum of the hand, at the highest point of the muscle bulge between the 1st and 2nd metacarpal bones.
Notes: *Yuan*-source point; eliminates external Wind (with LU-7), Cold and Heat; most important distal point for ENT disorders.

L.I.-20 **Location:** in the nasolabial groove, at the level of the midpoint of the lateral border of the ala nasi.
Notes: opens the nasal passages.

LU-11 **Location:** on the thumb, next to the radial corner of the nail.
Notes: clears Wind-Heat from the Lungs.

ST-36 **Location:** 1 cun lateral to the anterior crest of the tibia, 1.5 cun inferior to the lower border of the head of the fibula (G.B.-34).
Notes: *He*-sea point, master point of hormones; tonifies the Stomach, Spleen, *Qi*, Blood (*Xue*); calming and tonifying point.

ST-44 **Location:** on the interdigital fold between the 2nd and 3rd toes, near the metatarsophalangeal joint of the 2nd toe.
Notes: clears Heat from the Stomach and *Yang Ming*.

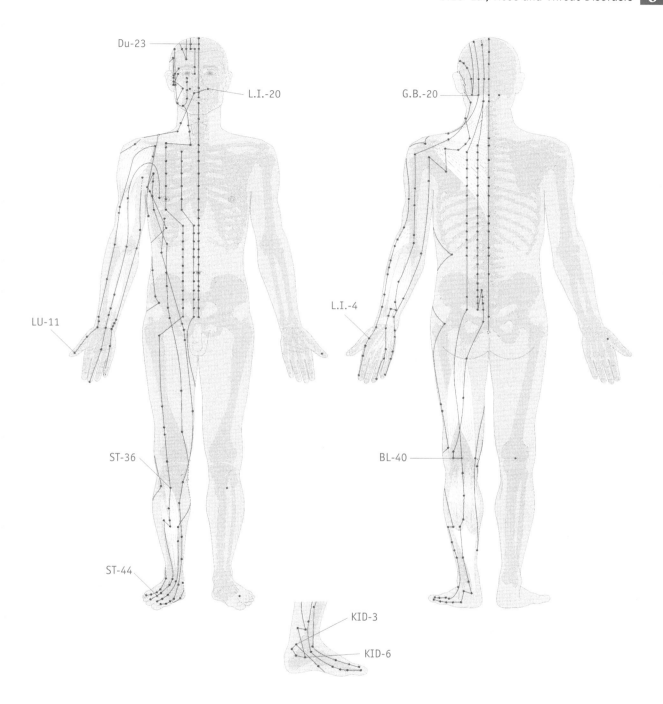

6.10.6 Tinnitus and deafness (1)

■ No indication for beginners!

According to TCM, tinnitus and deafness develop if the 'clear *Qi*' can't reach the ear. Failure of the 'clear *Qi*' to reach the ear can be caused by an obstruction due to emotions, Phlegm or noise (Excess). Tinnitus and deafness can also be the result of a deficiency of Essence (*Jing*), *Qi* or Blood. Maciocia differentiates according to syndromes, so that treatments vary considerably.

Basic point combination

T.B.-17, G.B.-2 or S.I.-19 or T.B.-21 (local points).

Individual point combination

From the points described below, choose only a few per treatment – preferably not more than seven.

Liver and Gall Bladder Fire

Symptoms: related to emotional state, sudden onset, loud, headaches, red face, dizziness, thirst; **tongue body:** red edges; **tongue coating:** yellow; **pulse:** tight, rapid.
Treatment principle: drain Liver Fire, calm the ears, the Spirit and the *Hun* (ethereal soul).
Points: T.B.-3, T.B.-5, T.B.-17, G.B.-8, G.B.-20, G.B.-43, LIV-2.

Phlegm Fire

Symptoms: tinnitus sounding like a cicada, deafness, tightness in the chest, expectorating Phlegm, thirst, dazed and dizzy.
Treatment principle: transform Phlegm, drain Fire, subdue Liver *Yang*, promote the rising of the clear *Qi* and the descending of the turbid *Qi*, tonify the Spleen.
Points: L.I.-4, ST-40, SP-9, S.I.-19, T.B.-3, T.B.-5, T.B.-21, BL-20, G.B.-2, G.B.-20, Ren-9, Ren-12.

Acupuncture points

BL-20   **Location:** 1.5 cun lateral to the spinous process of T11.
Notes: back-*Shu* point of the Spleen; together with ST-36 and Ren-12 tonifies the Spleen and promotes the transformation of Phlegm.

G.B.-2   **Location:** with the mouth open, in the depression anterior to the antitragic notch, posterior to the condyloid process of the mandible.
Notes: eliminates obstructions from the meridian, benefits the ears, expels external Wind; most important local point for tinnitus due to Kidney Essence (*Jing*) deficiency; promotes the rising of the clear *Qi* to the ear and the descending of the turbid *Qi* from the ear (see T.B.-21).

G.B.-8   **Location:** 1.5 cun superior to the apex of the ear.
Notes: eliminates Wind and obstructions; benefits/calms the ear.

G.B.-20   **Location:** posterior to the mastoid, between the trapezius and sternocleidomastoid muscles, on the lower border of the occiput.
Notes: subdues Liver *Yang*, benefits the eyes, supports the ears.

G.B.-43   **Location:** between the 4th and 5th toes, proximal to the margin of the web, closer to the metatarsophalangeal joint of the 4th toe.
Notes: *Ying*-spring point, sedation point; eliminates Liver Fire, subdues Liver *Yang*, cools the Blood (*Xue*), subdues internal Wind.

L.I.-4   **Location:** on the dorsum of the hand, at the highest point of the muscle bulge between the 1st and 2nd metacarpal bones.
Notes: *Yuan*-source point, metabolic point, command point of the face; regulates the rising of the clear *Qi* to the head and the descending of the turbid *Qi* from the head.

LIV-2   **Location:** between the 1st and 2nd toes, proximal to the margin of the web, at the lateral aspect of the metatarsophalangeal joint of the 1st toe.
Notes: *Ying*-spring point, sedation point; eliminates Liver Fire, subdues Liver *Yang*, cools Blood (*Xue*), subdues internal Wind.

Ren-9   **Location:** 1 cun superior to the umbilicus.
Notes: Phlegm, Dampness, pus.

Ren-12   **Location:** midway between the umbilicus and the xiphoid process.
Notes: front-*Mu* point of the Stomach; combined with ST-36 and BL-20 tonifies the Stomach and the Spleen, promotes the transformation of Phlegm.

S.I.-19   **Location:** with the mouth open, in the depression between the tragus and the temporomandibular joint; T.B.-21 is located superior to and G.B.-21 inferior to S.I.-19.
Notes: most important local point for tinnitus due to *Qi* deficiency in the Upper Burner; benefits the ears, promotes the rising of the clear *Qi* to the ear and the descending of the turbid *Qi* from the ear.

SP-9   **Location:** with the knee flexed in the depression inferior to the medial condyle of the tibia, at the same level as G.B.-34.
Notes: *He*-sea point; eliminates Heat, resolves Dampness/Phlegm.

ST-40   **Location:** at the midpoint of the distance between the highest prominence of the medial malleolus and the knee joint space, 2 cun lateral to the anterior crest of the tibia.
Notes: *Luo*-connecting point (connects with SP-3); eliminates Phlegm, Dampness, Heat – 'Mucosolvan of acupuncture'.

T.B.-3   **Location:** when a loose fist is made on the dorsum of the hand, between the 4th and 5th metacarpal bones, in the depression proximal to the metacarpophalangeal joints.
Notes: tonification point, *Shu*-stream point; eliminates Heat, dispels Wind, benefits the ears, subdues Liver *Yang*.

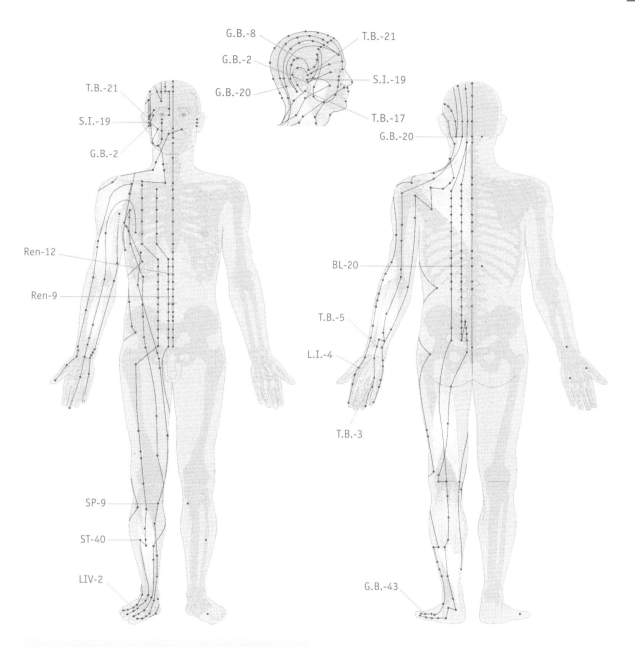

T.B.-5 **Location:** 2 cun proximal to the midpoint of the dorsal wrist crease, opposite P-6.
Notes: *Luo*-connecting point, opening point of the *Yang Wei Mai*; eliminates Wind-Heat and meridian obstructions, releases the surface, benefits the ears (meridian pathway!), subdues Liver *Yang*.

T.B.-17 **Location:** on the anterior border of the mastoid.
Notes: instantly unblocks the nasal passages!; eliminates Wind and unblocks the meridians and collaterals; benefits the ears.

T.B.-21 **Location:** at the level of the supratragic incisure, with the mouth open in the depression superior to the condyloid process of the mandible.
Notes: master point for the ears; most important local point for tinnitus due to Phlegm Fire; promotes the rising of the clear *Qi* to the ear and the descending of the turbid *Qi* from the ear – combine with S.I.-19 and G.B.-2.

6.10.6 *Tinnitus and deafness (2)*

Kidney Essence (*Jing*) deficiency – presbycusis with or without tinnitus

Symptoms: slow onset, quiet, intermittent, like rushing water, pain and weakness in the lumbar region and the knees, low sex drive, poor memory, sensation of 'emptiness' in the head, blurry vision. Caution: Kidney *Jing* deficiency can manifest with symptoms of either Kidney *Yin* or Kidney *Yang* deficiency. **Tongue body:** either pale or red; **pulse:** superficial or deep, but always a deficiency pulse!

Treatment principle: tonify Essence (*Jing*), the Sea of Marrow (brain), Kidney *Yang* and Kidney *Yin*; if necessary, harmonize the Heart and the Kidneys, subdue Liver *Yang*.

Points: SP-6, HE-6, BL-23, KID-3, KID-7, G.B.-2, LIV-3, Du-4, Ren-4.

Qi deficiency in the Upper Burner

Symptoms: slow onset, intermittent quiet tinnitus, tired, dyspnoea, spontaneous sweating or sweating after exertion; **complexion and tongue body:** pale, scalloped; pulse: empty.

Treatment principle: tonify Lung *Qi*, promote the rising of the pure *Qi* to the head.

Points: LU-9, S.I.-19, BL-13, T.B.-16, Du-20, Ren-6, Ren-17.

Heart Blood (*Xue*) deficiency

Symptoms: slow onset, intermittent quiet tinnitus; **complexion:** greyish-sallow pale, palpitations, insomnia, poor memory, anxious, low self-esteem; **tongue body:** pale, thin; **pulse:** empty, choppy.

Treatment principle: tonify the Heart, nourish the Blood.

Points: SP-6, S.I.-19, BL-15, P-6, Du-20, Ren-14.

Acupuncture points

BL-13 **Location:** 1.5 cun lateral to the spinous process of T3.
 Notes: back-*Shu* point of the Lungs; tonifies Lung *Qi* with LU-9 and Ren-17.

BL-15 **Location:** 1.5 cun lateral to the spinous process of T5.
 Notes: back-*Shu* point of the Heart; combined with Ren-14 tonifies the Heart.

BL-23 **Location:** 1.5 cun lateral to the spinous process of L2.
 Notes: back-*Shu* point of the Kidneys; tonifies the Kidneys and the Essence (*Jing*).

Du-4 **Location:** below the spinous process of L2, at the same level as BL-23 and BL-52.
 Notes: moxa has a tonifiying effect for Kidney *Yang* deficiency.

Du-20 **Location:** on a line connecting the apices of the ears, 7 cun superior the posterior hairline.
 Notes: universal meeting point; raises the clear *Qi* to the head.

G.B.-2 **Location:** with the mouth open, in the depression anterior to the antitragic notch, posterior to the condyloid process of the mandible.
 Notes: eliminates obstructions from the meridian, benefits the ears, expels external Wind, most important local point for tinnitus due to Kidney Essence (*Jing*) deficiency; promotes the rising of the clear *Qi* to the ear and the descending of the turbid *Qi* from the ear (see T.B.-21).

HE-6 **Location:** 0.5 cun proximal to HE-7.
 Notes: *Xi*-cleft point; tonifies and nourishes Heart *Yin*; combined with KID-7 harmonizes the Heart and the Kidneys.

KID-3 **Location:** between the highest prominence of the medial malleolus and the Achilles tendon.
 Notes: *Yuan*-source point, *Shu*-stream point; tonifies the Kidneys and Essence (*Jing*).

KID-7 **Location:** on the anterior border of the Achilles tendon, posterior to the flexor digitorum longus, 2 cun superior to the highest prominence of the medial malleolus.
 Notes: tonification point, *Jing*-river point; tonifies the Kidneys and Essence (*Jing*).

LIV-3 **Location:** on the dorsum of the foot, in the depression distal to the junction of the 1st and 2nd metatarsal bones.
 Notes: *Yuan*-source point and *Shu*-stream point; subdues Liver *Yang*, eliminates internal Wind, promotes the smooth flow of Liver *Qi*.

LU-9 **Location:** on the wrist crease, radial to the radial artery.
 Notes: *Shu*-stream point, *Yuan*-source point; combined with BL-13 and Ren-17, tonifies Lung *Qi* and *Yin*.

P-6 **Location:** on the anterior aspect of the forearm, 2 cun proximal to the midpoint of the wrist crease, between the tendons of the flexor carpi radialis and palmaris longus.
 Notes: opening point of the *Yin Wei Mai*, *Luo*-connecting point (connects with T.B.-4); regulates Heart Blood (*Xue*) and Triple Burner as well as Heart *Qi*.

Ren-4 **Location:** 2 cun superior to the upper border of the pubic symphysis (2/5 of the distance between the symphysis and the umbilicus).
 Notes: internal meeting point of the 3 *Yin* of the lower extremity, front-*Mu* point of the Small Intestine; tonifies the Kidneys and Essence (*Jing*).

Ren-6 **Location:** 1.5 cun inferior to the umbilicus.
 Notes: tonifies the Kidneys and original *Qi*.

Ren-14 **Location:** 2 cun inferior to the xiphoid process.
 Notes: front-*Mu* point of the Heart; combined with BL-15, tonifies the Heart.

Ren-17 **Location:** on the midline of the sternum, at the level of the 4th ICS; in men between the nipples.
 Notes: front-*Mu* point of the Pericardium, *Hui*-meeting point of the *Qi*/respiration; tonifies the Heart *Qi*.

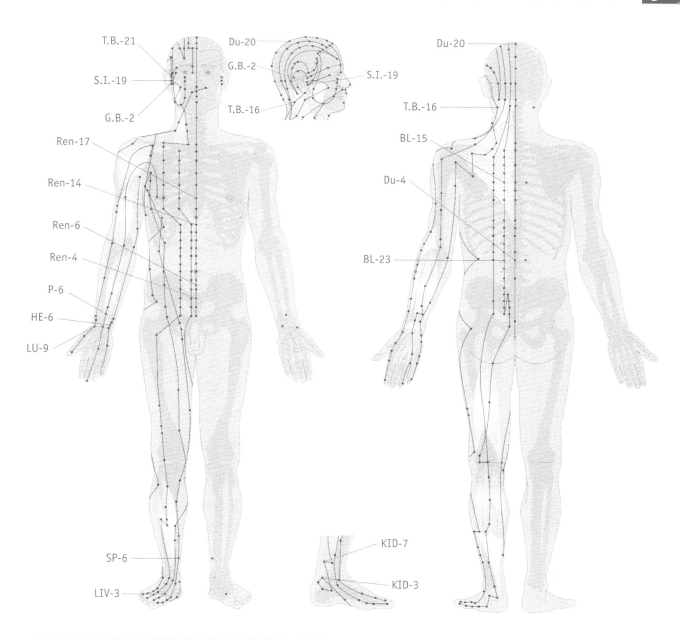

S.I.-19 **Location:** with the mouth open, in the depression between the tragus and the temporomandibular joint; T.B.-21 is located superior, G.B.-21 inferior, to S.I.-19.
Notes: most important local point for tinnitus due to *Qi* deficiency in the Upper Burner; benefits the ears, promotes the rising of the clear *Qi* to the ear and the descending of the turbid *Qi* from the ear.

SP-6 **Location:** 3 cun superior to the highest prominence of the medial malleolus, on the posterior border of the tibia.

Notes: as group *Luo*-connecting point (SP, LIV, KID), tonifies *Qi*, Blood (*Xue*) and *Yin*, nourishing point; eliminates Dampness.

T.B.-16 **Location:** on the posterior border of the sternocleidomastoid, at the level of the mandibular angle, inferior to T.B.-17,
Notes: especially useful for acute hearing loss!; raises the clear *Yang* to the head.

6.11 Disorder of the eyes

G.Kubiena, B. Sommer, J. Nepp

Some ophthalmic disorders lend themselves well to treatment with acupuncture. However, it is recommended that treatments should be discussed with the treating consultant. Within the framework of this book, only conjunctivitis is described in more detail; because other indications such as glaucoma or retinal detachment require intensive conventional therapy, acupuncture will not yield the expected results during the acute stage. As a genetic disorder, retinitis pigmentosa cannot be treated successfully with acupuncture, but its multiple accompanying symptoms can certainly be alleviated with treatments tailored to the individual symptoms.

TCM

The eye is associated with the Wood element (Liver/Gall Bladder); the Liver 'opens' into the eyes. One of the most important distal points is therefore LIV-3. A further important distal point is L.I.-4.

Method: it is self-evident that particular care is required when needling or applying laser to points close to the eyes.

Deep parabulbar needling is contraindicated owing to the risk of injuring the eyeball, especially as deep needling does not seem to give better results than superficial needling.

6.11.1 *Conjunctivitis (1)*

The points mentioned here can also be used for other irritations to the eye, such as irritated eyes due to wearing contact lenses. Generally, the results are good.

TCM

According to TCM, conjunctivitis is caused – apart from injuries, foreign objects and infections – by external pathogens (Wind, Heat, Dryness), rising Liver *Yang* or Liver Fire, Blood deficiency and *Yin* deficiency.

Basic point combination

L.I.-4, BL-1, G.B.-1, LIV-3, hand point 4 (*Yuan Dian*, eye point).

Vienna School of Acupuncture after Kubiena

Local points: 1–2 points around the eye (e.g. BL-1, BL-2, G.B.-14, Ex-HN-4 (*Yu Yao*), G.B.-1, T.B.-23, ST-1 [ST-4 Bi], ST-2 [ST-5 Bi] and Ex-HN-3 (*Yin Tang*) – depending on sensitivity to pressure.
Points according to organs involved: LIV-3, G.B.-41, T.B.-5 (LIV/G.B.), L.I.-4, LU-7 (LU/L.I.).

Acupuncture points

BL-1 **Location:** at the inner canthus of the eye – where glasses rest on the nose!
Notes: meeting point of the Bladder meridian, *Yang Qiao Mai* and *Yin Qiao Mai*; eliminates Wind and Heat, benefits the eyes, alleviates tearing, stops itching and pain.

BL-2 **Location:** at the junction of a vertical line through the medial end of the eyebrow (inner canthus) and the supraorbital foramen.
Notes: dispels Wind, benefits the eyes.

Ex-HN-3 **Location:** at the midpoint between the eyebrows.

Ex-HN-4 **Location:** at the midpoint of the eyebrows.
Notes: eliminates Heat, brightens the eyes.

G.B.-1 **Location:** 0.5 cun lateral to the outer canthus of the eye, in the depression lateral to the orbit.
Notes: dispels Wind-Heat, eliminates Fire, brightens the eyes.

G.B.-14 **Location:** 1 cun superior to the midpoint of the eyebrow, on the pupil line.
Notes: eliminates internal Wind.

G.B.-41 **Location:** in the depression distal to the junction of the 4th and 5th metatarsal bones.
Notes: opening point of the *Dai Mai*; eliminates Damp-Heat and Fire, improves vision.

L.I.-4 **Location:** on the dorsum of the hand, at the highest point of the muscle bulge between the 1st and 2nd metacarpal bones.
Notes: *Yuan*-source point, metabolic point; eliminates external pathogens, including Wind.

LIV-3 **Location:** on the dorsum of the foot, in the depression distal to the junction of the 1st and 2nd metatarsal bones.
Notes: *Yuan*-source point and *Shu*-stream point; subdues Liver *Yang*, eliminates internal Wind, smoothes the flow of *Qi*.

LU-9 **Location:** on the wrist crease, radial to the radial artery.
Notes: *Yuan*-source point; for Lung deficiency.

ST-1 **Location:** on the pupil line, on the between the eyeball and the infraorbital ridge.
Notes: local point.

ST-2 **Location:** on the pupil line, in the depression above the infraorbital foramen.
Notes: local point.

T.B.-5 **Location:** 2 cun proximal to the midpoint of the dorsal wrist crease, opposite P-6.
Notes: *Luo*-connecting point, opening point of the *Yang Wei Mai*; eliminates all external pathogens, especially Wind-Heat.

T.B.-23 **Location:** in a depression at the lateral end of the eyebrow.
Notes: for disorders of the eyes due to external Wind, Liver Yang, or Fire.

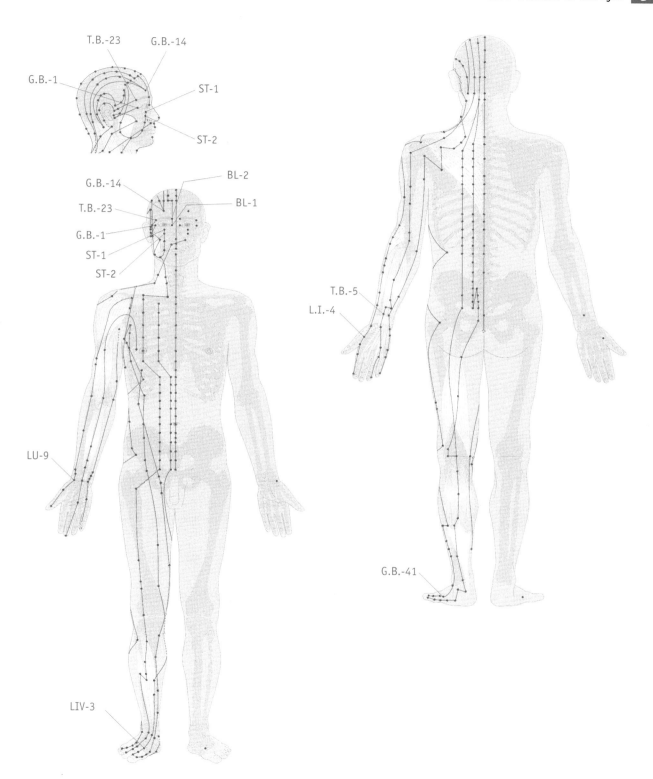

T.B.-23
G.B.-14
G.B.-1
ST-1
ST-2

G.B.-14
T.B.-23
G.B.-1
ST-1
ST-2
BL-2
BL-1

LU-9

LIV-3

T.B.-5
L.I.-4

G.B.-41

299

6.11.1 *Conjunctivitis (2)*

Individual point combinations

Key symptom: redness

ST-41, P-7, LIV-2, Ex-HN-2 (*Dang Yang*).

Key symptom: itching

G.B.-14.

Key symptom: tearing

S.I.-3, BL-67.

Conjunctivitis due to draught

G.B.-20.

Key symptom: pain

Ex-HN-3 (*Yin Tang*, 'point de merveille'), Ex-HN-4 (*Yu Yao*), Ex-HN-9 (*Nei Ying Xiang*).
Method: insert needle, remove immediately, no retention.

Conjunctivitis (sicca)

KID-6, KID-8, BL-31, Ren-5.

Conjunctivitis allergica

G.B.-1, G.B.-14, G.B.-20, G.B.-40, LIV-3, LIV-8.

Conjunctivitis due to psychological problems

BL-10, G.B.-20 (vegetative foundation), Du-20, Ex-HN-3 (*Yin Tang*, 'point de merveille'), ST-36.

Conjunctivitis due to rheumatoid disorders

G.B.-41, T.B.-5.

Acupuncture points

BL-10 **Location:** 1.5 cun lateral to the spinous process of T1.
BL-31 **Location:** over the 1st sacral foramen.
 Notes: master point for menopause.
BL-67 **Location:** on the 5th toe, at the lateral corner of the nail.
 Notes: eliminates Wind, benefits the eyes.
Du-20 **Location:** on a line connecting the apices of the ears, 7 cun superior the posterior hairline.
 Notes: universal meeting point.
Ex-HN-2 **Location:** on the forehead, on the pupil line, 1 cun superior to the anterior hairline.
 Notes: eliminates Wind and Heat.
Ex-HN-3 **Location:** at the midpoint between the eyebrows.
 Notes: eliminates Heat.
Ex-HN-9 **Location:** in the nasal cavity, at the junction of the bone and cartilage.
 Notes: for severe eye pain.
G.B.-1 **Location:** 0.5 cun lateral to the outer canthus of the eye, in the depression lateral to the orbit.
 Notes: dispels Wind-Heat, eliminates Fire, benefits the eyes.
G.B.-14 **Location:** 1 cun superior to the midpoint of the eyebrow, on the pupil line.
 Notes: eliminates internal Wind.
G.B.-20 **Location:** posterior to the mastoid, between the trapezius and sternocleidomastoid on the lower border of the occiput.
 Notes: for internal/external Wind and Liver *Yang*/Fire in the head; benefits the eyes.
G.B.-40 **Location:** on the junction of a horizontal line through the prominence of the lateral malleolus and a vertical line through the greatest circumference of the lateral malleolus, over the calcaneocuboidal joint.
 Notes: *Yuan*-source point.
G.B.-41 **Location:** in the depression distal to the junction of the 4th and 5th metatarsal bones.
 Notes: *Shu*-stream point, opening point of the *Dai Mai*, master point of the big joints.
KID-6 **Location:** below the prominence of the medial malleolus.
 Notes: opening point of the *Yin Qiao Mai*, metabolic point; combine with BL-62 for insomnia and pain that cannot be localized.
KID-8 **Location:** 2 cun superior to the highest prominence of the medial malleolus (2 cun superior to KID-3).
 Notes: *Xi*-cleft point of the *Yin Qiao Mai*, meeting point of the 3 *Yin* of the leg (KID, LIV, SP).
LIV-2 **Location:** between the 1st and 2nd toes, proximal to the margin of the web, at the lateral aspect of the metatarsophalangeal joint of the 1st toe.
 Notes: Fire point, *Ying*-spring point, sedation point; for rising Liver Fire and Liver *Yang*; for acute red eyes.
LIV-3 **Location:** on the dorsum of the foot, in the depression distal to the junction of the 1st and 2nd metatarsal bones.
 Notes: *Yuan*-source point and *Shu*-stream point.
LIV-8 **Location:** with the knee flexed, in the depression anterior to the medial end of the popliteal crease.
 Notes: *He*-sea point.
P-7 **Location:** on the anterior aspect of the wrist joint, between the tendons of the flexor carpi radialis and palmaris longus.
 Notes: *Yuan*-source point and *Shu*-stream point, sedation point; eliminates Heat/Fire.
Ren-5 **Location:** 2 cun inferior to the umbilicus.
 Notes: front-*Mu* point of the Triple Burner.
S.I.-3 **Location:** when a fist is made, on the dorsum of the hand, in the depression at the end of the most distal palmar crease.
 Notes: opening point of the *Du Mai*; eliminates Wind.

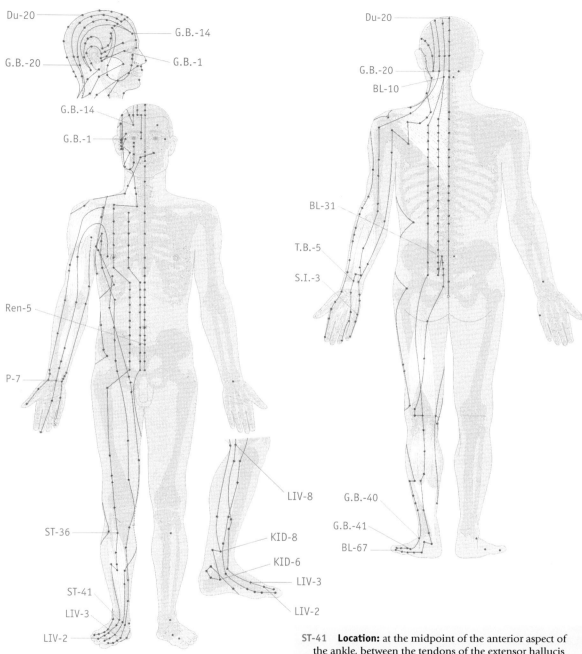

ST-36 **Location:** 1 cun lateral to the anterior crest of the tibia, 1.5 cun inferior to the lower border of the head of the fibula (G.B.-34).
Notes: *He*-sea point, master point of hormones, blood pressure.

ST-41 **Location:** at the midpoint of the anterior aspect of the ankle, between the tendons of the extensor hallucis longus and extensor digitorum longus.
Notes: Fire point.

T.B.-5 **Location:** 2 cun proximal to the midpoint of the dorsal wrist crease, opposite P-6.
Notes: *Luo*-connecting point, opening point of the *Yang Wei Mai*, master point of the small joints.

6.11.2 Atrophy of the optic nerve

Don't promise the patient any miracles. In China, acupuncture is the treatment of choice for atrophy of the optic nerve.

TCM

Atrophy of the optic nerve is always caused by a lack of nourishment of the eye with *Qi* and Blood (*Xue*). The key symptom is always blurry vision.

Basic point combination

G.B.-20, BL-1, BL-2, BL-10, scalp acupuncture after Zeitler: visual zone, G.B.-37, Du-20, Ex-HN-7 (*Qiu Hou*). Ear acupuncture: eye.

Individual point combination

Liver and Kidney *Yin* deficiency

LIV-3, KID-3, BL-18, BL-23 (herbal formula: *Qi Ju Di Huang Wan*).
TCM: Liver and Kidney *Yin* deficiency lead to Blood (*Xue*) and Essence (*Jing*) deficiency. **Symptoms:** dry eyes, blurry vision, lower back pain; **pulse:** thready, rapid; **tongue body:** red; **tongue coating:** little or none. Cause: overexertion, ageing.

Qi and Blood (*Xue*) deficiency

ST-36, SP-6; herbal formula: *Ba Zhen Tang* (plus *Fructus lycii*).
TCM: Symptoms: blurry vision, dyspnoea with exertion, reluctance to talk, dizziness, loss of appetite, loose stools; **pulse:** thready, forceless; **tongue:** pale, thin white tongue coating. **Example:** anaemia.

Liver *Qi* stagnation

LIV-14, LIV-3, G.B.-34 (herbal formula: *Hei Xiao Yao San*).
TCM: generally triggered by emotions. **Symptoms:** depression, dizziness, pain/pressure in the hypochondrium, bitter taste in the mouth, dry throat; **pulse:** tight/wiry.

Acupuncture points

BL-1 **Location:** at the inner canthus of the eye – where glasses rest on the nose!
Notes: meeting point of the Bladder meridian, *Yang Qiao Mai* and *Yin Qiao Mai*; eliminates Wind and Heat, benefits the eyes, alleviates tearing. In China, the most important point for eye disorders, but caution: danger of haematoma (angular vein), therefore in the West BL-2 is often used as an alternative.

BL-2 **Location:** at the junction of a vertical line through the medial end of the eyebrow (inner canthus) and the supraorbital foramen.
Notes: eliminates Wind, benefits the eyes.

BL-10 **Location:** at the external occipital protuberance, on the lateral aspect of the trapezius insertion.
Notes: eliminates Wind, locally unblocks the meridians; vagotonic point.

BL-18 **Location:** 2 cun lateral to the spinous process of T9.
Notes: back-*Shu* point of the Liver; benefits the Liver, Gall Bladder and the eyes.

BL-23 **Location:** 1.5 cun lateral to the spinous process of L2.
Notes: tonifies Kidney *Yin*, strengthens Essence (*Jing*), the brain and marrow, benefits the Spirit, brightens the eyes.

Du-20 **Location:** on a line connecting the apices of the ears, 7 cun superior the posterior hairline.
Notes: universal meeting point; connects with an internal branch of the Liver and the eyes, therefore particularly effective when combined with LIV-3.

Ex-HN-7 **Location:** on the lower margin of the orbit, at the junction of the lateral 1/4 and the medial 3/4.
Notes: specific point for disorders of the eyes: neuritis and atrophy of the optic nerve, glaucoma.

G.B.-20 **Location:** posterior to the mastoid, between the trapezius and sternocleidomastoid on the lower border of the occiput.
Notes: benefits the eyes, eliminates Wind and Heat.

G.B.-34 **Location:** with the knee flexed, in the depression anterior and inferior to the head of the fibula.
Notes: *He*-sea point, smoothes the flow of Liver *Qi*, subdues rebellious *Qi*.

G.B.-37 **Location:** 5 cun superior to the lateral malleolus, on the anterior border of the fibula.
Notes: *Luo*-connecting point (connects with LIV-3); benefits the eyes.

KID-3 **Location:** between the highest prominence of the medial malleolus and the Achilles tendon.
Notes: *Yuan*-source point, *Shu*-stream point; tonifies the Kidneys, Essence (*Jing*), combined with BL-23 also Kidney *Yin*.

LIV-3 **Location:** on the dorsum of the foot, in the depression distal to the junction of the 1st and 2nd metatarsal bones.
Notes: *Yuan*-source point and *Shu*-stream point; subdues Liver *Yang*, eliminates internal Wind, smoothes the flow of *Qi*.

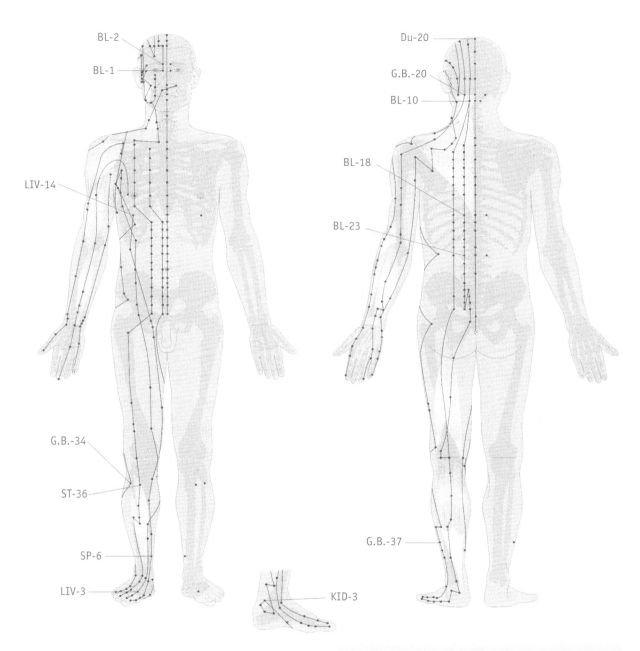

LIV-14   **Location:** on the midclavicular line, in the 6th ICS, directly below the nipple.
   Notes: front-*Mu* point of the Liver; promotes the smooth flow of *Qi*.
SP-6   **Location:** 3 cun superior to the highest prominence of the medial malleolus, on the posterior border of the tibia.

Notes: group *Luo*-connecting point for the 3 *Yin* of the leg; tonifies the Spleen, Kidney and Liver – *Qi*, *Yin* and Blood (*Xue*).
ST-36   **Location:** 1 cun lateral to the anterior crest of the tibia, 1.5 cun inferior to the lower border of the head of the fibula (G.B.-34).
   Notes: *He*-sea point; tonifies the Spleen, *Qi*, Blood (*Xue*) and the body, benefits the eyes.

6.12 Disorders of the teeth, mouth and jaw

U.Völkel

In dentistry, acupuncture is mainly used for analgesic purposes. Inflammatory disorders of the teeth, periodontium or temporomandibular joint can also be treated with acupuncture.

 The accompanying treatment by a dentist is, of course, important in order to determine the cause of the pain and the root of any inflammation.

We can distinguish therapeutic and purely analgesic forms of acupuncture. The pain-relieving effect of the latter will subside once needle stimulation has ended.

6.12.1 Toothache

Acupuncture analgesia is indicated for toothache and dental interventions when conventional local or superficial anaesthesia is contraindicated for a particular patient, for example due to:

- Allergies to local anaesthetics
- Disorders of the respiratory organs
- Cardiac decompensation
- Severe metabolic disorders
- Fear of medication
- Danger of collapse.

In these cases, acupuncture analgesia presents an advantageous alternative as it is much less taxing for the cardiovascular and respiratory systems.

Method: the needles have to be stimulated for the whole duration of the dental treatment.

Specific treatment methods for toothache

Acupressure

Use the acupressure analgesia point at the midpoint of the posterior border of the ramus of the mandible. Add ST-6 or S.I.-18 depending on the location of the affected tooth. Strong pressure is applied with the fingertip for approximately 1–2 minutes. The analgesic effect tends to be sufficient for a short intervention (e.g. extraction of loose teeth or first teeth), so that the requirement for a local anaesthetic becomes redundant.

Electroacupuncture

Although electroacupuncture increases the analgesic effect, there are side-effects that have to be considered, even with so-called constant current devices:

- The direct current component of the impulses causes harmful electrolysis.
- There should be no current through the heart, so heart function has to be monitored.
- Possible reactions of the brain triggered by the electric current have to be monitored.

6.12.1 Toothache (1)

Basic point combination

Upper jaw, frontal section (incisors and canines)

Du-26, L.I.-20.

Upper jaw, lateral section (premolars and molars)

ST-2, S.I.-18, ST-7, Ex-HN-5 (*Tai Yang*).

Lower jaw, frontal section (incisors and canines)

Ren-24.

Lower jaw, lateral section (premolars and molars)

ST-6, ST-5, T.B.-17.

Molars (upper and lower jaw)

T.B.-23, G.B.-2.

Distal points for toothache

L.I.-1 (can also be massaged), L.I.-4, ST-40, BL-60.

Extra points for toothache

Ex-UE-9 (*Ba Xie*), Ex-LE-9 (*Wai Huai Jian*).
Ear acupuncture: 7 analgesia point for the teeth of the upper jaw.

Individual point combination

Hyperaemia of the pulpa

Local points will alleviate the hyperaemia of the affected area (see point combinations above).
Distal points: L.I.-4, ST-44.

Post-extraction pain

L.I.-4 (strong stimulation by twisting the needle for about 3–5 minutes without interruption); L.I.-1 (can also be massaged), ST-40, BL-60, Ex-UE-9 (*Ba Xie*), Ex-LE-9 (*Wai Huai Jian*).

For inflammation

T.B.-5, LU-5.

Acupuncture points

BL-60   **Location:** in the depression between the Achilles tendon and the lateral malleolus.
   Notes: master point for pain.

Du-26   **Location:** at the junction of the upper and middle third of the philtrum.
   Notes: local analgesic point.

Ex-HN-5   **Location:** on the temple, in a depression approximately 1 cun lateral to the midpoint of a line connecting the lateral extremity of the eyebrow and the outer canthus of the eye.
   Notes: local point.

Ex-LE-9   **Location:** on the prominence of the lateral malleolus.
   Notes: specific point for toothache (this point is located on the BL meridian and the teeth pertain to the BL/KID).

Ex-UE-9   **Location:** when a loose fist is made, 4 points on the dorsum of each hand, slightly proximal to the margins of the webs between the heads of the 1st to 5th metacarpal bones.
   Notes: the *Ba Xie* points eliminate Heat.

G.B.-2   **Location:** with the mouth open, in the depression anterior to the antitragic notch, posterior to the condyloid process of the mandible.

KID-3   **Location:** between the highest prominence of the medial malleolus and the Achilles tendon.
   Notes: *Yuan*-source point; tonifies the Kidney *Yin*; specific point for toothache due to Kidney *Yin* deficiency.

L.I.-1   **Location:** on the index finger, next to the radial corner of the nail.
   Notes: master point for toothache.

L.I.-4   **Location:** on the dorsum of the hand, at the highest point of the muscle bulge between the 1st and 2nd metacarpal bones.
   Notes: *Yuan*-source point; universal point for any tooth problems.

L.I.-20   **Location:** in the nasolabial groove, level with the midpoint of the lateral border of the ala nasi.
   Notes: local point; specific effect for deficiency, stagnation and Heat in the *Yang Ming* (L.I./ST).

LU-5   **Location:** on the cubital crease, radial to the tendon of the biceps.
   Notes: sedation point, *He*-sea point; has an effect on the face, eliminates Lung Heat and Phlegm.

Ren-24   **Location:** in the centre of the mentolabial groove.
   Notes: local point for the lower jaw.

S.I.-18   **Location:** on the anterior border of the insertion of the masseter on the maxilla. Ask the patient to clench their teeth or open the mouth.
   Notes: local point, master point for trismus.

ST-2   **Location:** on the pupil line, in the depression above the infraorbital foramen.
   Notes: local point.

ST-5   **Location:** on the anterior border of the mandibular insertion of the masseter; ask the patient to blow their cheeks – the point is where the facial artery can be felt.
   Notes: local point.

ST-6   **Location:** 1 cun anterior and superior to the mandibular angle.
   Notes: local point.

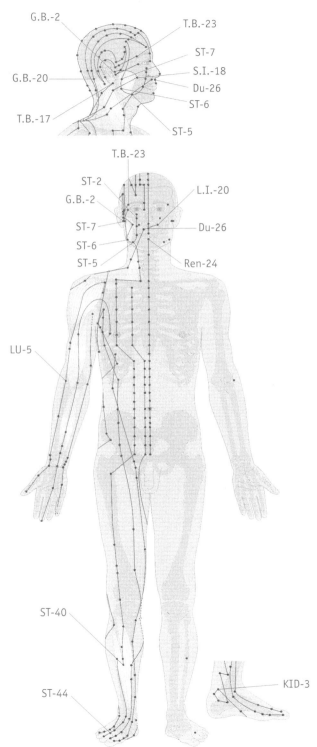

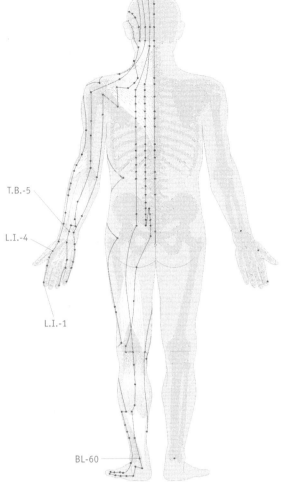

ST-7 **Location:** at the midpoint of the lower border of the zygomatic arch.
Notes: local point.

ST-40 **Location:** at the midpoint of the distance between the medial malleolus and the knee joint space, 2 cun lateral to the anterior crest of the tibia.
Notes: *Luo-connecting* point.

ST-44 **Location:** on the interdigital fold between the 2nd and 3rd toes, near the metatarsophalangeal joint of the 2nd toe.
Notes: eliminates heat from the Stomach and *Yang Ming*.

T.B.-5 **Location:** 2 cun proximal to the midpoint of the dorsal wrist crease, opposite P-6.
Notes: eliminates all external pathogens.

T.B.-17 **Location:** on the anterior border of the mastoid.
Notes: local point.

T.B.-23 **Location:** in a depression at the lateral end of the eyebrow.
Notes: local point.

6.12.1 Toothache (2)

Acupuncture according to TCM diagnosis (for subsiding pain)

Full heat in the *Yang Ming*

Intermittent pain, yellow tongue coating; foul breath.
ST-3, ST-44, T.B.-5, G.B.-20.
Local points: see point combinations for toothache (1).
Ear acupuncture: 7 analgesia point for the teeth of the upper jaw.

Yin deficiency with tense *Yang*

No foul breath.
KID-3. **Upper jaw:** ST-3, **lower jaw:** ST-5 or ST-6.

Acupuncture points

G.B.-20 **Location:** posterior to the mastoid, between the trapezius and sternocleidomastoid on the lower border of the occiput.
Notes: eliminates Wind and Heat.

KID-3 **Location:** between the highest prominence of the medial malleolus and the Achilles tendon.
Notes: *Yuan*-source point; tonifies the Kidney *Yin*: specific point for toothache due to deficient Kidney *Yin*.

ST-3 **Location:** at the intersection of the pupil line and a horizontal line level with the lower border of the ala nasi.
Notes: local point.

ST-5 **Location:** on the anterior border of the mandibular insertion of the masseter; ask the patient to blow their cheeks – the point is where the facial artery can be felt.
Notes: local point.

ST-6 **Location:** 1 cun anterior and superior to the mandibular angle.
Notes: local point.

ST-44 **Location:** on the interdigital fold between the 2nd and 3rd toes, near the metatarsophalangeal joint of the 2nd toe.
Notes: eliminates Heat from the Stomach and *Yang Ming*.

T.B.-5 **Location:** 2 cun proximal to the midpoint of the dorsal wrist crease, opposite P-6.
Notes: eliminates all external pathogens.

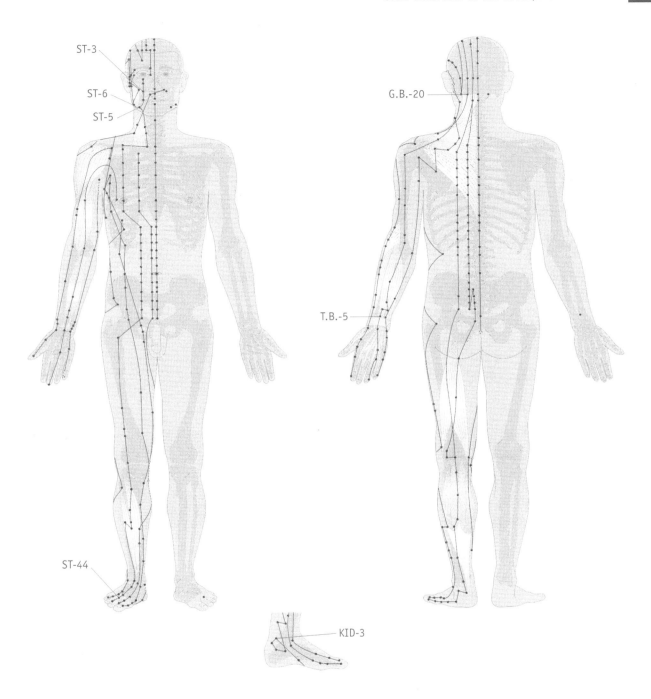

ST-3
ST-6
ST-5
ST-44
G.B.-20
T.B.-5
KID-3

6.12.2 Stomatitis

The following can cause periodontal disorders:
- Inflammations such as gingivitis (stomatitis and marginal periodontitis)
- Dystrophies such as atrophy due to inactivity, occlusal trauma, gingivosis, periodontosis, metabolic disorders, side-effects of medication.

Basic point combination

Pressure-sensitive local points; also ST-7, Du-26, Ren-24.
One or two of the following distal points: P-6, L.I.-4, LU-7, ST-36.

Individual point combination

With pain

L.I.-4, ST-44, S.I.-3.

With purulent inflammation

T.B.-5, L.I.-11, LU-5.

Aphthous stomatitis

L.I.-4, ST-44, BL-23, LIV-8, Ren-12 and local soft-laser application.

Stomatitis secondary to gastritis or gastrointestinal disorders

ST-36, P-6, SP-4, LIV-13, S.I.-19, Ren-12.

Acupuncture points

BL-23 Location: 1.5 cun lateral to L2, level with Du-4.
Notes: back-*Shu* point of the Kidneys; tonifies the *Qi*, *Yin*, *Yang* and Essence (*Jing*) of the Kidneys.
Du-19 Location: 5.5 cun superior the occipital hairline.
Notes: psychologically harmonizing.
Du-26 Location: at the junction of the upper and middle third of the philtrum.
Notes: local analgesic point.
L.I.-4 Location: on the dorsum of the hand, at the highest point of the muscle bulge between the 1st and 2nd metacarpal bones.
Notes: *Yuan*-source point; universal point for any tooth problems.

L.I.-11 Location: with the arm fully flexed at the radial end of the cubital crease.
Notes: *He*-sea point, tonification point; eliminates Damp-Heat and Wind.
LIV-8 Location: with the knee flexed, in the depression anterior to the medial end of the popliteal crease.
Notes: for toothache due to Liver *Yin* deficiency.
LIV-13 Location: on the lower border of the free end of the 11th rib.
Notes: front-*Mu* point of the Spleen; benefits the Stomach and Spleen, harmonizes the Liver and the Spleen/Stomach.
LU-5 Location: on the cubital crease, radial to the tendon of the biceps.
Notes: sedation point, *He*-sea point; has an effect on the face, eliminates Lung Heat and Phlegm.
LU-7 Location: 1.5 cun proximal to the wrist crease, superior to the radial artery.
Notes: *Luo*-connecting point, opening point of the *Ren Mai*, master point for stagnation; dispels pathogenic factors.
P-6 Location: 2 cun proximal to the midpoint of the palmar wrist crease, between the tendons of the flexor carpi radialis and palmaris longus.
Notes: opening point for the *Yin Wei Mai*, master point for nausea; harmonizes the Stomach, calming.
Ren-12 Location: midway between the umbilicus and the xiphoid process.
Notes: front-*Mu* point of the Stomach; combined with ST-36, also tonifies the Spleen.
Ren-24 Location: in the centre of the mentolabial groove.
Notes: local point.
S.I.-3 Location: when a fist is made, on the dorsum of the hand, in the depression at the end of the most distal palmar crease.
Notes: opening point of the *Du Mai* – the *Du Mai* ends in the gingiva of the upper jaw.
SP-4 Location: in the depression at the junction of the base and shaft of the 1st metatarsal bone, at the junction of the red and white skin.
Notes: opening point for the *Chong Mai*; tonifies the Stomach and the Spleen.
ST-7 Location: at the midpoint of the lower border of the zygomatic arch.
Notes: local point.
ST-36 Location: 0.5 cun lateral to the anterior crest of the tibia, 1.5 cun inferior to the lower border of the head of the fibula (G.B.-34).
Notes: *He*-sea point; tonifies the Spleen and Stomach, strengthening, psychologically harmonizing.
ST-44 Location: on the interdigital fold between the 2nd and 3rd toes, near the metatarsophalangeal joint of the 2nd toe.
Notes: eliminates Heat from the Stomach and *Yang Ming*.
T.B.-5 Location: 2 cun proximal to the midpoint of the dorsal wrist crease, opposite P-6.
Notes: eliminates all external pathogens.

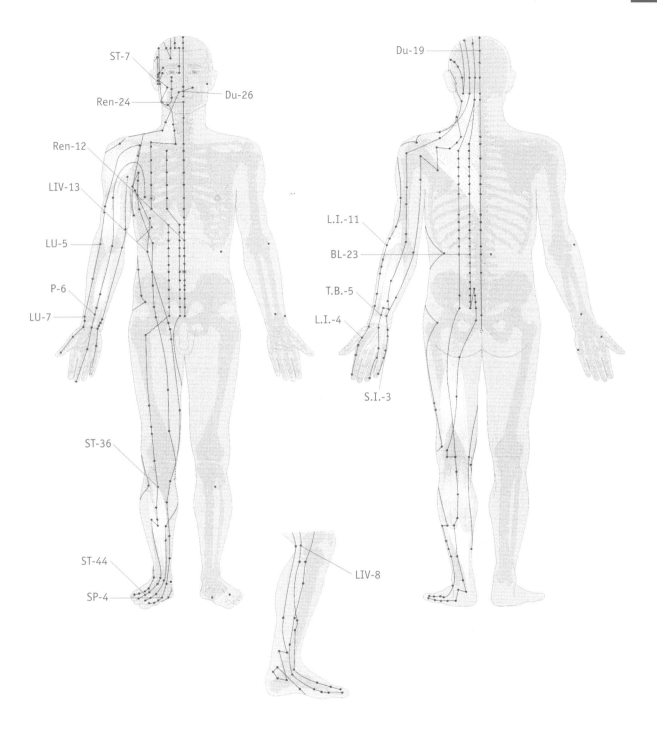

ST-7
Ren-24
Du-26
Ren-12
LIV-13
LU-5
P-6
LU-7
ST-36
ST-44
SP-4

Du-19
L.I.-11
BL-23
T.B.-5
L.I.-4
S.I.-3
LIV-8

6.12.3 Temporomandibular joint disorders (1)

In cases of monoarticular disorders it is important to consider a focal inflammation or infection:

- Tonsillar scars
- Infected teeth
- Impacted or displaced wisdom teeth
- Retained roots
- Periodontal pockets
- Pronounced periodontal changes
- Chronic otitis
- Operative scars following otitis media surgery
- Scars due to occipital furuncles and carbuncles
- Sinus infections.

Occlusal disorders may also cause longstanding non-physiological strain of one or both joints and the chewing muscles.

> In cases of true polyarthritis rheumatica, needles should be used very sparingly with intervals of 2–3 weeks between treatments to avoid triggering of a rheumatic flare-up.

Psychological factors can also have a damaging influence on the chewing musculature and result in a traumatic injury to the jaws (for example, grinding one's teeth during sleep or in stressful situations).

Basic point combination

According to the Five Phases, the bones are governed by the Kidneys, whereas the tendons and ligaments pertain to the Liver. For this reason, the *He*-sea points and the *Xi*-cleft points of the Liver, Kidney, Bladder and Gall Bladder are often selected in the treatment of TMJ disorders.

Individual point combination

Inflammatory, rheumatic processes

Method: during the acute stage, daily treatments; for chronic cases, every other day. Retain the needles for 15–20 minutes.
Local points: S.I.-18, ST-7 [ST-2 Bi], G.B.-2, G.B.-20, T.B.-15, BL-10.
Distal points of the hand: L.I.-3, S.I.-3, T.B.-5.
Distal points of the legs: ST-36, G.B.-34, LIV-6, BL-63.

Acupuncture points

BL-10 **Location:** at the external occipital protuberance, on the lateral aspect of the trapezius insertion.
  Notes: eliminates Wind, locally unblocks the meridians, vagotonic point (vegetative foundation with G.B.-20).

BL-63 **Location:** in the depression between the calcaneus and the cuboid bones, approximately 1 cun anterior and inferior to BL-62.
  Notes: *Xi*-cleft point of the Bladder.

G.B.-2 **Location:** with the mouth open, in the depression anterior to the antitragic notch, posterior to the condyloid process of the mandible.

G.B.-20 **Location:** posterior to the mastoid, between the trapezius and sternocleidomastoid muscles, on the lower border of the occiput.
  Notes: eliminates Wind from the head, subdues internal and external Wind.

G.B.-34 **Location:** with the knee flexed, in the depression anterior and inferior to the head of the fibula.
  Notes: *He*-sea point of the Gall Bladder, *Hui*-meeting point of the tendons, master point of the musculature; relaxes the tendons, promotes the smooth flow of Liver *Qi*.

L.I.-4 **Location:** on the dorsum of the hand, at the highest point of the muscle bulge between the 1st and 2nd metacarpal bones.
  Notes: *Yuan*-source point; universal point for any tooth problems.

LIV-6 **Location:** 7 cun superior to the medial malleolus, slightly posterior to the medial border of the tibia.
  Notes: promotes the harmonious flow of Liver *Qi*.

S.I.-3 **Location:** when a fist is made, on the dorsum of the hand, in the depression at the end of the most distal palmar crease.
  Notes: tonification point, opening of the *Du Mai* (CNS), spasmolytic point; has an effect on the mucosa.

S.I.-18 **Location:** on the anterior border of the insertion of the masseter on the maxilla. Ask the patient to clench their teeth or open the mouth.
  Notes: local point, master point for trismus.

ST-7 **Location:** at the midpoint of the lower border of the zygomatic arch.
  Notes: local point.

ST-36 **Location:** 0.5 cun lateral to the anterior crest of the tibia, 1.5 cun inferior to lower border of the head of the fibula (G.B.-34).
  Notes: *He*-sea point; tonifies the Spleen and Stomach, strengthening, psychologically harmonizing.

T.B.-5 **Location:** 2 cun proximal to the midpoint of the dorsal wrist crease, opposite P-6.
  Notes: eliminates all external pathogens.

T.B.-15 **Location:** in the suprascapular fossa, midway between G.B.-21 (highest point on the shoulder, midway between the acromion and the spinous process of C7) and S.I.-13 (in the medial section of the supraspinous fossa, at the curved medial end of the scapular spine).
  Notes: adjacent point.

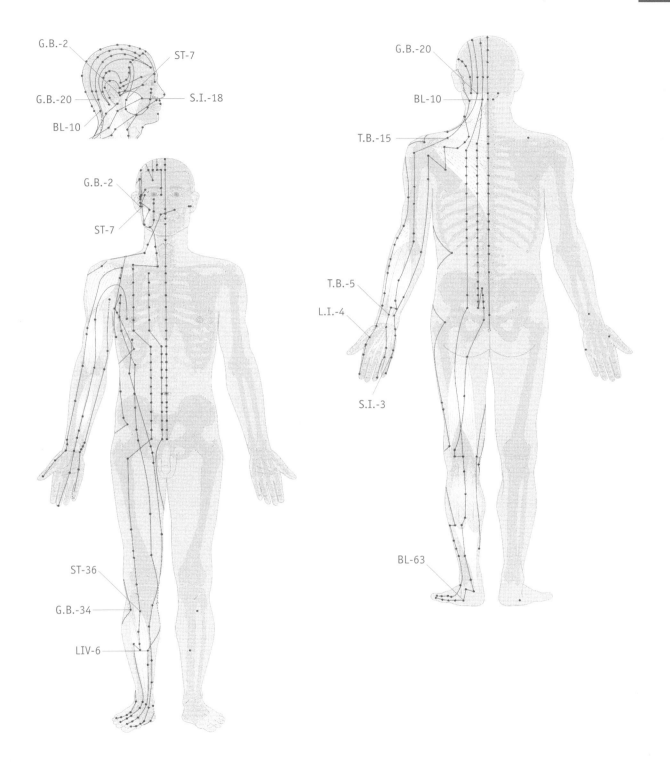

G.B.-2
ST-7
G.B.-20
S.I.-18
BL-10

G.B.-2
ST-7

ST-36
G.B.-34
LIV-6

G.B.-20
BL-10
T.B.-15

T.B.-5
L.I.-4
S.I.-3

BL-63

6.12.3 *Temporomandibular joint disorders (2)*

Grinding one's teeth

Ren-15, Du-19, ST-3, HE-3, ST-36, L.I.-4.

Trismus ('lock-jaw')

The most common cause of trismus are inflammatory processes near the 2nd and 3rd molars with frequently oedematous swellings that quickly affect the surrounding chewing muscles, often resulting in a complete inability to open the jaw. In addition, all other TMJ disorders, as well as inflammatory and neoplastic processes of the tonsils, the neighbouring lymph glands and salivary glands may lead to lock-jaw.

Local points: S.I.-18, ST-6 [ST-3 Bi], T.B.-17, G.B.-20.
Distal points on the hands: L.I.-4, T.B.-5.
Soft-laser (stoma laser) on the affected area (wisdom teeth or at site of local inflammation).

Acupuncture points

Du-19   **Location:** 5.5 cun superior the occipital hairline.
Notes: Du-20 is now much more commonly used; balances the autonomic nervous system.

G.B.-20   **Location:** posterior to the mastoid, between the trapezius and sternocleidomastoid muscles, on the lower border of the occiput.
Notes: eliminates Wind from the head; subdues internal and external Wind.

HE-3   **Location:** with the elbow fully flexed, between the medial end of the cubital crease and the medial epicondyle.
Notes: *He*-sea point, master point for depression; eliminates Heat, psychologically uplifting.

L.I.-4   **Location:** on the dorsum of the hand, at the highest point of the muscle bulge between the 1st and 2nd metacarpal bones.
Notes: *Yuan*-source point; universal point for any tooth problems.

Ren-15   **Location:** 1 cun inferior to the xiphoid process.
Notes: combined with Du-19 or 20 harmonizes the autonomic nervous system.

S.I.-18   **Location:** on the anterior border of the insertion of the masseter on the maxilla. Ask the patient to clench their teeth or open the mouth.
Notes: local point; master point for trismus.

ST-3   **Location:** at the intersection of the pupil line and a horizontal line level with the lower border of the ala nasi.
Notes: local point.

ST-6   **Location:** 1 cun anterior and superior to the mandibular angle.
Notes: local point.

ST-36   **Location:** 0.5 cun lateral to the anterior crest of the tibia, 1.5 cun inferior to the lower border of the head of the fibula (G.B.-34).
Notes: *He*-sea point; tonifies the Spleen and Stomach, strengthening, psychologically harmonizing.

T.B.-5   **Location:** 2 cun proximal to the midpoint of the dorsal wrist crease, opposite P-6.
Notes: eliminates all external pathogens.

T.B.-17   **Location:** on the anterior border of the mastoid.
Notes: eliminates Wind; local point.

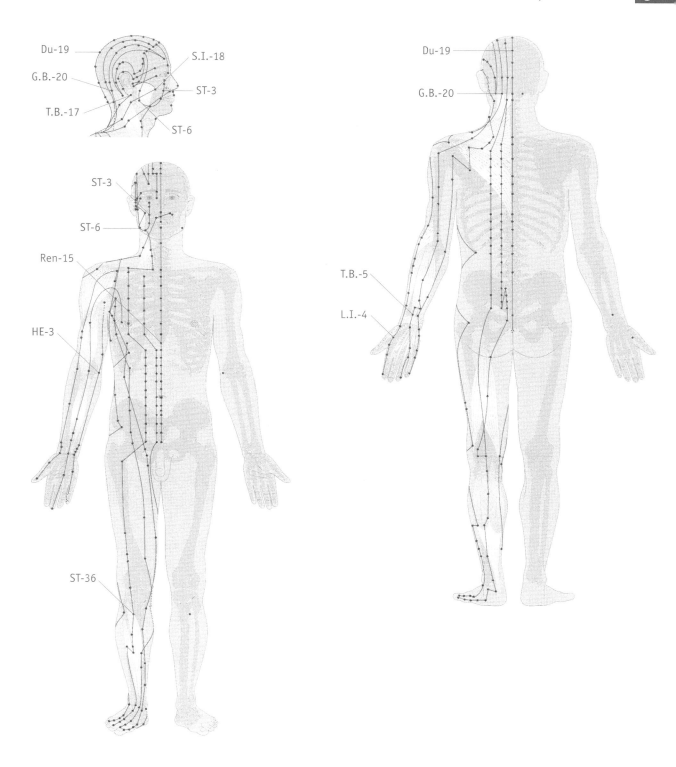

6.13 Musculoskeletal disorders

G. Kubiena, B. Sommer

Musculoskeletal disorders respond extremely well to acupuncture. Even for arthrosis an improvement can be expected. Although acupuncture cannot reverse any pathological changes, it can eliminate pain and swelling. In general the following rule of thumb applies: the shorter the duration of the disorder, the better the prognosis.

TCM

As acupuncture moves the *Qi* and pain is caused by *Qi* and Blood (*Xue*) stagnation, even a basic acupuncture treatment will, in most cases, show good results.

Fundamental treatment principles for musculoskeletal disorders

> The **location** of the pain determines the **location** of the treatment. The **type** of pain determines the **type** of treatment.

Primary criterion: location of the pain

See also Table 4.1 → overview of the 72 meridians.

- Determine the affected meridian: ask the patient to show the exact site of pain.
- Select distal, adjacent and local points on the affected or its paired meridian.
- Acute pain: check the medical history for the presence of an external pathogen (e.g. draught); key symptom: a superficial pulse signifying that a pathogen acutely obstructs the sinew meridian. **Therapy:** ipsilateral needling with shallow insertion of the *A-Shi* point (painful point) on the affected sinew meridian and the *Jing*-well point; light bleeding or excretion of serous fluid is desirable.
- Unilateral pain occurring regularly at the same time of day, accompanied by an 'organ sensation', is often connected to a problem at the level of the divergent meridians (psychosomatic component). **Therapy:** contralateral needling of the *Jing*-well point and *He*-sea point of the affected meridian, as well as Du-20.
- Acute pain, onset only a few hours previously. **Therapy:** use microsystems (ear, hand, scalp) and/or contralateral distal points on the corresponding meridian; ask the patient to move the painful joint during stimulation of the distal point; subsequently needle local points.
- Acute pain, onset a few days previously. **Therapy:** as above, but ipsilateral needling of the distal points.
- Chronic pain. **Therapy:** mainly use local points; in addition, determine the cause of the pain and treat accordingly – 'Rule of Three' of the Vienna School: Which meridian? Any organ involvement? Accompanying circumstances? (see below).
- General chronic pain. **Therapy:** SP-21, BL-17.
- Individual joints or areas of the body. **Therapy:** needling around the affected area using both local and distal points.
- Lateral–medial rule: treat pain on the lateral aspect of the joint by also needling its medial aspect, and vice versa.
- Anterior–posterior rule: treat pain on the anterior aspect by also needling points on the posterior aspect, and vice versa.

Secondary criterion: cause of the pain – 'accompanying circumstances'

Qi stagnation as well as *Qi* and Blood (*Xue*) stagnation can have various causes:

- 'Excess' signifies the presence of external pathogens – predominantly Wind, Cold and Dampness – which have to be eliminated. For external Wind, select 'Wind points' such as G.B.-20, T.B.-17 and G.B.-31; Cold requires application of moxa; for Dampness, SP-9 is a particularly effective point.
- 'Deficiency' refers to a lack of substrate: deficient defensive *Qi* (*Wei Qi*) allows external pathogens to invade the body; *Qi* and Blood deficiency can lead to diffuse pain; *Yin*, *Yang* or Essence (*Jing*) deficiency are often the underlying cause of lumbar pain, as the lumbar region represents the 'House of the Kidneys' and thus the abode of *Yin* and *Yang*.
- Cold always requires treatment with moxibustion. In cases of external excess-Cold, combine with a sedating needling technique; for deficiency-Cold (= *Yang* deficiency), combine with tonifying techniques. A combination of *Yang* deficiency triggered by external Cold – a common pattern – should be treated with moxa and neutral stimulation.

- Heat or Fire requires points that drain Heat and Fire. **Basic point prescription:** L.I.-4, L.I.-11, Du-14; Heat points: the 1st or 2nd most distal point on the affected meridian – in severe cases even bloodletting at Ex-UE-11 (*Shi Xuan*) and/or Ex-LE-12 (*Qi Duan*). In cases of deficiency Fire (= *Yin* deficiency plus Fire), Heat has to be eliminated, but more importantly *Yin* has to be tonified: BL-23, KID-3 KID-8/MP-6. A reminder: owing to its relationship with Heat, Fire is considered to be one of the 6 external pathogens; however, in contrast to the other 5 pathogens, it is not related to a particular season and can form at any time as a result of the combination of 2 pathogenic factors (external or internal, or mixed), for example a flare-up of chronic rheumatism.

Bi syndrome

TCM refers to muscle and joint pain as '*Bi*', which means 'meridian obstruction'. *Bi* syndromes affecting the musculoskeletal system are caused predominantly by Cold, Wind and Dampness, particularly if there is an existing predisposition. TCM differentiates *Bi* syndromes based on two systems:

Differentiation of Bi *syndromes according to stages and pathogens*

The main criterion is the nature of the pathogen:

- 'Wandering *Bi*' ('Wind *Bi*'): pain moves around, not localized, susceptible to weather changes, infections. Predisposition: Blood deficiency.
  Special points: sedate G.B.-20 as well as other Wind points; BL-17, SP-10.
- 'Cold *Bi*' ('painful *Bi*'): soft tissue rheumatism, pain without signs of inflammation, desire for warmth. Predisposition: *Qi* or *Yang* deficiency.
  Special points: BL-23, Ren-4. Primarily moxibustion, secondarily acupuncture: deep needling, long needle retention.
- 'Damp *Bi*' ('fixed *Bi*'): rheumatism affecting the joints, geloses, sensation of heaviness, localized pain, desire for warmth, worse with dampness. Predisposition: Spleen *Qi* or *Yang* deficiency.
  Special points: Ren-4, SP-9, Ren-9 moxa, cupping; ST-36, Ren-12, BL-20.
- 'Heat *Bi*': arthritis, gout, fever, redness, swelling; worse with warmth. Pathogenesis: combination of several pathogenic factors.
  Special points: Du-14, L.I.-11; no moxa.

Differentiation of Bi *syndromes according to levels*

The criterion here is the depth that the pathogenic factor has reached within body; which parts of the body are affected – the skin, muscles, tendons, joints, vessels?

- Skin *Bi*: psoriasis
- Muscle *Bi*: soft tissue rheumatism
- Tendon *Bi*: contractures, arthritic psoriasis. Therapy: sedate G.B.-34, moxa, cupping
- Bone *Bi*: bones – deformed joints: arthrosis with exophytes, spondylosis, gout. Therapy: BL-11, G.B.-39. Acupuncture, moxa cupping
- Vessel *Bi*: rheumatoid endocarditis, vasculitis.

Fundamental treatment principles for pareses and atrophies – *Wei* syndrome

TCM

Muscle paresis and atrophy are always caused by a deficient or disruptive diet (*Yin* and Blood deficiency) or by a lack of moistening (Essence [*Jing*] deficiency).

Basic point combination

Primarily points on the *Yang Ming* meridians (L.I., ST), which promote the circulation of *Qi* and Blood in the meridians as well as 'nourishment' of the muscles and tendons; add G.B.-34 and G.B.-39.

TCM mentions 4 causes of paresis and muscular atrophy:

- Excess-Heat in the Lungs – for example, poliomyelitis injures the Essence (*Jing*) and therefore the Body Fluids.
  Special points: LU-5, BL-13.
- Damp-Heat causes chronic *Qi* and Blood stagnation in the meridians, resulting in impaired nourishment of the muscles and tendons.
  Special points: BL-20, SP-9.
- Liver and Kidney *Yin* deficiency: impaired nourishment of the muscles, tendons and bones.
  Special points: BL-18, BL-23.
- Trauma: injury to the spine.
  Special points: *Hua Tuo* points in the affected area.

Individual point combinations

- Upper extremity: L.I.-15, L.I.-11, L.I.-4, T.B.-5
- Lower extremity: ST-31, G.B.-30, G.B.-34, G.B.-39, SP-10, ST-41

- Urinary incontinence: Ren-3, SP-6
- Faecal incontinence: BL-25, BL-32.

In contrast to other disorders of the musculoskeletal system, signs and symptoms of an arthritic nature are interpreted as Heat and are therefore treated differently. Major points: L.I.-11 and Du-14 [Du-13 Bi].

The more acute the case, the more distal points are selected, the more chronic, the more local points are needled. Ear acupuncture is particularly relevant for acute conditions.

6.13.1 Cervical pain

Basic point combination

Local points: BL-10, G.B.-20, Du-14 [Du-13 Bi].
Distal points: S.I.-3, T.B.-5, G.B.-34.
Ear acupuncture: cervical spine.
Hand points: hand point 14 (occiput).
Extra points: Ex-HN-15 (*Jing Bai Lao*).

Individual point combination

Moving pain

TCM: moving pains are attributed to Wind.
BL-17, SP-10.

Localized pain

Worse with cold.
Moxa.

Difficulty nodding the head (saying 'yes')

S.I.-3, BL-60, BL-10, G.B.-20.

Difficulty shaking the head (saying 'no')

T.B.-5, G.B.-41, G.B.-20, BL-10, T.B.-15.

Acute pain, occipital stiffness

Ear acupuncture: 37 cervical spine, 29 occiput, 26 brain-stem, hypothalamus; hand point 14 *Jing Xiang Dian*, Ex-HN-15 (*Jing*) *Bai Lao*.

Acupuncture points

BL-10 **Location:** at the external occipital protuberance, on the lateral aspect of the trapezius insertion.
Notes: local point for tonifying the parasympathetic nervous system; combined with GB-20 harmonizes the autonomic nervous system.

BL-17 **Location:** 1.5 cun lateral to the spinous process of T7.
Notes: back-*Shu* point of the diaphragm, relaxes the diaphragm; *Hui*-meeting point of the Blood (*Xue*), nourishes and invigorates the Blood (*Xue*).

BL-60 **Location:** in the depression between the Achilles tendon and the lateral malleolus.
Notes: *Jing*-river point, master point for pain along the meridian pathway.

Du-14 **Location:** below the spinous process of C7.
Notes: meeting point of all *Yang* meridians; eliminates pathogens (especially Wind-Cold) from the surface; for Heat/fever, combine with L.I.-4 and L.I.-11.

Ex-HN-15 **Location:** 2 cun superior to the lower border of the spinous process of C7 and 1 cun lateral to the midline.
Notes: local point.

G.B.-20 **Location:** posterior to the mastoid, between the trapezius and sternocleidomastoid muscles, on the lower border of the occiput.
Notes: local point, major point for Wind in the upper half of the body; with BL-10 harmonizes the autonomic nervous system.

G.B.-34 **Location:** with the knee flexed, in the depression anterior and inferior to the head of the fibula.
Notes: *He*-sea point of the Gall Bladder, *Hui*-meeting point of the tendons, master point of the musculature.

G.B.-41 **Location:** in the depression distal to the junction of the 4th and 5th metatarsal bones.
Notes: *Shu*-stream point, opening point of the *Dai Mai*, master point of the big joints.

Hand point 14 **Location:** on the dorsum of the hand, between the metacarpophalangeal joints of the 2nd and 3rd fingers, closer to the 2nd finger.
Notes: for acute cervical pain.

S.I.-3 **Location:** when a fist is made, on the dorsum of the hand, in the depression at the end of the most distal palmar crease.
Notes: tonification point, opening point of the *Du Mai* – meridian pathway!

S.I.-9 **Location:** with the arm adducted, 1 cun superior to the end of the posterior axillary fold.
Notes: local point; eliminates Wind.

SP-10 **Location:** with the knee flexed, 2 cun superior to the upper patellar border, medial to the vastus medialis.
Notes: 'Sea of Blood'; tonifies and cools the Blood (*Xue*); moves the *Qi* and Blood (*Xue*), thus eliminating Wind.

T.B.-5 **Location:** 2 cun proximal to the midpoint of the dorsal wrist crease, opposite P-6.
Notes: *Luo*-connecting point, opening point of the *Yang Wei Mai*, master point of the small joints; dispels all *Yang* pathogenic factors.

T.B.-15 **Location:** in the suprascapular fossa, midway between G.B.-21 (highest point on the shoulder, midway between the acromion and the spinous process of C7) and S.I.-13 (in the medial section of the supraspinous fossa, at the curved medial end of the scapular spine).
Notes: meeting point with the *Yang Wei Mai*, master point for the upper extremities; for pathogenic Wind and susceptibility to changes in the weather.

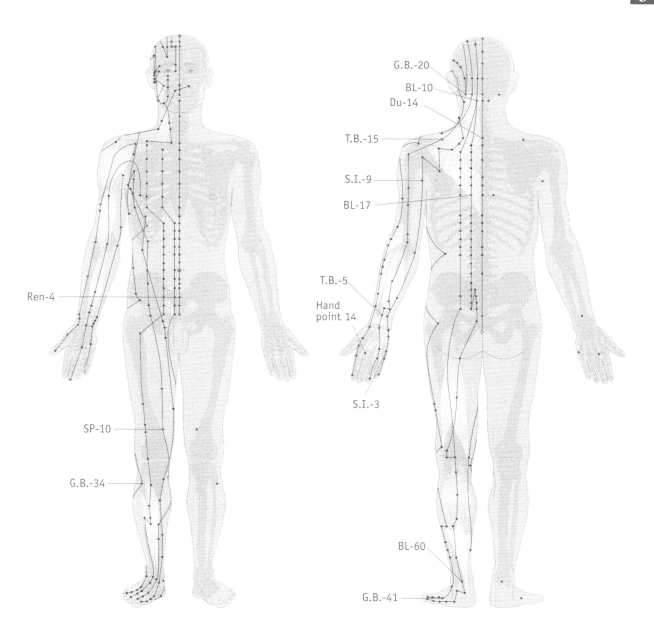

G.B.-20
BL-10
Du-14
T.B.-15
S.I.-9
BL-17

T.B.-5
Hand
point 14

S.I.-3

Ren-4

SP-10

G.B.-34

BL-60

G.B.-41

6.13.2 Segmental thoracic pain

Once the possibility of a heart disorder has been eliminated, local and distal points are selected based on the site of the pain and the meridian pathway. Heart disease can often lead to vertebral blockages at the level of T4 and T5. If the patient is also receiving any form of manual therapy, it is advisable to have acupuncture first in order to relax the muscles.

Ear acupuncture is recommended especially if the relevant ear points are active.

Basic point combination

Segmental pressure-sensitive points on the *Hua Tuo* line (Ex-B-2).

Ear acupuncture: pressure-sensitive points on the thoracic zone.

Individual point combination

Pain on the anterior aspect of the thorax

Ren-17, distal points: P-6, LU-7, HE-7.

Pain on the posterior aspect

Local points: BL meridian (→ back-*Shu* points, 5.2.1 and 5.6) or segmental points on the *Hua Tuo* line (Ex-B-2).
Distal points: pain on the medial border of the scapula: S.I.-3; pain on the lateral border of the scapula: S.I.-6.

Check the back-*Shu* points and corresponding *Yuan*-source points of the affected area.

Lateral pain

G.B.-24, BL-14 to BL-21, SP-21, P-1, HE-1. Distal points: G.B.-40, T.B.-6.

Acupuncture points

> **BL-14** **Location:** 1.5 cun lateral to the spinous process of T4.
> **Notes:** back-*Shu* point of the Pericardium.
> **BL-15** **Location:** 1.5 cun lateral to the spinous process of T5.
> **Notes:** back-*Shu* point of the Heart.
> **BL-16** **Location:** 1.5 cun lateral to the spinous process of T6.
> **Notes:** back-*Shu* point of the *Du Mai*.
> **BL-17** **Location:** 1.5 cun lateral to the spinous process of T7, approximately level with the inferior angle of the scapula.
> **Notes:** *Hui*-meeting point of the Blood (*Xue*); nourishes and invigorates the Blood (*Xue*); back-*Shu* point of the diaphragm, relaxes the diaphragm.

> **BL-18** **Location:** 2 cun lateral to the spinous process of T9.
> **Notes:** back-*Shu* point of the Liver, promotes the smooth flow of *Qi*.
> **BL-19** **Location:** 1.5 cun lateral to the spinous process of T10.
> **Notes:** back-*Shu* point of the Gall Bladder.
> **BL-20** **Location:** 1.5 cun lateral to the spinous process of T11.
> **Notes:** back-*Shu* point of the Spleen.
> **BL-21** **Location:** 1.5 cun lateral to the spinous process of T12.
> **Notes:** back-*Shu* point of the Stomach, master point for the Stomach.
> **Ex-B-2** **Location:** 17 point pairs, 0.5 cun lateral to the lower borders of the spinous processes of T1 to L5; medial to the inner Bladder line.
> **G.B.-24** **Location:** on the midclavicular line, in the 7th ICS.
> **Notes:** front-*Mu* point of the Gall Bladder; mobilizes Liver *Qi* stagnation.
> **G.B.-40** **Location:** on the junction of a horizontal line through the prominence of the lateral malleolus and a vertical line through the greatest circumference of the lateral malleolus, over the calcaneocuboidal joint.
> **Notes:** *Yuan*-source point; 'miracle point' for lateral thoracic pain! Tonifies and mobilizes *Qi* along the meridian pathway, particularly for stagnation due to deficiency.
> **HE-1** **Location:** in the centre of the axilla, medial to the axillary artery.
> **Notes:** local point, tonifies the Heart *Yin*.
> **HE-7** **Location:** on the ulnar aspect of the wrist crease, on the radial aspect of the pisiform bone.
> **Notes:** *Shu*-stream point, *Yuan*-source point, sedation point; resolves stagnation in the meridians of the chest.
> **LU-7** **Location:** 1.5 cun proximal to the wrist crease, superior to the radial artery.
> **Notes:** *Luo*-connecting point and opening point of the *Ren Mai*, master point for stagnation; promotes the descending and dispersing function of the Lung, therefore effective for chronically rebellious or stagnated Lung *Qi*.
> **P-1** **Location:** in the 4th ICS, 1 cun lateral to the midclavicular line (1 cun lateral to the nipple).
> **Notes:** local point; removes *Qi* stagnation from the Heart, Liver and Lung; resolves Heart Blood (*Xue*) stagnation.
> **P-6** **Location:** 2 cun proximal to the midpoint of the palmar wrist crease, between the tendons of the flexor carpi radialis and palmaris longus.
> **Notes:** *Luo*-connecting point and opening point of the *Yin Wei Mai*; has an effect on Heart function, unbinds the thorax.
> **Ren-17** **Location:** on the midline of the sternum, at the level of the 4th ICS, between the nipples (in men).
> **Notes:** front-*Mu* point of the Pericardium, *Hui*-meeting point of the respiratory system; unbinds the thorax.

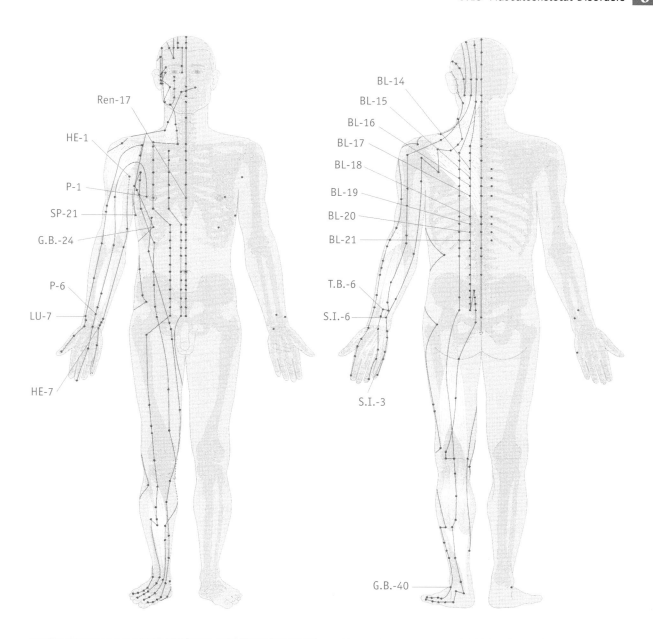

Ren-17

HE-1

P-1

SP-21

G.B.-24

P-6

LU-7

HE-7

BL-14
BL-15
BL-16
BL-17
BL-18
BL-19
BL-20
BL-21

T.B.-6

S.I.-6

S.I.-3

G.B.-40

S.I.-3 **Location:** when a fist is made, on the dorsum of the hand, in the depression at the end of the most distal palmar crease.
Notes: *Shu*-stream point, therefore effective for musculoskeletal disorders, particularly when due to Dampness; as tonification point and opening point of the *Du Mai*, influences the spine and central nervous system.
S.I.-6 **Location:** in a depression just proximal and radial to the styloid process of the ulna.

Notes: *Xi*-cleft point; for acute upper back pain, especially lateral to the scapula.
SP-21 **Location:** on the midaxillary line, in the 6th ICS.
Notes: has a connection to all collaterals, therefore for pain in the whole body; here used as a local point.
T.B.-6 **Location:** 3 cun proximal to the midpoint of the dorsal wrist crease.
Notes: *Jing*-river point; regulates the thoracic *Qi*, mobilizes *Qi* stagnation in the 3 Burners.

6.13.3 Shoulder pain

In patients with shoulder and arm pain it is important to eliminate coronary heart disease and gall bladder disorders. Ear acupuncture is recommended in most cases.

Basic point combination

Distal point: ST-38 – very effective for any type of shoulder pain.

Local points: L.I.-15, T.B.-14, S.I.-9.

Acute points: these are not identical to *Xi*-cleft points but are empirical points below the knee that are located on the corresponding meridian. Shoulder in general: ST-38; anterior shoulder pain: add SP-9; posterior shoulder pain: G.B.-34; scapular pain: BL-40 [BL-54 Bi].

Ear acupuncture: 64 shoulder joint.

Hand acupuncture: hand point 5, shoulder.

Individual point combination

Anterior shoulder pain (Large Intestine meridian)

L.I.-15, LU-2; distal point: L.I.-4; acute points: ST-38, SP-9.

Posterior shoulder pain (Triple Burner meridian)

T.B.-14, T.B.-15, S.I.-9, S.I.-10; distal point: L.I.-4; acute point: G.B.-34.

Scapular pain (Small Intestine meridian)

Among the following select pressure-sensitive points: S.I.-9, S.I.-10, S.I.-11, S.I.-12, S.I.-13, BL-43 [BL-38 Bi], T.B.-14; distal points: S.I.-3, BL-62 or BL-60; acute point: BL-40 [BL-54 Bi].

Acupuncture points

> **BL-40** **Location:** in the centre of the popliteal crease, between the tendons of the semitendinosus and the biceps femoris.
> **Notes:** *He*-sea point, metabolic point, reactive test point for gonarthralgia, command point for the back.
>
> **BL-43** **Location:** 3 cun lateral to the spinous process of T4, lateral to BL-14.
> **Notes:** local point; tonifies *Qi*, deficiency, Essence (*Jing*) and Lung *Yin*.

> **BL-60** **Location:** in the depression between the Achilles tendon and the lateral malleolus.
> **Notes:** master point for pain along the pathway of the Bladder meridian; strengthens the back.
>
> **BL-62** **Location:** below the prominence of the lateral malleolus.
> **Notes:** opens the *Yang Qiao Mai* (it is its opening point), increases the effect of S.I.-3.
>
> **G.B.-34** **Location:** with the knee flexed, in the depression anterior and inferior to the head of the fibula.
> **Notes:** *He*-sea point of the Gall Bladder, *Hui*-meeting point of the tendons, master point of the musculature.
>
> **Hand point 5** **Location:** at the metacarpophalangeal joint of the index finger, at the junction of the red and white skin, between L.I.-2 and L.I.-3.
> **Notes:** for acute shoulder pain.
>
> **L.I.-4** **Location:** on the dorsum of the hand, at the highest point of the muscle bulge between the 1st and 2nd metacarpal bones.
> **Notes:** *Yuan*-source point; regulates the L.I. meridian for pain of the hand and arm.
>
> **L.I.-15** **Location:** with the arm abducted, in the anterior of the two depressions inferior to the acromioclavicular joint, between the anterior and medial third of the deltoid (T.B.-14 is located in the posterior depression).
> **Notes:** master point for pareses of the upper extremity, meeting point with the *Yang Wei Mai*.
>
> **LU-2** **Location:** on the lower border of the clavicle, 6 cun lateral to the anterior midline. Caution: pneumothorax!
> **Notes:** local point, especially for chronic disorders.
>
> **S.I.-3** **Location:** when a fist is made, on the dorsum of the hand, in the depression at the end of the most distal palmar crease.
> **Notes:** tonification point, opening point of the *Du Mai*; has an effect on the spine and CNS.
>
> **S.I.-9** **Location:** with the arm adducted, 1 cun superior to the end of the posterior axillary fold.
> **Notes:** local point; eliminates Wind and obstructions in the meridian.
>
> **S.I.-10** **Location:** on the lower border of the scapular spine, perpendicularly superior to S.I.-9.
> **Notes:** important local point; meeting point with the *Yang Qiao Mai* (BL-62) and *Yang Wei Mai* (T.B.-5).
>
> **S.I.-11** **Location:** in the centre of the infraspinous fossa, at the level of the spinous process of T5.
> **Notes:** local point.
>
> **S.I.-12** **Location:** with the arm abducted, in a depression in the centre of the suprascapular fossa.
>
> **S.I.-13** **Location:** in the medial section of the supraspinous fossa, where the scapular spine curves upwards (name!).
>
> **SP-9** **Location:** with the knee flexed, in the depression inferior to the medial condyle of the tibia, at the same level as G.B.-34.
> **Notes:** *He*-sea point; here used as point for acute pain around LU-2 – SP-9 is located on the corresponding meridian (*Tai Yin*).

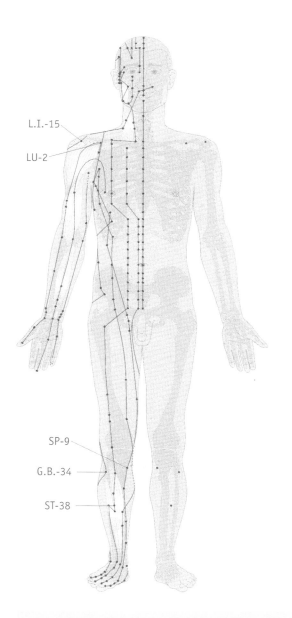

ST-38 **Location:** 1 cun lateral to the anterior crest of the tibia, 7 cun inferior to the lower border of the head of the fibula, at the midpoint of the distance between the highest prominence of the medial malleolus and the knee joint space.

Notes: most important empirical point for acute pain of the whole shoulder region.

T.B.-5 **Location:** 2 cun proximal to the midpoint of the dorsal wrist crease, opposite P-6.

Notes: *Luo*-connecting point, opening point of the *Yang Wei Mai*, master point of the small joints; dispels all *Yang* pathogenic factors.

T.B.-14 **Location:** with the arm abducted, in the depression posterior and inferior to the acromion, between the medial and posterior fibres of the deltoid (L.I.-15 lies anterior to T.B.-14).

Notes: local point.

T.B.-15 **Location:** in the suprascapular fossa, midway between G.B.-21 (highest point on the shoulder, midway between the acromion and the spinous process of C7) and S.I.-13 (in the medial section of the supraspinous fossa, at the curved medial end of the scapular spine).

Notes: meeting point with the *Yang Wei Mai*, master point for the upper extremities; for pathogenic Wind and susceptibility to changes in the weather.

6.13.4 *Elbow pain*

In chronic elbow pain, the focus of the disorder might be located in the cranial area.

Ear acupuncture is often beneficial here.

Basic point combination

L.I.-11, HE-3, T.B.-10; don't forget to needle ulnar points for radial pain, and vice versa!
Ear acupuncture: 66 elbow.

Individual point combination

Radial pain

L.I.-10 or L.I.-11, T.B.-10; distal point: L.I.-4.

Ulnar pain

HE-3, P-3, S.I.-8; distal point: S.I.-3.

Acupuncture points

HE-3   **Location:** with the elbow fully flexed, between the medial end of the cubital crease and the medial epicondyle.
Notes: *He*-sea point and master point for depression.

L.I.-4   **Location:** on the dorsum of the hand, at the highest point of the muscle bulge between the 1st and 2nd metacarpal bones.
Notes: *Yuan*-source point; regulates the L.I. meridian for pain of the hand and arm.

L.I.-10   **Location:** on the radial aspect of the forearm, 3 cun distal to L.I.-11, on the belly of the extensor muscles.
Notes: for disorders along the pathway of the L.I. meridian; eliminates swellings.

L.I.-11   **Location:** with the arm fully flexed, at the radial end of the cubital crease.
Notes: *He*-sea point and tonification point; local point; supports the tendons and joints.

P-3   **Location:** with the elbow flexed, on the cubital crease, ulnar to the tendon of the biceps (LU-5 is located radial to the tendon).
Notes: *He*-sea point.

S.I.-3   **Location:** when a fist is made, on the dorsum of the hand, in the depression at the end of the most distal palmar crease.
Notes: as *Shu*-stream point for joint disorders due to Dampness.

S.I.-8   **Location:** with the elbow flexed, in the depression between the olecranon process of the ulna and the medial epicondyle of the humerus, 0.5 cun from the tip of the olecranon.
Notes: *He*-sea point and sedation point.

T.B.-10   **Location:** with the elbow slightly flexed, in the depression 1 cun superior to the olecranon.
Notes: *He*-sea point.

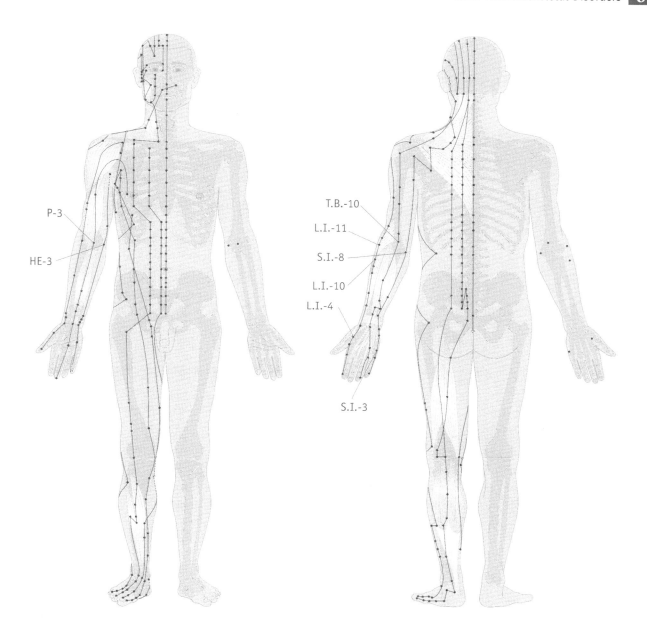

P-3

HE-3

T.B.-10

L.I.-11

S.I.-8

L.I.-10

L.I.-4

S.I.-3

6.13.5 *Hand and wrist pain*

The points around the wrist form a 'ring', which can also be successfully needled for diffuse pain. Ear acupuncture is often beneficial.

Basic point combination

Local 'ring' of points around the wrist: LU-9, L.I.-5, T.B.-4, S.I.-5, HE-7, P-7.
Ear acupuncture: 67 wrist.

Individual point combination

Distal point for ulnar pain

BL-62.

Distal point for radial pain

ST-42.

Acupuncture points

BL-62 **Location:** below the prominence of the lateral malleolus.
Notes: opening point of the *Yang Qiao Mai*, located on the corresponding meridian (*Tai Yang*).

HE-7 **Location:** on the ulnar aspect of the wrist crease, on the radial aspect of the pisiform bone.
Notes: *Shu*-stream point, *Yuan*-source point, sedation point; drains Heat.

L.I.-5 **Location:** on the radial aspect of the wrist crease, in a depression between the tendons of the extensor pollicis brevis and extensor carpi radialis longus. Tip: hold the patient's wrist between two fingers and ask them to flex the wrist. This is the best way to locate the wrist crease. S.I.-5 is on its ulnar aspect, L.I.-5 on its radial aspect.
Notes: *Jing*-river point.

LU-9 **Location:** on the wrist crease, radial to the radial artery.
Notes: *Shu*-stream point, *Yuan*-source point, tonification point, *Hui*-meeting point and master point of the vessels.

P-7 **Location:** on the palmar aspect of the wrist joint, between the tendons of the flexor carpi radialis and palmaris longus.
Notes: *Shu*-stream point, *Yuan*-source point, sedation point; drains Heat; specific point for carpal tunnel syndrome.

S.I.-5 **Location:** on the ulnar aspect of the wrist crease, distal to the styloid process of the ulna and proximal to the triquetrum bone.
Notes: *Jing*-river point, Fire point.

ST-42 **Location:** on the highest point of the dorsum of the foot (dorsalis pedis artery).
Notes: *Yuan*-source point on the corresponding meridian (*Yang Ming*).

T.B.-4 **Location:** on the wrist crease, in the depression lateral to the tendon of the extensor digitorum longus.
Notes: *Yuan*-source point.

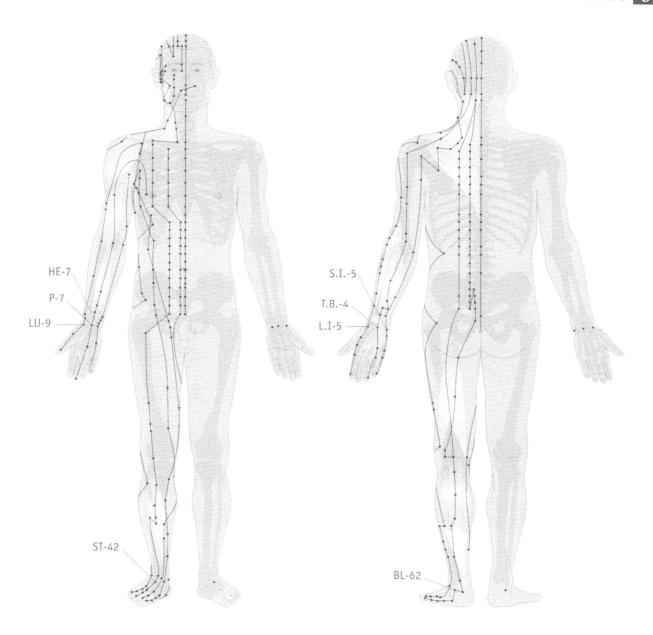

HE-7

P-7

LU-9

ST-42

S.I.-5

T.B.-4

L.I-5

BL-62

6.13.6 *Lower back pain*

With lower back pain there will always be underlying *Qi* stagnation or *Qi* and Blood stagnation. Triggers are trauma, external pathogens, suppressed emotions (clinically more common in men than in women) as well as deficiency patterns. For the latter, a differential diagnosis is particularly important.

Basic point combination

Local points: pressure-sensitive points, BL-23, BL-31, Du-3. Distal points: BL-60, BL-40 [BL-54 Bi].
Ear acupuncture: 54 lumbar spine, 55 *Shen Men*.
Hand points: hand point 1 (*Yao Tui Dian*, lumbar/leg point).

Individual point combination

Pain triggered by Cold or due to deficiency-Cold (*Yang* deficiency)

BL-23 **M**, for excess – external Cold, neutral stimulation; for *Yang* deficiency, tonifying stimulation.

Pain with *Yin* deficiency

Worse during the night and with tiredness.
BL-23, KID-3 or SP-6 with tonifying method, no moxa!

Pain in the iliosacral joint

Acute point S.I.-3.

Pain with twisting movement

BL-23, BL-52 [BL-47 Bi], G.B.-26, G.B.-27, G.B.-28; distal points: G.B.-41, T.B.-5; acute point: T.B.-3.

Pain with bending forward

BL-23, BL-31, BL-32, Du-4, Ex-B-2 – local *Hua Tuo* points; acute points: S.I.-3, BL-62 or BL-60.

Pain radiating to the groin

G.B.-27, G.B.-28, ST-36.

Acute lower back pain, sciatica, trauma

Du-26, Ex-B-6 (*Yao Yi*); method: needling or moxa for 10–20 minutes.
Ear acupuncture: lumbar spine, *Shen Men*, thalamus; hand point 1 *Yao Tui Dian* (lumbar region/leg).

Acupuncture points

BL-23 **Location:** 1.5 cun lateral to L2, level with Du-4.
Notes: back-*Shu* point of the Kidney; strengthens the lumbar region, tonifies Kidney *Yin* and *Yang;* use moxa only with Cold symptoms, for *Yin* deficiency use tonifying acupuncture.

BL-31 **Location:** over the 1st sacral foramen.
Notes: local point, master point for menopause.

BL-32 **Location:** over the 2nd sacral foramen.
Notes: see BL-31.

BL-40 **Location:** in the centre of the popliteal crease, between the tendons of the semitendinosus and the biceps femoris.
Notes: *He*-sea point, command point for the back.

BL-52 **Location:** 3 cun lateral to the spinous process of L2, lateral to BL-23.
Notes: local point; has a connection with the soul of the Kidneys (willpower, *Zhi*).

BL-60 **Location:** in the depression between the Achilles tendon and the lateral malleolus.
Notes: *Jing*-river point, master point for pain along the meridian pathway.

BL-62 **Location:** below the prominence of the lateral malleolus.
Notes: opening point of the *Yang Qiao Mai* – meridian pathway!

Du-3 **Location:** below the spinous process of L4.
Notes: by influencing the lower part of the spine, Du-3 also has an effect on its upper part.

Du-4 **Location:** below the spinous process of L2.
Notes: complements Kidney *Yin*, firms the Essence (*Jing*), strengthens Kidney *Yang*, the lower back and the knees.

Du-26 **Location:** at the junction of the upper and middle third of the philtrum.
Notes: empirically an effective point for acute lumbar pain.

Ex-B-2 **Location:** 17 point pairs, 0.5 cun lateral to the lower borders of the spinous processes of T1 to L5; medial to the inner Bladder line.
Notes: very effective local points.

Ex-B-6 **Location:** 3 cun lateral to the spinous process of L4.
Notes: for acute lower back pain.

G.B.-26 **Location:** on the anterior axillary line, anterior to the highest point of the anterior superior iliac spine (ASIS), level with the umbilicus.
Notes: local point.

G.B.-27 **Location:** 3 cun inferior to the umbilicus (level with Ren-4), anterior to the ASIS.
Notes: local point.

G.B.-28 **Location:** 0.5 cun inferior to the ASIS.
Notes: local point.

G.B.-41 **Location:** in the depression distal to the junction of the 4th and 5th metatarsal bones.
Notes: *Shu*-stream point, opening point of the *Dai Mai*, master point of the big joints.

Hand point 1 *(Yao Tui Dian)*
Notes: point for the lower back and the leg.

KID-3 **Location:** between the highest prominence of the medial malleolus and the Achilles tendon.
Notes: tonifies the Kidneys, the lumbar region and the knees; benefits the Essence (*Jing*), the Kidney *Yin* as well as the *Yang*.

KID-7 **Location:** on the anterior border of the Achilles tendon, posterior to the flexor digitorum longus, 2 cun superior to the highest prominence of the medial malleolus.
Notes: *Jing*-river point and tonification point; with moxa tonifies specifically Kidney *Yang*.

S.I.-3 **Location:** when a fist is made, on the dorsum of the hand, in the depression at the end of the most distal palmar crease.
Notes: as *Shu*-stream point, effective for musculoskeletal disorders, particularly those due to Dampness; as tonification point and opening point of the *Du Mai*, influences the spine and the CNS – meridian pathway!

SP-6 **Location:** 3 cun superior to the highest prominence of the medial malleolus, on the posterior border of the tibia.
Notes: as group *Luo*-connecting point (Spleen, Liver, Kidneys), tonifies the *Qi*, Blood (*Xue*), and *Yin* – nourishing point; eliminates Dampness.

ST-36 **Location:** 0.5 cun lateral to the anterior crest of the tibia, 1.5 cun inferior to the lower border of the head of the fibula (G.B.-34).
Notes: *He*-sea point, here used to direct the effect of the acupuncture towards the inguinal region.

T.B.-3 **Location:** when a loose fist is made, on the dorsum of the hand, between the 4th and 5th metacarpal bones, in the depression proximal to the metacarpophalangeal joints.
Notes: as *Shu*-stream point for pain of the musculoskeletal system.

T.B.-5 **Location:** 2 cun proximal to the midpoint of the dorsal wrist crease, opposite P-6.
Notes: *Luo*-connecting point, opening point of the *Yang Wei Mai* – see pathway of the T.B. meridian!; master point of the small joints; dispels all *Yang* pathogenic factors.

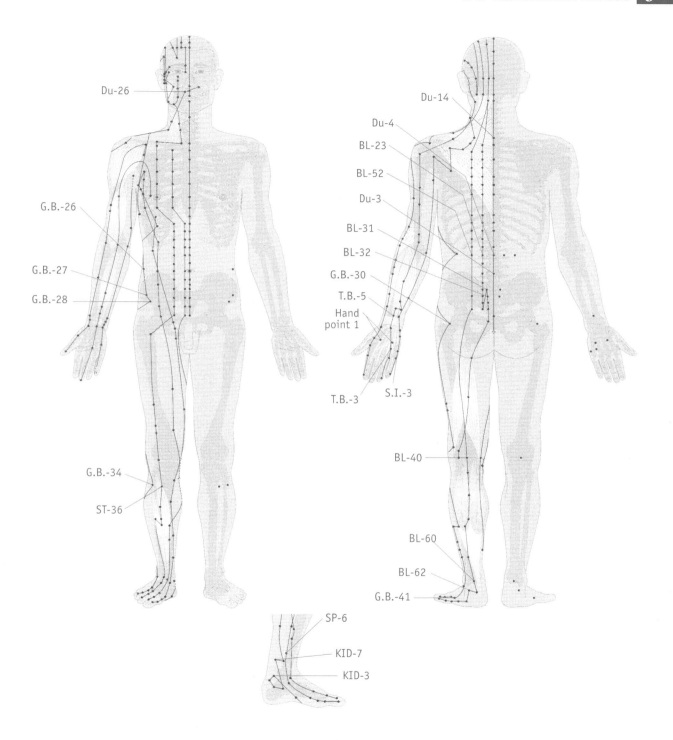

6.13.7 Hip pain

As pain of the hip joint tends to affect the adjacent joints as well, points for the lumbar region and the knee joint are also often indicated. Ear acupuncture is particularly important for coxarthrosis.

Basic point combination

Local point: G.B.-30.
Adjacent point: G.B.-26, G.B.-34, BL-23, BL-25, BL-31.
Distal points: G.B.-41, T.B.-5.
Ear acupuncture: 57 hip, *Shen Men*.

Acupuncture points

BL-23 **Location:** 1.5 cun lateral to L2, level with Du-4.
Notes: back-*Shu* point of the Kidneys; strengthens the lumbar region.

BL-25 **Location:** 1.5 cun lateral to the lower border of the spinous process of L4.
Notes: back-*Shu* point of the Large Intestine; local point for the sacroiliac joint.

BL-31 **Location:** over the 1st sacral foramen.
Notes: local point; master point for menopause.

G.B.-26 **Location:** on the anterior axillary line, anterior to the highest point of the ASIS, level with the umbilicus.
Notes: local point, point on the *Dai Mai*.

G.B.-30 **Location:** on a line connecting the greater trochanter and the sacral hiatus, at the junction of the lateral and medial third.
Notes: meeting point with the Bladder meridian, master point for sciatica and paresis of the lower extremities.

G.B.-34 **Location:** with the knee flexed, in the depression anterior and inferior to the head of the fibula.
Notes: *He*-sea point of the Gall Bladder, *Hui*-meeting point of the tendons, master point of the musculature.

G.B.-41 **Location:** in the depression distal to the junction of the 4th and 5th metatarsal bones.
Notes: *Shu*-stream point, opening point of the *Dai Mai* – meridian pathway!; master point of the big joints, particularly effective if combined with its partner point, T.B.-5.

T.B.-5 **Location:** 2 cun proximal to the midpoint of the dorsal wrist crease, opposite P-6.
Notes: *Luo*-connecting point, opening point of the *Yang Wei Mai* – meridian pathway!; master point of the small joints; dispels all *Yang* pathogenic factors.

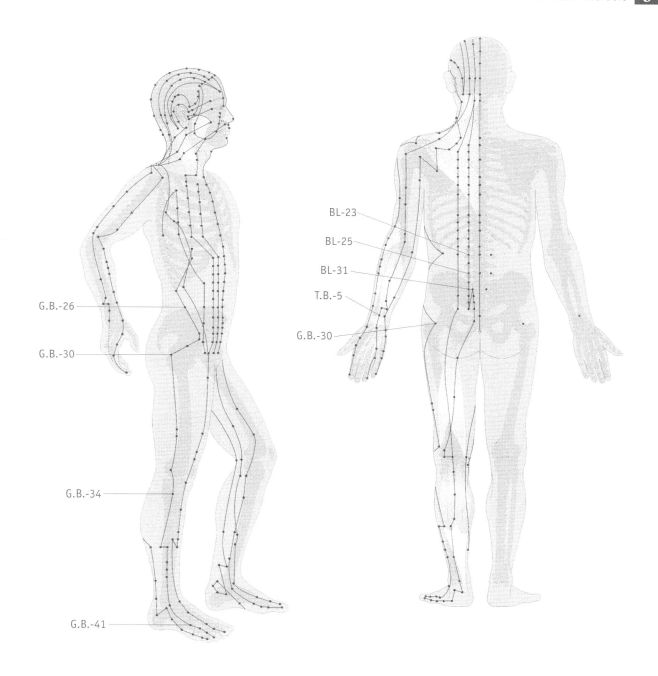

G.B.-26

G.B.-30

G.B.-34

G.B.-41

BL-23

BL-25

BL-31

T.B.-5

G.B.-30

6.13.8 *Knee joint pain*

Again, always include adjacent joints – here the hip and ankle joint – in the treatment. Select the relevant point based on the pathway of the affected meridian. Ear acupuncture is particularly important for gonarthrosis.

Basic point combination

BL-40 [BL-54 Bi], ST-36, SP-9, G.B.-34.
Knee points after Bachmann: Ex-LE-2 (*He Ding*), Ex-LE-4 (*Xi Yan*).
Distal points: G.B.-41, T.B.-5, SP-6.
Ear acupuncture: 49 knee, 55 *Shen Men*.

Acupuncture points

Bachmann knee points   Location: one point at the highest point of the patella, two points medial and lateral to the patellar tendon and a further point in the centre of the patella.
Notes: local points.

BL-40   Location: in the centre of the popliteal crease, between the tendons of the semitendinosus and the biceps femoris.
Notes: *He*-sea point, metabolic point, testing point for gonarthralgia, command point for the back.

Ex-LE-2   Location: at the centre of the upper patellar border.
Notes: local point.

Ex-LE-4   Location: with the knee flexed, the inner eye of the knee lies medial to the tendon, the outer eye (which is identical with ST-35) lies lateral to the tendon.
Notes: local points.

G.B.-34   Location: with the knee flexed, in the depression anterior and inferior to the head of the fibula.
Notes: *He*-sea point of the Gall Bladder, *Hui*-meeting point of the tendons, master point of the musculature.

G.B.-41   Location: in the depression distal to the junction of the 4th and 5th metatarsal bones.
Notes: *Shu*-stream point, opening point of the *Dai Mai*, master point of the big joints.

SP-6   Location: 3 cun superior to the highest prominence of the medial malleolus, on the posterior border of the tibia.
Notes: as group *Luo*-connecting point, strengthens the Spleen, Liver and Kidneys, and therefore *Qi*, Blood (*Xue*) and *Yin*; nourishing point; eliminates Dampness.

SP-9   Location: with the knee flexed, in the depression inferior to the medial condyle of the tibia, at the same level as G.B.-34.
Notes: *He*-sea point; regulates Fluids and Dampness, tonifies Spleen *Qi*.

ST-36   Location: 0.5 cun lateral to the anterior crest of the tibia, 1.5 cun inferior to the lower border of the head of the fibula (G.B.-34).
Notes: *He*-sea point of the Stomach; epithet: Great Healer of the Feet and Knees; master point of hormones.

T.B.-5   Location: 2 cun proximal to the midpoint of the dorsal wrist crease, opposite P-6.
Notes: *Luo*-connecting point, opening point of the *Yang Wei Mai*, master point of the small joints; dispels all *Yang* pathogenic factors.

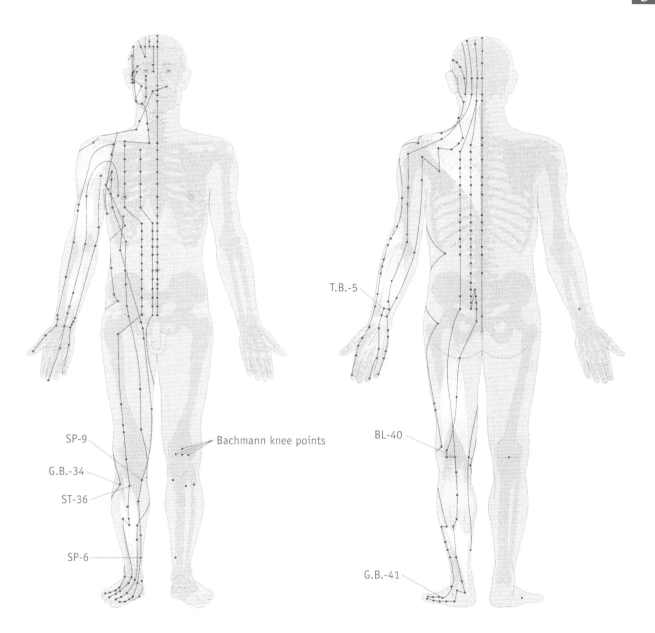

SP-9

G.B.-34

ST-36

SP-6

Bachmann knee points

T.B.-5

BL-40

G.B.-41

6.13.9 Ankle, toes and achillodynia

Again, the same rule applies as above: always involve adjacent areas into the treatment. Knee points of the affected meridian are also indicated. Ear acupuncture is also beneficial for disorders of the ankle.

Basic point combination

Local points: BL-60, BL-62, KID-3, KID-6, G.B.-40, SP-5, ST-41, Ex-LE-8 (*Nei Huai Dian*) – choose points depending on the location of the disorder.
Distal point: T.B.-5.
Ear acupuncture: 55 *Shen Men*, 48 ankle.
Hand points: hand point 2 (*Huai Dian*/ankle).

Individual point combination

Achillodynia

BL-60, KID-3, BL-57.

Joints of the toes

Ex-LE-10 (*Ba Feng*/Eight Winds).

Acupuncture points

BL-57 Location: in the depression below the two bellies of the gastrocnemius; on tiptoes; midway between BL-40 and BL-60.
Notes: relaxes the tendons; special point for calf cramps.

BL-60 Location: in the depression between the Achilles tendon and the lateral malleolus.
Notes: *Jing*-river point, master point for pain along the meridian pathway.

BL-62 Location: below the prominence of the lateral malleolus.
Notes: opening point of the *Yang Qiao Mai*; local point.

Ex-LE-8 Location: on the prominence of the medial malleolus.
Notes: local point.

Ex-LE-10 Location: 4 points on the dorsum of the foot, 0.5 cun proximal to the interdigital folds.
Notes: relax the tendons, dispel Wind-Cold, invigorate the Blood (*Xue*).

G.B.-40 Location: on the junction of a horizontal line through the prominence of the lateral malleolus and a vertical line through the greatest circumference of the lateral malleolus, over the calcaneocuboidal joint.
Notes: *Yuan*-source point, 'miracle point' for lateral thoracic pain! Tonifies and mobilizes *Qi* along the meridian pathway, particularly for stagnation due to deficiency.

Hand point 2 Location: on the radial aspect of the metacarpophalangeal joint of the thumb, at the junction of the palm and the dorsum of the hand.
Notes: for acute ankle pain.

KID-3 Location: between the highest prominence of the medial malleolus and the Achilles tendon.
Notes: *Shu*-stream point and *Yuan*-source point, local point.

KID-6 Location: below the prominence of the medial malleolus.
Notes: opening point of the *Yin Qiao Mai*, local point.

SP-5 Location: with the foot in dorsiflexion, in the depression between the tendons of the tibialis anterior and the medial malleolus, on to the navicular bone.
Notes: *Jing*-river point, sedation point, master point for connective tissue.

ST-41 Location: at the midpoint of the anterior aspect of the ankle, between the tendons of the extensor hallucis longus and extensor digitorum longus.
Notes: local point for the ankle; *Jing*-river point and tonification point; eliminates *Qi* stagnation from the leg.

T.B.-5 Location: 2 cun proximal to the midpoint of the dorsal wrist crease, opposite P-6.
Notes: *Luo*-connecting point, opening point of the *Yang Wei Mai*, master point of the small joints; dispels all *Yang* pathogenic factors.

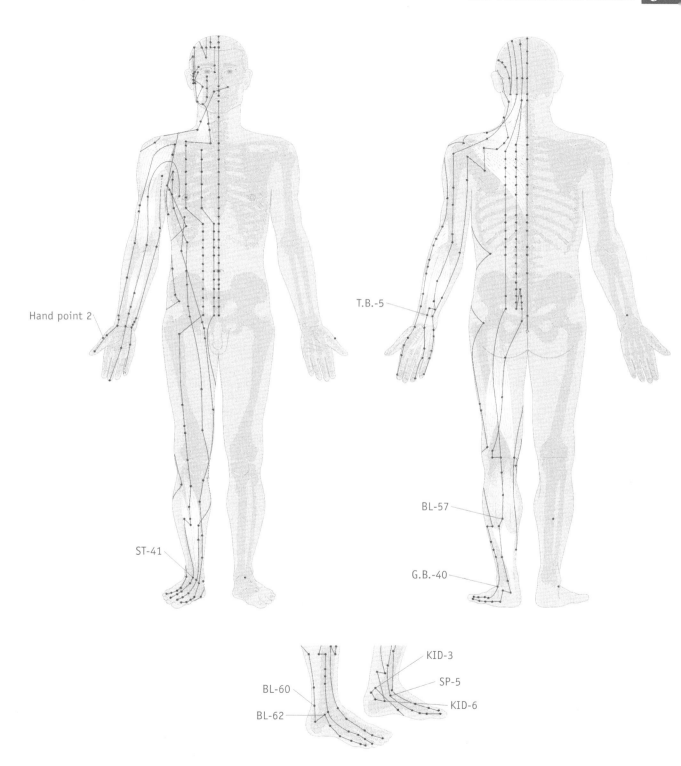

Hand point 2

T.B.-5

BL-57

G.B.-40

ST-41

BL-60

BL-62

KID-3

SP-5

KID-6

6.14 Connective tissue/oedema

G. Kubiena

6.14.1 Descensus, ptosis, varicosities, haemorrhoids (1)

The cause of the above disorders is Spleen *Qi* deficiency and sinking Spleen *Qi*.

The Spleen and the Stomach are the main producers of postnatal *Qi*, whereas the Kidney provides original *Qi* derived from the Essence (*Jing*).

The Spleen *Qi* holds the organs in their place. A prolapse of the uterus is not only a sign of Spleen *Qi* deficiency but also indicates an instability of the *Ren Mai* and *Chong Mai*, as well as an insufficiency of the *Dai Mai*, for example with Essence (*Jing*) deficiency due to several childbirths.

Basic point combination

ST-36+ **M**, Ren-4+ **M**, Ren-6+ **M**, Du-20 **M**.

Individual point combination

Rectal prolapse

ST-36+, Du-20 M, BL-25+ M, Du-1, Ren-8 M (fill the umbilicus with salt, place a ginger slice and a moxa cone on top).
With faecal incontinence: BL-25+, BL-31+.

Uterine descensus, uterine prolapse

Qi deficiency: ST-36+ **M**, Ren-12+ **M**, BL-20 **M**, Du-20 **M**, ST-29+.
Kidney deficiency: Ren-4+ **M**, Ex-CA-1 (*Zi Gong*), LIV-8+ **M** [Bi LIV-9], KID-6.

Acupuncture points

BL-20 **Location:** 1.5 cun lateral to the spinous process of T11.
Notes: back-*Shu* point of the Spleen.

BL-25 **Location:** 1.5 cun lateral to the lower border of the spinous process of L4.
Notes: promotes the functioning of the Large Intestine, eliminates stagnation in the meridian.

BL-31 **Location:** over the 1st sacral foramen.
Notes: BL-31–BL-35 strengthen the Kidneys, lumbar region, genitals and Essence (*Jing*).

Du-1 **Location:** between the coccyx and the anus.
Notes: raises the rectum/perineum; regulates the *Du Mai* and *Ren Mai*, eliminates Damp-Heat.

Du-20 **Location:** on a line connecting the apices of the ears.
Notes: raises sinking organ *Qi*, tonifies *Yang*, promotes the raising function of the Spleen, dispels internal Wind.

Ex-CA-1 **Location:** on the abdomen, 1 cun superior to the upper border of the pubic symphysis (level of Ren-3) and 3 cun lateral to the midline.
Notes: has a specific action on the uterus, hence its name 'Palace of the Child'.

KID-6 **Location:** below the prominence of the medial malleolus.
Notes: combined with LIV-8, tonifies and supports the uterus.

LIV-8 **Location:** with the knee flexed, in the depression anterior to the medial end of the popliteal crease.
Notes: 'nourishes' Liver Blood (*Xue*), relaxes the tendons; specific point for exhaustion.

Ren-4 **Location:** 2 cun superior to the upper border of the pubic symphysis.
Notes: tonifies *Qi*, strengthens the Kidneys, restores *Yang Qi*.

Ren-6 **Location:** 1.5 cun inferior to the umbilicus.
Notes: strengthens and moves *Qi* in the Lower Burner, strengthens the Kidneys and original *Qi*, activates *Yang Qi*, benefits the uterus.

Ren-8 **Location:** in the centre of the umbilicus.
Notes: strengthens Spleen and Stomach *Qi* as well as original *Qi*, regulates the function of the intestines, stops diarrhoea. Do not needle! Only moxibustion.

Ren-12 **Location:** midway between the umbilicus and the xiphoid process.
Notes: strengthens Stomach and Spleen *Qi*.

ST-29 **Location:** 2 cun lateral to the midline and 4 cun inferior to the umbilicus, level with Ren-3 and KID-12.
Notes: raises the uterus.

ST-36 **Location:** 0.5 cun lateral to the anterior crest of the tibia, 1.5 cun inferior to the lower border of the head of the fibula (G.B.-34).
Notes: benefits the Stomach and the Spleen, tonifies *Ying Qi* and *Wei Qi*, raises the *Yang* for ptosis (moxa – combine with Du-20 and Ren-6), regulates the circulation of *Qi* and Blood (*Xue*).

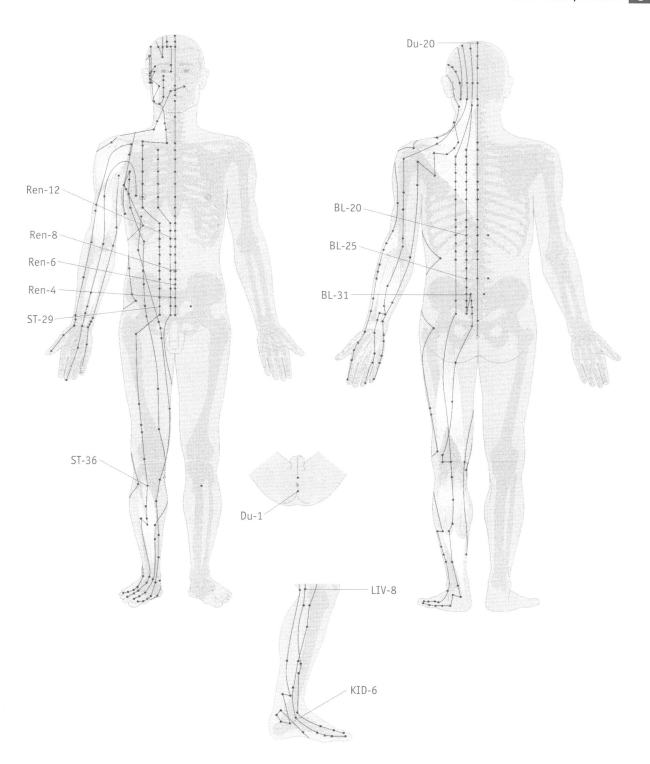

Ren-12

Ren-8

Ren-6

Ren-4

ST-29

ST-36

Du-1

Du-20

BL-20

BL-25

BL-31

LIV-8

KID-6

6.14.1 Descensus, ptosis, varicosities, haemorrhoids (2)

Individual point combination

Varicose veins

Qi and Blood (Xue) stagnation, sinking Spleen Qi, Damp-Heat (thrombophlebitis).
SP-6+, ST-36+ M, BL-40-, BL-58; opening points: SP-4, P-6.
Thrombophlebitis: plus SP-9–.
Painful varicosities: SP-5.
Leg ulcer: plus LIV-3, LIV-8 [LIV-9 Bi], BL-40–, BL-58.

Haemorrhoids

Du-1, Du-20 M, BL-30.
Individual combination: SP-6, LIV-3, Du-4, BL-31, BL-32, BL-57, KID-7; opening points: SP-4, P-6.
Bleeding: SP-1 – for deficiency bleeding, moxa; for bleeding due to Heat (inflammation), reducing method.

Acupuncture points

BL-30 **Location:** 1.5 cun lateral to the posterior midline, at the level of the 4th sacral foramen.
Notes: 'white precious ring' (perineum) that holds the Essence (Jing, also includes sperm) and Qi.
BL-31 **Location:** over the 1st sacral foramen.
Notes: BL-31–BL-35 strengthen the Kidneys, lumbar region, genitals and Essence (Jing).
BL-32 **Location:** over the 2nd sacral foramen.
Notes: see BL-31.
BL-40 **Location:** in the centre of the popliteal crease, between the tendons of the semitendinosus and the biceps femoris.
Notes: resolves Blood (Xue) stagnation, cools the Blood (Xue).
BL-57 **Location:** in the depression below the two bellies of the gastrocnemius; on tiptoes; midway between BL-40 and BL-60.
Notes: invigorates the Blood (Xue), eliminates Heat; specific point for calf cramps, lower back pain, haemorrhoids.
BL-58 **Location:** 1 cun distal and lateral to BL-57, on the lateral border of the gastrocnemius, on the soleus. On a cross-section through the lower leg at 7.30 and 4.30 respectively.
Notes: adds a 'spring to the step', hence its name 'Soaring Upwards'.
Du-1 **Location:** between the coccyx and the anus.
Notes: raises the rectum/perineum; regulates the Du Mai and Ren Mai, eliminates Damp-Heat.

Du-4 **Location:** below the spinous process of L2.
Notes: complements Kidney Yin, firms the Essence (Jing), strengthens the Kidney Yang, the lower back and the knees; tonifies in general.
Du-20 **Location:** on a line connecting the apices of the ears.
Notes: raises sinking organ Qi, tonifies Yang, promotes the raising function of the Spleen, dispels internal Wind.
KID-7 **Location:** on the anterior border of the Achilles tendon, posterior to the flexor digitorum longus, 2 cun superior to the highest prominence of the medial malleolus.
Notes: Jing-river point and tonification point.
LIV-3 **Location:** on the dorsum of the foot, in the depression distal to the junction of the 1st and 2nd metatarsal bones.
Notes: promotes the smooth flow of Qi, spasmolytic.
LIV-8 **Location:** with the knee flexed, in the depression anterior to the medial end of the popliteal crease.
Notes: 'nourishes' Liver Blood (Xue), relaxes the tendons; specific point for exhaustion.
P-6 **Location:** 2 cun proximal to the midpoint of the palmar wrist crease, between the tendons of the flexor carpi radialis and palmaris longus.
Notes: as its paired opening point, it increases the effect of SP-4.
SP-1 **Location:** on the big toe, next to the medial corner of the nail.
Notes: strengthens the Spleen, regulates Blood (Xue) – stops any bleeding (uterus, haemorrhoids, nose), calms the Spirit.
SP-4 **Location:** in the depression at the junction of the base and shaft of the 1st metatarsal bone, at the junction of the red and white skin.
Notes: strengthens the Stomach and the Spleen, regulates the Chong Mai.
SP-5 **Location:** with the foot in dorsiflexion, in the depression between the tendons of the tibialis anterior and the medial malleolus, on the navicular bone.
Notes: strengthens the Stomach and the Spleen, eliminates Dampness; specific point for varicose-related pain.
SP-6 **Location:** 3 cun superior to the highest prominence of the medial malleolus, on the posterior border of the tibia.
Notes: strengthens the Spleen, eliminates Blood (Xue) stagnation – hence for disorders affecting the circulation in the lower extremities; regulates the uterus.
SP-9 **Location:** with the knee flexed in the depression inferior to the medial condyle of the tibia, at the same level as G.B.-34.
Notes: eliminates Damp-Heat.
ST-36 **Location:** 0.5 cun lateral to the anterior crest of the tibia, 1.5 cun inferior to the lower border of the head of the fibula (G.B.-34).
Notes: benefits the Stomach and the Spleen, tonifies nutritive Qi (Ying Qi) and defensive Qi (Wei Qi), raises the Yang for ptosis (moxibustion with Du-20 and Ren-6), regulates the circulation of Qi and Blood (Xue).

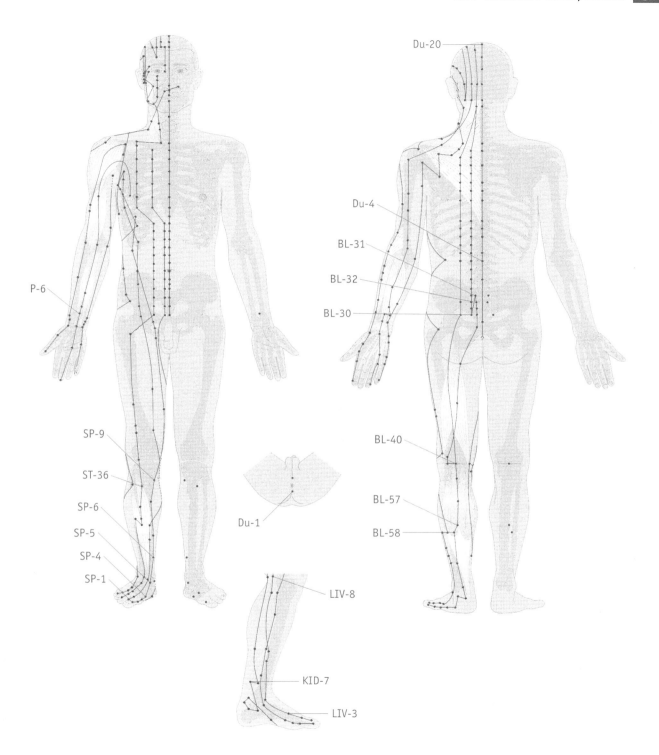

Du-20

Du-4

BL-31

BL-32

BL-30

BL-40

BL-57

BL-58

P-6

SP-9

ST-36

SP-6

SP-5

SP-4

SP-1

Du-1

LIV-8

KID-7

LIV-3

6.14.2 Oedema

According to TCM, oedema is caused either by the invasion of pathogenic Wind and Dampness from outside, or by organ disharmonies. TCM distinguishes between *Yang* and *Yin* oedema as described below.

Individual point combination

Yang oedema, high-altitude pulmonary oedema (Monk's disease), facial oedema with common cold

LU-7, L.I.-4, L.I.-6, SP-9, BL-39 [BL-53 Bi], Du-26.
TCM: fluid accumulation in the interior of the body, exacerbated by external Wind. Sudden onset, oedema in the upper half of the body, especially facial oedema, swelling of the eyelids, fever, chills, thirst, asthmatic cough, scanty urine; **tongue coating:** white, thin; **pulse:** slippery, rapid.

Yin oedema, secondary oedema (e.g. due to cardiac insufficiency or liver failure)

BL-20 **M**, BL-23 **M**, Ren-9, Ren-4 **M**, KID-7 **M**, ST-36+, G.B.-41, SP-5.
TCM: disharmony between the internal organs. Spleen and Kidney *Yang* deficiency lead to a (relative) excess of *Yin* (water), which the *Qi* cannot cope with. Hence oedema in the lower part of the body; cold sensation, cold extremities, lower back pain (Kidney *Yang* deficiency), possibly feeling of fullness in the epigastrium (Spleen *Yang* deficiency); loose stools; **face:** pale or sallow; **tongue body:** pale; **tongue coating:** white; **pulse:** deep, thready.

Acupuncture points

BL-20 **Location:** 1.5 cun lateral to T11.
Notes: back-*Shu* point of the Spleen; strengthens the Spleen, eliminates Dampness.

BL-23 **Location:** 1.5 cun lateral to L2, level with Du-4.
Notes: back-*Shu* point of the Kidneys; strengthens Kidney *Yin* and *Yang*.

BL-39 **Location:** lateral (*Yang*) to BL-40 (*Wei Zhong*), at the medial side of the tendon of the biceps femoris.
Notes: lower *He*-sea point of the Triple Burner; opens the water passages of the Triple Burner.

Du-26 **Location:** at the junction of the upper and middle third of the philtrum.
Notes: local point for facial oedema.

G.B.-41 **Location:** in the depression distal to the junction of the 4th and 5th metatarsal bones.
Notes: *Shu*-stream point; local point for oedema of the dorsum of the foot.

KID-7 **Location:** on the anterior border of the Achilles tendon, posterior to the flexor digitorum longus, 2 cun superior to the highest prominence of the medial malleolus.
Notes: *Jing*-river point and tonification point; specifically strengthens Kidney *Yang* with moxa.

L.I.-4 **Location:** on the dorsum of the hand, at the highest point of the muscle bulge between the 1st and 2nd metacarpal bones.
Notes: *Yuan*-source point and command point of the face; eliminates external Wind (combined with LU-7).

L.I.-6 **Location:** on the radial aspect of the forearm, on the lateral border of the radius, 3 cun proximal to the wrist crease. Tip: cross the thumbs so that the interdigital webs touch; with the index finger reach round the dorsum of the hand to the radial pulse; the tip of the index finger will point to LU-7, the tip of the middle finger to L.I.-6.
Notes: *Luo*-connecting point; opens the water passages of the Lung – specific point for oedema of the face and hands due to external pathogens.

LU-7 **Location:** 1.5 cun proximal to the wrist crease, superior to the radial artery.
Notes: master point for stagnation; moves, descends and disperses Lung *Qi*; combined with L.I.-4, eliminates external pathogens.

Ren-4 **Location:** 2 cun superior to the upper border of the pubic symphysis.
Notes: combined with Ren-9 promotes the circulation of Fluids; with moxibustion tonifies original *Qi*.

Ren-9 **Location:** 1 cun superior to the umbilicus.
Notes: promotes the transformation of Fluids and Dampness.

SP-5 **Location:** with the foot in dorsiflexion, in the depression between the tendons of the tibialis anterior and the medial malleolus, on the navicular bone.
Notes: master point of connective tissue; local point for the dorsum of the foot.

SP-9 **Location:** with the knee flexed, in the depression inferior to the medial condyle of the tibia, at the same level as G.B.-34.
Notes: *He*-sea point; eliminates Dampness and Heat, regulates the water passages.

ST-36 **Location:** 0.5 cun lateral to the anterior crest of the tibia, 1.5 cun inferior to the lower border of the head of the fibula (G.B.-34).
Notes: *He*-sea point; strengthens the transporting and transforming function of the Spleen and Stomach, normalizes the distribution of Fluids.

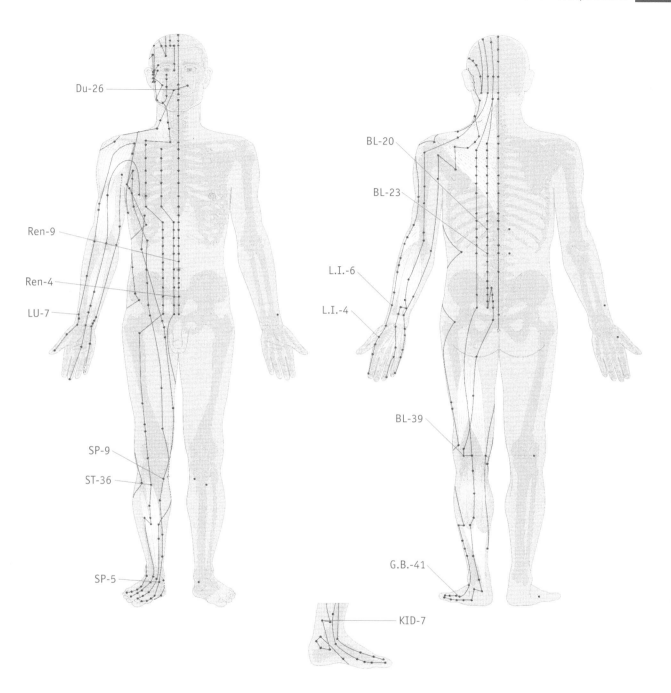

Du-26

Ren-9

Ren-4

LU-7

SP-9

ST-36

SP-5

BL-20

BL-23

L.I.-6

L.I.-4

BL-39

G.B.-41

KID-7

6.15 Treatment of pain

A. Meng

6.15.1 Treatment of pain with acupuncture: introduction

Differential diagnosis

A basic form of diagnosis consists of determining the affected meridian system, organ system and the modifying circumstances (the 'Rule of Three' of the Vienna School: Where? Where? How?). The point combinations presented below are based on *Bian Zheng*, and can also be applied as modules to other disorders (*Bian Bing*).

The diagnosis and resulting basic therapy should always follow the principles of evidence-based medicine (EBM). Chinese herbal medicine and acupuncture/tuina can be used as adjunctive therapies.

Since 1983 the neurological department of the Lainz Hospital in Vienna has successfully administered body acupuncture and auricular therapy, including the use of intradermal needles, TENS and, to a lesser extent, laser acupuncture. While initially limited to the treatment of pain, acupuncture is now also applied for early post-stroke treatment and chronic neurological disorders.

Meridian + organ + accompanying circumstances = simplified TCM diagnosis

Rule 1: Which meridian is affected? – Where to treat?

Any stimuli that excite the receptors are further processed as nerve impulses by the nervous system. These processes require the close interaction between the autonomic and peripheral nervous system, the endocrine system and the meridian system. The organism's response is either physiological or pathophysiological.

The meridian system has the task of providing a network of channels for the transport of *Qi* and Blood (*Xue*), and also the communication between the organs. The meridian system (channel system) is located in the subcutaneous zone and at varying depths between the muscles.

> Example: lower back pain radiating down the posterior aspect of the thigh and the lateral aspect of the lower leg is typical of sciatica with the root at L5/S1. This pattern of pain distribution corresponds exactly to the pathway of the Bladder meridian.

Rule 2: Which organ is affected? – Where to treat?

Select points relevant to the affected organ or segment.

Rule 3: What type of pain is it? What are its circumstances? – How to treat?

In addition to the questions 'What is the pain like? How long have you had the pain? How intense is the pain?', it is important to find out the following:

● Does the pain occur at a particular time?
● What makes it better or worse. What can trigger or influence the pain?
● What is the quality of the pain?

The character of the pain, its intensity, the overall condition of the patient (their nutritional status) and triggers (pathogenic factors) determine the treatment techniques (intensity of needle stimulation, stimulation method).

Pathogenic factors – Wind, Cold, Heat, Dampness, Dryness (bioclimatic factors) – are the triggers of a disharmony; they characterize and determine the nature of the disorder.

Treatment

For practical reasons, the preferred method of classifying pain is according to its location. The individual circumstances of each case have to be considered carefully.

● Organ pain (determine the affected organ)
● Pain of the extremities (determine the affected meridian)
● Cranial pain (determine the affected meridian)
● Pain of the torso (determine the affected meridian/segment)

Assign to the individual circumstances (description of the disorder)

> There should always be a clear Western diagnosis prior to treating with acupuncture.

It is always beneficial to use psychologically effective points; for example:

● Du-20 (Hundred Meetings)
● Du-24 (Spirit Court)
● G.B.-13 (Root of the Spirit)
● HE-7 (Spirit Gate).

I also recommend the points *Si Shen Cong* (Four Alert Spirit, Ex-HN-1). Also very effective are ST-36, P-6, P-7,

BL-15. If the pain occurs in a rhythmic pattern, it is often helpful to consider the organ clock ($\rightarrow$ Fig. 2.3) in the treatment plan.

Organ pain

Pain of the thoracic organs (Lung and Heart), the abdominal organs (Liver, Gall Bladder, Spleen, Stomach, intestines) and the pelvic organs (Kidneys, Bladder) may be a primary or secondary symptom caused by an organ disorder. Here, TCM differential diagnosis is based mainly on determining the affected organ and meridian. Accompanying signs and symptoms help to differentiate the diagnosis further.

Acute organ pain

Mainly excess symptoms, acute onset, severe.
Treatment principle: symptomatic treatment in order to reduce the pain quickly. Circulation of the Blood (*Xue*) and the vital energy *Qi* within the meridians will return to normal.

Local pain points, *Xi*-cleft points, *He*-sea points and *Luo*-connecting points are frequently used in these situations.

Chronic organ pain

Often characterized by deficiency symptoms lasting for more than 6 weeks; the character of the pain is dull, irritating and recurring. Differentiation of accompanying signs and symptoms is of great importance for good results.
Treatment principle: treatment of the root is in the foreground; therefore more segmental points (back-*Shu* points and front-*Mu* points) should be selected.

The organ pain is interpreted as a result of a disharmony of *Qi* and Blood (*Xue*) at an organ level.

For Cold symptoms: choose the relevant *Rong* points (*Ying*-spring points; the second most distal point of each meridian).
If there are signs of Blood (*Xue*) stasis and *Qi* stagnation: L.I.-4, SP-6.

Organ disorders may also manifest with referred pain on the back or the front of the torso. Positive findings may include changes in skin colour, pressure pain, gelosis, myogelosis, swellings. Such zones often respond well to acupuncture or acupressure.

Pain of the extremities

Pain of the extremities refers to both soft tissue and joint pain on the extremities. Differentiation according to the meridian is highly important. The term *Bi* syndrome corresponds to rheumatism in Western medicine.

Pain along the extremity (e.g. neuralgia)

Needle 1–3 points on the affected meridian. For the upper extremity, the points L.I.-11, L.I.-4 and HE-1 often prove to be beneficial.

For the lower extremity, the points ST-36, G.B.-30, G.B.-34 and BL-40 [BL-54 Bi] often lead to good results. On these points the *De Qi* sensation can be obtained easily. If the patient is not very sensitive to needling (difficult to obtain *Qi*), several points along the meridian should be needled in order to elicit the sensation of the *Qi* spreading along the meridian.

Pain in a fixed location (e.g. tendinopathy)

This often indicates a disharmony of the sinew channels.

Mainly local points should be used.

Acute pain

For acute pain, local needling may increase the Blood (*Xue*) and *Qi* disharmony; therefore distal points should be used.

After obtaining the *Qi* sensation, the patient is asked to move the affected joint. If there is still local tension and tightness, this should be needled with gentle, superficial insertions. The rule of opposites is here indicated.

Chronic pain

In chronic pain there is always underlying Blood (*Xue*) and *Qi* stagnation, so needling of predominantly local points is indicated. If more than one meridian is involved or the location of the pain keeps changing, points with an overall regulating effect should be selected (mainly distal to the elbow and knee).

Joint pain

L.I.-4 and LIV-3 (pain within the framework of depression and *Qi* stagnation).

Pain due to disharmony between Qi and Blood (Xue)

L.I.-11 and ST-36.

Pain due to muscular tightness and tendon problems

G.B.-34 and T.B.-5.

Pain that flares up chronically

Du-14 [Du-13 Bi] for the head, thorax and shoulder girdle; Du-4 for the abdomen and pelvic girdle; Ren-4, Ren-6 and Ren-8 have a tonifying effect on the *Yin*.

Psychosomatic pain

Points on the head and back-*Shu* points have a calming, anxiolytic and analgesic effect: G.B.-20, BL-10, Du-24, *Si Shen Cong* (Four Alert Spirit, Ex-HN-1), BL-15 (back-*Shu* point of the Heart), BL-18 (back-*Shu* point of the Liver) and BL-20 (back-*Shu* point of the Spleen).

Pain in the head

Any disorder, either local or distal, can cause pain in the cranial region. A TCM differential diagnosis should be based on the Rule of Three (see above): distal points (distal to the knee and elbow).

For an organ-related treatment, the back-*Shu* points and the main points on the back generally lead to good results.

Pain in the torso

Pain in the torso is differentiated according to location – anterior, posterior or lateral:

- Anterior aspect: *Yang Ming* meridians – ST/L.I. (ST-44, L.I.-4, SP-6)
- Lateral aspect: *Shao Yang* meridians – G.B./T.B. (LIV-3, G.B.-34, T.B.-7)
- Posterior aspect: *Tai Yang* meridians – S.I./BL (BL-60, S.I.-6, KID-3).

The distal points are selected according to the meridian affected and supplemented by local points.

> The more acute the pain, the more distal points should be selected; the more chronic, the more local points should be needled.

The basic point prescription for chronic lower back pain comprises the following points: BL-23, BL-52 [BL-47 Bi], G.B.-34, G.B.-39, Du-4.

Modifying factors

Wind as trigger, modifying circumstance or factor causing a change of symptoms

Symptomatology with quickly changing signs and symptoms: select meridian points that are indicated for Wind.

Therapy: BL-12, Du-14 [Du-13 Bi], Du-16, G.B.-20, G.B.-31, all with reducing method and moxibustion.

External Cold as trigger, modifying circumstance or factor causing a change of symptoms

External Cold lodges in the deep levels of the body, cramping, stagnates the circulation in the meridians.
Therapy: Du-14 [Du-13 Bi], BL-12 and L.I.-11 with reducing method and moxibustion.
Additionally, needle L.I.-4 with tonifying method and KID-7 with reducing method in order to expel the Cold in the superficial layers of the body by promoting sweating.

BL-60 combined with KID-3 promotes the 'expulsion of Cold from the surface of the body'.

Dampness as trigger, modifying circumstance or factor causing a change of symptoms

Lingering, fixed pain, often with localized oedema.
Therapy: ST-36; SP-9 promotes diuresis through digestion. L.I.-4 and LIV-3 support the elimination of oedema by improving the liver function (*Qi Ji*).

Also use SP-6 and ST-28 (*Shui Dao*), G.B.-34, Du-14 [Du-13 Bi], Ren-12.

With depression as modifying circumstance

TCM associates the Liver with depression; the Liver governs spreading (*Shu Xie*).

There will be a slowing down, stagnation sets in, 'knotting' and tension occur. In such a scenario, pain or depression can present as the key symptoms.
Therapy: BL-18 with reducing method, LIV-14.
Also G.B.-34, LIV-3 and/or P-6.

Dysfunction of the vital energy Qi as modifying circumstance

The physiological direction of the flow of *Qi* has become disturbed (*Qi Ji*) with symptoms such as cough, hiccups, stenocardia, thoracic pain, epigastric pain, vomiting, diarrhoea, dysmenorrhoea, etc.
Therapy: ST-36 and P-6 (abdomen), Ren-17 (thorax), Ren-6 (lower abdomen).

Blood stasis (Xue Yu) as modifying circumstance

Trauma, overexertion, etc. can lead to local microhaematoma or macrohaematoma, which may cause stabbing, localized pain.

Therapy: SP-10, BL-17, SP-6, all with reducing method; bloodletting at BL-54 [BL-54 Bi].
Add local pain points.

Internal Cold as trigger, modifying circumstance or factor causing a change of symptoms

Weak, chronically ill patients with epigastric, abdominal, hypochondriacal and back pain, as well as dysmenorrhoea.
Therapy: ST-25, ST-36, Ren-6, Ren-12 with tonifying method and moxibustion.
Add the back-*Shu* points of the affected organs.

Digestive problems as modifying circumstance of the pain

The retention of food in the gastrointestinal tract causes abdominal pain.
Therapy: ST-25 and Ren-6, Ren-12 with reducing method, longer needle retention.
For diarrhoea: ST-39.
For constipation: add ST-37.

Excess Liver Yang as modifying circumstance

Yin deficiency or Liver stagnation can lead to the pattern of 'Fire and Wind in the Liver', manifesting with symptoms such as migraine, headaches with hypertonic crisis.
Therapy: L.I.-4, G.B.-20, LIV-3, DU-20 and Ex-HN-5 (*Tai Yang*).
To stabilize the condition, add SP-6 and KID-3.
The presence of Fire can indicate a local inflammation or a reactive arthrosis: sedating needling method at the tips of the fingers and toes (e.g. for tonsillitis, LU-11 and L.I.-1).

Deficiency of the vital energy Qi and Blood (Xue) as modifying circumstance

Frequently seen in elderly or chronically ill patients, recurring pain, worse with exertion (*Qi* deficiency) and rest (Blood [*Xue*] deficiency):
Apart from a symptomatic treatment, also give a tonifying treatment to strengthen the *Qi* and the Blood (*Xue*).
Therapy: tuina or acupuncture at ST-36, BL-17, BL-20, Du-20, Ren-4, Ren-6, all with tonifying method and moxibustion.

6.15.2 Sciatica

The pathway of the sciatic nerve (L4–S3) corresponds to the Bladder meridian, the longest meridian.

The sciatic nerve is the largest and strongest of the peripheral nerves. Injuries to its trunk are generally a result of direct trauma. Chinese medicine recognizes pathogenic factors such as Wind, Cold and Dampness, as well as Heat, as further causes. Degenerative disorders with a deficiency of *Qi* and Blood (*Xue*) also play a role.

Individual point combination

Type A: pain along the Bladder meridian: BL-23, BL-25, BL-36 [BL-50 Bi], BL-40 [BL-54 Bi], BL-57, BL-60 and local pressure-sensitive points.
Type B: pain along the Gall Bladder meridian: G.B.-30, G.B.-31, G.B.-34, G.B.-39, G.B.-40 and local pressure-sensitive points.
Type C: pain along the Stomach meridian: ST-31, ST-32, ST-36, ST-41 and local pressure-sensitive points.
During the acute stage it is important to get appropriate physical rest. For good treatment results, obtaining a *De Qi* sensation is also important.

Acupuncture points

BL-23 **Location:** 1.5 cun lateral to L2, level with Du-4.
  Notes: back-*Shu* point of the Kidneys.
BL-25 **Location:** 1.5 cun lateral to the lower border of the spinous process of L4.
  Notes: back-*Shu* point of the Large Intestine.
BL-36 **Location:** in the centre of the transverse gluteal crease.
  Notes: local point.
BL-40 **Location:** in the centre of the popliteal crease, between the tendons of the semitendinosus and the biceps femoris.
  Notes: *He*-sea point, command point for the back; eliminates Blood (*Xue*) stagnation.
BL-57 **Location:** in the depression below the two bellies of the gastrocnemius; on tiptoes; midway between BL-40 and BL-60.

  Notes: for calf cramps!
BL-60 **Location:** in the depression between the Achilles tendon and the lateral malleolus.
  Notes: *Jing*-river point, master point for any pain along the meridian pathway.
G.B.-30 **Location:** on a line connecting the greater trochanter and the sacral hiatus, at the junction of the lateral and medial third.
  Notes: meeting point with the Bladder meridian, master point for sciatica and paresis of the legs.
G.B.-31 **Location:** on the lateral aspect of the thigh; with the arms hanging down, the middle finger will indicate this point.
  Notes: for pain susceptible to Wind and to changes in the weather.
G.B.-34 **Location:** with the knee flexed, in the depression anterior and inferior to the head of the fibula.
  Notes: *He*-sea point of the Gall Bladder, *Hui*-meeting point of the tendons, master point of musculature.
G.B.-39 **Location:** 3 cun superior to the lateral malleolus, on the posterior border of the fibula.
  Notes: *Hui*-meeting point of the marrow (of the bones and spinal cord)! Group *Luo*-connecting point of the 3 lower *Yang*: ST, G.B., BL.
G.B.-40 **Location:** on the junction of a horizontal line through the prominence of the lateral malleolus and a vertical line through the greatest circumference of the lateral malleolus, over the calcaneocuboidal joint.
  Notes: *Yuan*-source point.
ST-31 **Location:** at the level of the perineum, on a line connecting the anterior superior iliac spine and the lateral upper border of the patella.
  Notes: local point; strengthens the *Qi* and Blood (*Xue*).
ST-32 **Location:** 6 cun superior to the patella, on the rectus femoris muscle.
  Notes: meeting point of the arteries and veins.
ST-36 **Location:** 0.5 cun lateral to the anterior crest of the tibia, 1.5 cun inferior to the lower border of the head of the fibula (G.B.-34).
  Notes: *He*-sea point, master point of hormones; alternative name: 'Great Healer of the Feet and Knees'.
ST-41 **Location:** at the midpoint of the anterior aspect of the ankle, between the tendons of the extensor hallucis longus and extensor digitorum longus.
  Notes: *Jing*-river point and tonification point.

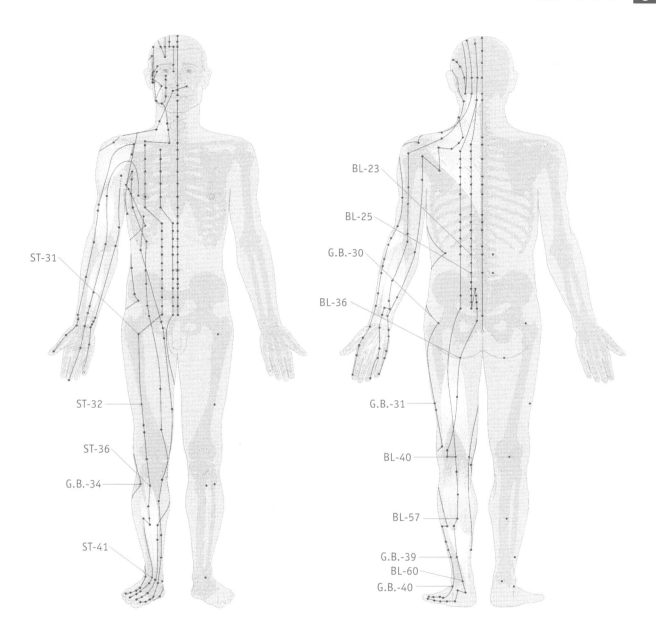

ST-31

ST-32

ST-36

G.B.-34

ST-41

BL-23

BL-25

G.B.-30

BL-36

G.B.-31

BL-40

BL-57

G.B.-39

BL-60

G.B.-40

6.15.3 *Meralgia paraesthetica*

Pain due to an injury to the lateral femoral cutaneous nerve (L2/L3), it passes deep to the inguinal ligament, medial to the anterior superior iliac spine, where mechanical injury can occur to this sensitive nerve. If avoidance of external strain and infiltration do not lead to an improvement of the condition, acupuncture might be the treatment of choice.

Basic point combination

ST-31, ST-32, G.B.-31, G.B.-32, G.B.-34.

Individual point combination

Changing, severe pain

SP-10, BL-17.

Paraesthesia of the skin

ST-36, SP-5.

Exhaustion

BL-23, Ren-4.
Local therapy covering a large surface area is the main approach.

Acupuncture points

BL-17 **Location:** 1.5 cun lateral to the spinous process of T7, approximately level with the inferior angle of the scapula.
Notes: *Hui*-meeting point of the Blood, back-*Shu* point of the diaphragm; tonifies the Blood, moves Blood (*Xue*) stagnation.

BL-23 **Location:** 1.5 cun lateral to L2, level with Du-4.
Notes: back-*Shu* point of the Kidneys; tonifies Kidney *Yin, Yang* and Essence (*Jing*).

G.B.-31 **Location:** on the lateral aspect of the thigh; with the arms hanging down, the middle finger will indicate this point.
Notes: Wind point.

G.B.-32 **Location:** 1 cun inferior to G.B.-31.
Notes: local point.

G.B.-34 **Location:** with the knee flexed, in the depression anterior and inferior to the head of the fibula.
Notes: *He*-sea point of the Gall Bladder, *Hui*-meeting point of the tendons, master point of the musculature.

Ren-4 **Location:** 2 cun superior to the upper border of the pubic symphysis.
Notes: internal meeting point of the 3 lower *Yin* meridians (SP, LIV, KID), front-*Mu* point of the Small Intestine; nourishing – tonifies Essence (*Jing*), *Qi, Yang*, Blood (*Xue*) and *Yin*.

SP-5 **Location:** with the foot in dorsiflexion, in the depression between the tendons of the tibialis anterior and the medial malleolus, superior to the navicular bone.
Notes: *Jing*-river point and sedation point, master point of connective tissue.

SP-10 **Location:** with the knee flexed, 2 cun superior to the upper patellar border, medial to the vastus medialis.
Notes: 'Sea of Blood (*Xue*)'; nourishes and cools the Blood (*Xue*), moves *Qi* and Blood (*Xue*), thus eliminating Wind.

ST-31 **Location:** at the level of the perineum, on a line connecting the anterior superior iliac spine and the lateral upper border of the patella.
Notes: local point, strengthens *Qi* and Blood (*Xue*).

ST-32 **Location:** 6 cun superior to the patella, on the rectus femoris.
Notes: meeting point of the arteries and veins.

ST-36 **Location:** 0.5 cun lateral to the anterior crest of the tibia, 1.5 cun inferior to the lower border of the head of the fibula (G.B.-34).
Notes: *He*-sea point, master point of hormones; alternative name: 'Great Healer of the Feet and Knees'.

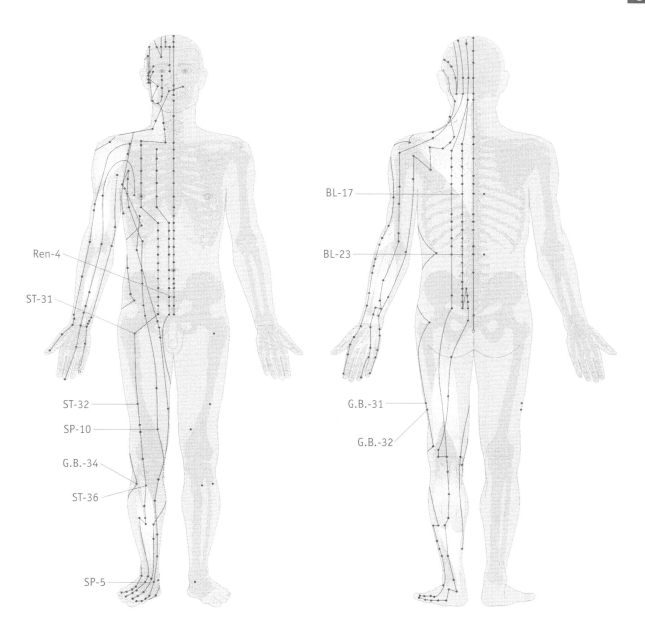

Ren-4

ST-31

ST-32

SP-10

G.B.-34

ST-36

SP-5

BL-17

BL-23

G.B.-31

G.B.-32

6.15.4 *Polyneuropathy*

Generally, polyneuropathy affects a number of peripheral nerves in a more or less bilateral pattern, usually starting at the distal aspect of the lower extremities. Symptoms include uncomfortable sensations, weak to missing reflexes, and generally tend to be worse at night. Besides causative therapy and physiotherapy, acupuncture presents an adjunctive therapy with, in less severe cases, often good results.

Basic point combination

LU-5, L.I.-4, L.I.-11, L.I.-15, ST-36, SP-6, BL-40 [BL-54 Bi], BL-60, T.B.-5, LIV-3, G.B.-39, Ex-UE-9 (*Ba Xie*), Ex-LE-10 (*Ba Feng*).
Caution: electroacupuncture may exacerbate the symptoms.

Acupuncture points

BL-40 **Location:** in the centre of the popliteal crease, between the tendons of the semitendinosus and the biceps femoris.
Notes: *He*-sea point, command point of the back; eliminates Blood (*Xue*) stagnation and Heat, relaxes the tendons.

BL-60 **Location:** in the depression between the Achilles tendon and the lateral malleolus.
Notes: *Jing*-river point, master point for any pain along the meridian pathway.

Ex-LE-10 **Location:** 4 points on the dorsum of the foot, 0.5 cun proximal to the interdigital folds.
Notes: relax the tendons, dispel Wind and Dampness, invigorate the Blood (*Xue*).

Ex-UE-9 **Location:** when a loose fist is made, 4 points on the dorsum of each hand, slightly proximal to the margins of the webs between the heads of the 1st to 5th metacarpal bones.
Notes: relax the tendons, dispel Wind and Dampness, invigorate the Blood (*Xue*).

G.B.-39 **Location:** 3 cun superior to the lateral malleolus, on the posterior border of the fibula.

Notes: *Hui*-meeting point of the marrow (of the bones and spinal cord)! Group *Luo*-connecting point of the 3 lower *Yang*: ST, G.B., BL.

L.I.-4 **Location:** on the dorsum of the hand, at the highest point of the muscle bulge between the 1st and 2nd metacarpal bones.
Notes: *Yuan*-source point, metabolic point; combined with L.I.-11, eliminates Wind-Heat, Blood (*Xue*) Heat, Blood (*Xue*) stagnation, Fire toxins, Damp-Heat and Blood (*Xue*) deficiency.

L.I.-11 **Location:** with the arm fully flexed, at the radial end of the cubital crease.
Notes: *He*-sea point and tonification point; eliminates external Wind, Heat and Dampness, particularly when combined with L.I.-4 and Du-14.

L.I.-15 **Location:** with the arm abducted, in the anterior of the two depressions inferior to the acromioclavicular joint, between the anterior and medial third of the deltoid (T.B.-14 is located in the posterior depression).
Notes: master point for pareses of the upper extremity, meeting point with the *Yang Qiao Mai*; dispels Wind from the four extremities.

LIV-3 **Location:** on the dorsum of the foot, in the depression distal to the junction of the 1st and 2nd metatarsal bones.
Notes: *Shu*-stream point and *Yuan*-source point; promotes the smooth the flow of *Qi*, spasmolytic; subdues Liver *Yang*, eliminates internal Wind.

LU-5 **Location:** on the cubital crease, radial to the tendon of the biceps.
Notes: *He*-sea point and sedation point; has an effect on the face, as water point for Heat, tonifies *Yin*.

SP-6 **Location:** 3 cun superior to the highest prominence of the medial malleolus, on the posterior border of the tibia.
Notes: as group *Luo*-connecting point (SP, LIV, KID), tonifies *Qi*, Blood (*Xue*) and *Yin*, nourishing point; eliminates Dampness.

ST-36 **Location:** 0.5 cun lateral to the anterior crest of the tibia, 1.5 cun inferior to the lower border of the head of the fibula (G.B.-34).
Notes: *He*-sea point, master point of hormones, blood pressure; tonifies *Qi* and Blood (*Xue*).

T.B.-5 **Location:** 2 cun proximal to the midpoint of the dorsal wrist crease, opposite P-6.
Notes: *Luo*-connecting point, opening point of the *Yang Wei Mai*, master point of the small joints; can eliminate any pathogen, particularly Wind-Heat.

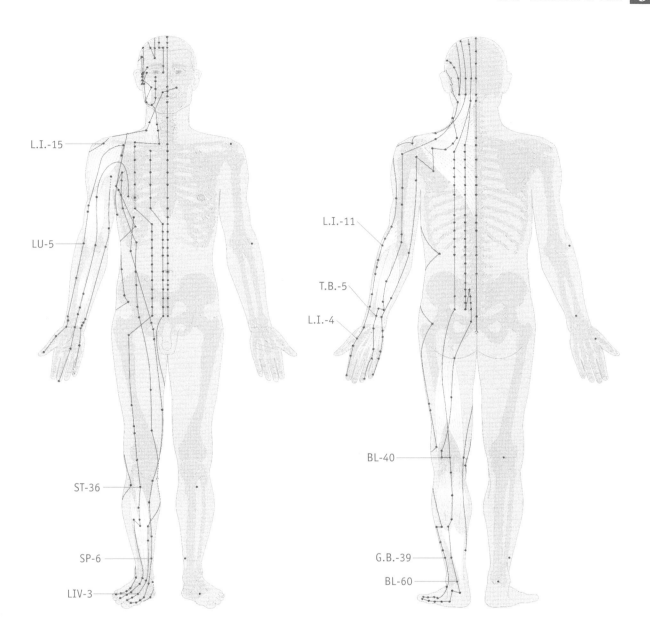

L.I.-15

LU-5

ST-36

SP-6

LIV-3

L.I.-11

T.B.-5

L.I.-4

BL-40

G.B.-39

BL-60

6.15.5 *Heel spur pain*

Heel spurs tend to respond well to acupuncture.

Basic point combination

KID-3, BL-57, BL-60, P-7.

Acupuncture points

BL-57 **Location:** in the depression below the two bellies of the gastrocnemius; on tiptoes; midway between BL-40 and BL-60.
Notes: local point; relaxes the tendons; specific point for calf cramps.

BL-60 **Location:** in the depression between the Achilles tendon and the lateral malleolus.
Notes: *Jing*-river point, master point for any pain along the meridian pathway.

KID-3 **Location:** between the highest prominence of the medial malleolus and the Achilles tendon.
Notes: *Shu*-stream point, *Yuan*-source point; local point.

P-7 **Location:** on the palmar aspect of the wrist joint, between the tendons of the flexor carpi radialis and palmaris longus.
Notes: *Shu*-stream point, sedation point, *Yuan*-source point; treats the corresponding joint on the lower extremity.

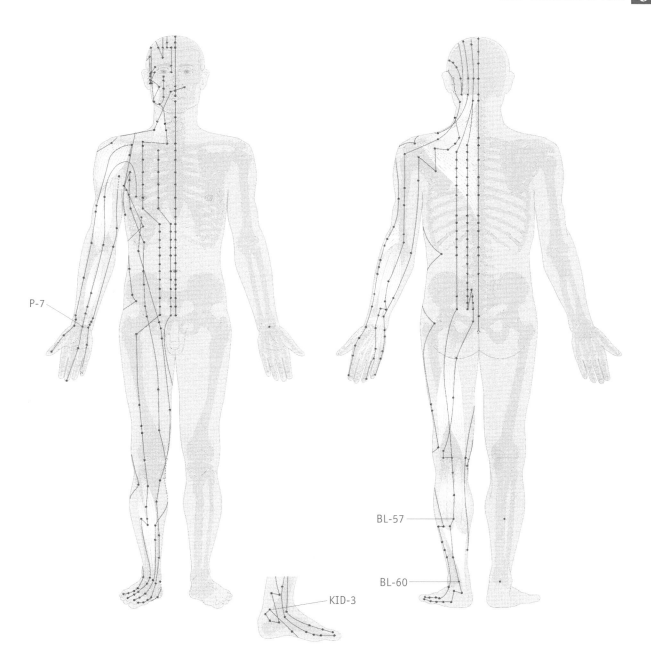

P-7

KID-3

BL-57

BL-60

6.15.6 *Sudeck syndrome, algodystrophy, reflex sympathetic dystrophy*

Stage I: severe spontaneous pain, oedema, painful dystrophy
Stage II: typical X-ray changes, atrophy
Stage III: contracture, pain subsiding.
Acupuncture can be used during any stage in addition to conventional treatment.

Local treatment is contraindicated during stage I and should be applied only from stage II (this applies in particular to interdigital points). Distal points are selected according to the affected meridians.

Individual point combination

Upper extremity

Distal points: LU-5, L.I.-11, L.I.-10, P-6.
Local points: L.I.-4, S.I.-3, P-6, T.B.-3, T.B.-5.

Lower extremity

Distal points: ST-36, SP-9, SP-10, G.B.-31, G.B.-34.
Local points: ST-41, SP-6, BL-60, KID-3, G.B.-41, LIV-3.

Acupuncture points

BL-60 **Location:** in the depression between the Achilles tendon and the lateral malleolus.
Notes: *Jing*-river point, master point for any pain along the meridian pathway.

G.B.-31 **Location:** on the lateral aspect of the thigh; with the arms hanging down, the middle finger will indicate this point.
Notes: Wind point.

G.B.-34 **Location:** with the knee flexed, in the depression anterior and inferior to the head of the fibula.
Notes: *He*-sea point of the Gall Bladder, *Hui*-meeting point of the tendons, master point of musculature; promotes the smooth flow of Liver *Qi*, eliminates Damp-Heat.

G.B.-41 **Location:** in the depression distal to the junction of the 4th and 5th metatarsal bones.
Notes: *Shu*-stream point and opening point of the *Dai Mai*, master point of the large joints; eliminates Damp-Heat, promotes the harmonious flow of Liver *Qi*.

KID-3 **Location:** between the highest prominence of the medial malleolus and the Achilles tendon.
Notes: *Shu*-stream point and *Yuan*-source point; tonifies Kidney *Yang* and, particularly, Kidney *Yin*. The bones pertain to the Kidneys!

L.I.-4 **Location:** on the dorsum of the hand, at the highest point of the muscle bulge between the 1st and 2nd metacarpal bones.
Notes: *Yuan*-source point, metabolic point; combined with L.I.-11 eliminates Wind-Heat, Blood (*Xue*) Heat, Blood (*Xue*) stagnation, Fire toxins, Damp-Heat and Blood (*Xue*) deficiency.

L.I.-10 **Location:** on the radial aspect of the forearm, 3 cun distal to L.I.-11, on the belly of the extensor muscles.
Notes: treats disorders along the pathway of the meridian; eliminates swellings.

L.I.-11 **Location:** with the arm fully flexed, at the radial end of the cubital crease.
Notes: *He*-sea point and tonification point; eliminates Damp-Heat and Wind, benefits the tendons and joints.

LIV-3 **Location:** on the dorsum of the foot, in the depression distal to the junction of the 1st and 2nd metatarsal bones.
Notes: *Shu*-stream point and *Yuan*-source point; smoothes the flow of *Qi*, spasmolytic; subdues Liver *Yang*, eliminates internal Wind.

LU-5 **Location:** on the cubital crease, radial to the tendon of the biceps.
Notes: *He*-sea point and sedation point; has an effect on the face, as water point for Heat, tonifies *Yin*.

P-6 **Location:** 2 cun proximal to the midpoint of the palmar wrist crease, between the tendons of the flexor carpi radialis and palmaris longus.
Notes: *Luo*-connecting point and opening point of the *Yin Wei Mai*; mobilizes the Blood (*Xue*), *Qi* and Phlegm stagnation.

S.I.-3 **Location:** when a fist is made, on the dorsum of the hand, in the depression at the end of the most distal palmar crease.
Notes: tonification point and opening point of the *Du Mai*; dispels external and internal Wind from the *Du Mai*, benefits the tendons, eliminates Dampness.

SP-6 **Location:** 3 cun superior to the highest prominence of the medial malleolus, on the posterior border of the tibia.
Notes: as group *Luo*-connecting point (SP, LIV, KID), tonifies *Qi*, Blood (*Xue*) and *Yin*; nourishing point; eliminates Dampness.

SP-9 **Location:** with the knee flexed, in the depression inferior to the medial condyle of the tibia, at the same level as G.B.-34.
Notes: *He*-sea point; regulates the Fluids and Dampness, tonifies Spleen *Qi*.

SP-10 **Location:** with the knee flexed, 2 cun superior to the upper patellar border, medial to the vastus medialis.
Notes: 'Sea of Blood (*Xue*)'; nourishes and cools the Blood (*Xue*), moves *Qi* and Blood (*Xue*), eliminates Wind and Heat.

ST-36 **Location:** 0.5 cun lateral to the anterior crest of the tibia, 1.5 cun inferior to the lower border of the head of the fibula (G.B.-34).
Notes: *He*-sea point, master point of hormones, hypertension; tonifies *Qi* and Blood (*Xue*).

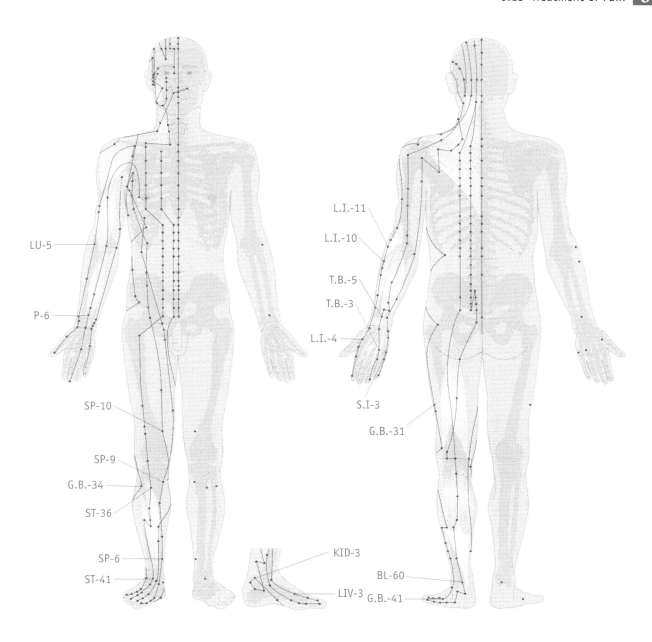

LU-5

P-6

SP-10

SP-9

G.B.-34

ST-36

SP-6

ST-41

L.I.-11

L.I.-10

T.B.-5

T.B.-3

L.I.-4

S.I-3

G.B.-31

KID-3

BL-60

LIV-3 G.B.-41

ST-41 **Location:** at the midpoint of the anterior aspect of the ankle, between the tendons of the extensor hallucis longus and extensor digitorum longus.
Notes: *Jing*-river point and tonification point; local point.

T.B.-3 **Location:** with the hand formed to a loose fist, on the dorsum of the hand, between the 4th and 5th metacarpal bones, in the depression proximal to the metacarpophalangeal joints.

Notes: *Shu*-stream point, tonification point; clears Heat, dispels Wind, promotes the flow of Qi in the meridian.

T.B.-5 **Location:** 2 cun proximal to the midpoint of the dorsal wrist crease, opposite P-6.
Notes: *Luo*-connecting point, opening point of the *Yang Wei Mai*, master point of the small joints; can eliminate any pathogen, particularly Wind-Heat.

6.15.7 *Phantom pain*

Phantom pain signals from amputated limbs often occur when the weather is changing.

Basic point combination

L.I.-4, ST-36, BL-60, P-6.
In addition, needle the painful meridian points on the unaffected side; for example, if there is phantom pain on the left big toe, needle SP-2 and LIV-2 on the right side.
Ear acupuncture: 55 *Shen Men* and 95 Kidney.
Also apply intradermal needles or press balls on the relevant projection zone of the ear. Instruct the patient to press these firmly, 2–3 times daily for 2–3 minutes, until warmth, heat or pain can be felt. Remove the press balls after 10 days.

Acupuncture points

BL-60 **Location:** in the depression between the Achilles tendon and the lateral malleolus.
Notes: *Jing*-river point, master point for any pain along the meridian pathway.

L.I.-4 **Location:** on the dorsum of the hand, at the highest point of the muscle bulge between the 1st and 2nd metacarpal bones.
Notes: *Yuan*-source point, metabolic point; combined with L.I.-11 eliminates Wind-Heat, Blood (*Xue*) Heat, Blood (*Xue*) stagnation, Fire toxins and Damp-Heat.

LIV-2 **Location:** on the web between the 1st and 2nd toes, at the lateral aspect of the metatarsophalangeal joint of the 1st toe.
Notes: *Ying*-spring point and sedation point; eliminates Liver Fire and Liver Wind, spasmolytic; here, symptomatic local point.

P-6 **Location:** 2 cun proximal to the midpoint of the palmar wrist crease, between the tendons of the flexor carpi radialis and palmaris longus.
Notes: *Luo*-connecting point and opening point of the *Yin Wei Mai*; mobilizes the Blood (*Xue*), *Qi* and Phlegm stagnation.

SP-2 **Location:** in the medial joint space of the metatarsophalangeal joint of the big toe, at the junction of the red and white skin.
Notes: *Ying*-spring point and tonification point; see LIV-2.

ST-36 **Location:** 0.5 cun lateral to the anterior crest of the tibia, 1.5 cun inferior to the lower border of the head of the fibula (G.B.-34).
Notes: *He*-sea point, master point of hormones, hypertension.

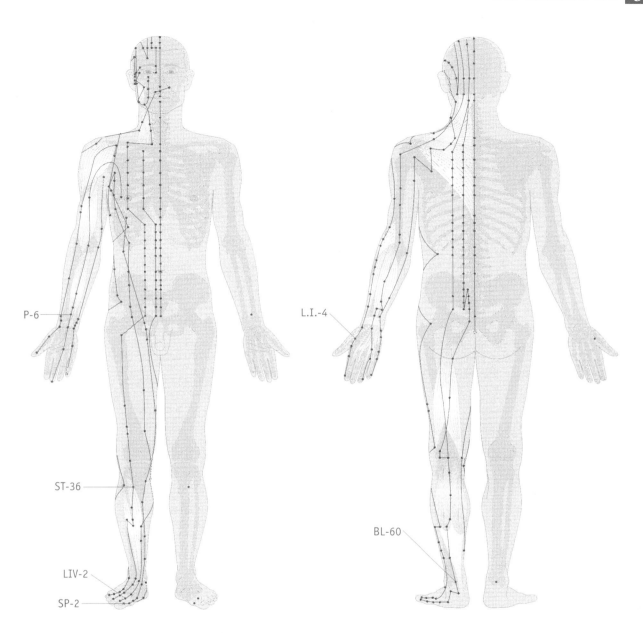

6.15.8 Multiple sclerosis (1)

Multiple sclerosis (MS) or encephalomyelitis disseminata is an inflammatory disease of the brain and spinal cord that typically occurs in episodes. Symptoms include paralysis, anaesthesia, pain, optic nerve lesions, spasticity, cerebellar symptoms, impaired ocular motility, loss of control of bowel and bladder, as well as psychoemotional difficulties.

Infusion therapy with steroids during episodes is now generally recognized. Conventional therapy uses a number of immunosuppressive substances and immune-stimulating treatments (e.g. β-interferon).

Acupuncture, tuina and Chinese herbal medicine, as well as physiotherapy, can be applied as symptomatic, adjunctive methods. Regarding Chinese medicine, the acupuncture point prescription, needling technique and herbal formulae have to be adapted to the patient's condition.

TCM

TCM attributes MS to the Liver and Kidney: generally MS manifests with symptoms indicative of *Yin* deficiency, Liver/Kidney deficiency and Kidney *Yang* deficiency (muscular atrophy).

Individual point combination

Liver/Kidney deficiency

SP-6, HE-7, BL-2, BL-18, BL-23, G.B.-20, LIV-3, Ex-HN-5 (*Tai Yang*).

Upper extremity

L.I.-4, L.I.-11, L.I.-14, L.I.-15, LU-5.

Acupuncture points

BL-2   **Location:** at the junction of the vertical line through the medial end of the eyebrow (inner canthus) and the supraorbital foramen.
Notes: dispels Wind, benefits the eyes; for neuritis of the optic nerve.

BL-18   **Location:** 2 cun lateral to the spinous process of T9.
Notes: back-*Shu* point of the Liver.

BL-23   **Location:** 1.5 cun lateral to L2, level with Du-4.
Notes: back-*Shu* point of the Kidneys; tonifies the *Qi*, *Yang*, *Yin* and Essence (*Jing*) of the Kidneys.

Ex-HN-5   **Location:** on the temple, in a depression approximately 1 cun lateral to the midpoint of a line connecting the lateral extremity of the eyebrow and the outer canthus of the eye.
Notes: local point for headaches; has an affinity to the G.B. and the T.B.

G.B.-20   **Location:** posterior to the mastoid, between the trapezius and sternocleidomastoid on the lower border of the occiput.
Notes: main point for Wind in the upper half of the body; combine with BL-10 to treat harmonize the sympathetic and parasympathetic nervous system.

HE-7   **Location:** on the ulnar aspect of the wrist crease, on the radial aspect of the pisiform bone.
Notes: *Shu*-stream point and *Yuan*-source point, sedation point; tonifies the Heart Blood, cools Heat, Fire and *Yin*.

L.I.-4   **Location:** on the dorsum of the hand, at the highest point of the muscle bulge between the 1st and 2nd metacarpal bones.
Notes: *Yuan*-source point, metabolic point; combined with L.I.-11, eliminates Wind-Heat, Blood (*Xue*) Heat, Blood (*Xue*) stagnation, Fire toxins, Damp-Heat and Blood (*Xue*) deficiency.

L.I.-1   **Location:** with the arm fully flexed at the radial end of the cubital crease.
Notes: *He*-sea point and tonification point; eliminates Damp-Heat and Wind, benefits the tendons and joints.

L.I.-14   **Location:** on the lateral aspect of the upper arm, slightly superior and anterior to the insertion of the deltoid.
Notes: meeting point with the Stomach and Large Intestine meridian and the *Yang Qiao Mai*; local point.

L.I.-15   **Location:** with the arm abducted, in the anterior of the two depressions inferior to the acromioclavicular joint, between the anterior and medial third of the deltoid (T.B.-14 is located in thse posterior depression).
Notes: master point for paresis of the upper extremity.

LIV-3   **Location:** on the dorsum of the foot, in the depression distal to the junction of the 1st and 2nd metatarsal bones.
Notes: *Shu*-stream point and *Yuan*-source point; subdues rising Liver *Yang* and Liver Wind, harmonizes the flow of Liver *Qi*.

LU-5   **Location:** on the cubital crease, radial to the tendon of the biceps.
Notes: *He*-sea point and sedation point; bloodletting eliminates *Qi* and Blood (*Xue*) stagnation.

SP-6   **Location:** 3 cun superior to the highest prominence of the medial malleolus, on the posterior border of the tibia.
Notes: as group *Luo*-connecting point (SP, LIV, KID), tonifies *Qi*, Blood (*Xue*) and *Yin*; nourishing point; eliminates Dampness.

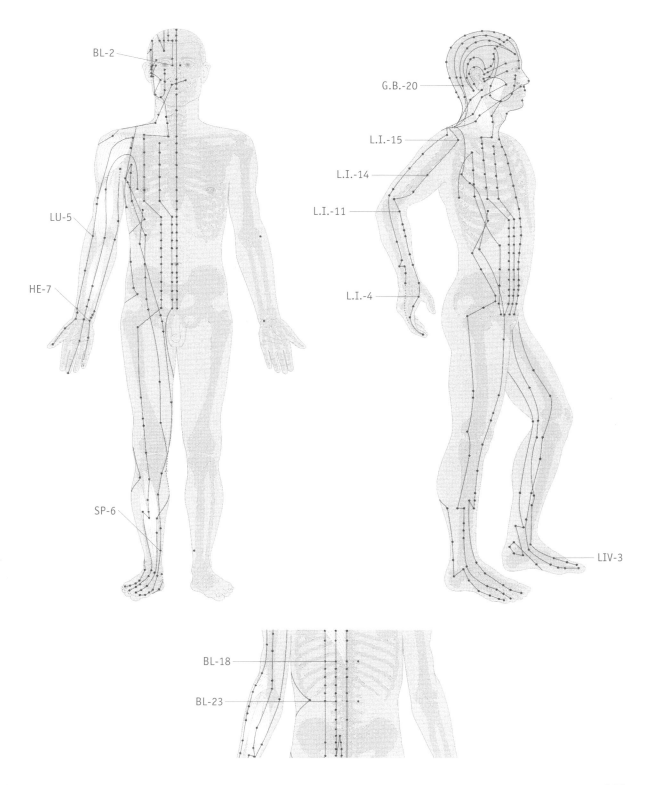

BL-2

G.B.-20

L.I.-15

L.I.-14

LU-5

L.I.-11

HE-7

L.I.-4

SP-6

LIV-3

BL-18

BL-23

6.15.8 Multiple sclerosis (2)

Lower extremity

ST-31, ST-32, ST-36, G.B.-30, G.B.-34, G.B.-39.

Difficulty with/loss of bladder and bowel function

SP-9, SP-10, BL-28, Ren-2, Ren-4, Ren-6.
Also add points according to the 'Rule of Three' (Alexander Meng)

Acupuncture points

BL-28   **Location:** 1.5 cun lateral to the posterior midline, at the level of the 2nd sacral foramen.
Notes: back-*Shu* point of the Bladder.

G.B.-30   **Location:** on a line connecting the greater trochanter and the sacral hiatus, at the junction of the lateral and medial third.
Notes: meeting point with the Bladder meridian, master point for sciatica and paresis of the legs.

G.B.-34   **Location:** with the knee flexed, in the depression anterior and inferior to the head of the fibula.
Notes: *He*-sea point of the Gall Bladder, *Hui*-meeting point of the tendons, master point of the musculature.

G.B.-39   **Location:** 3 cun superior to the lateral malleolus, on the posterior border of the fibula.
Notes: *Hui*-meeting point of the marrow (of the bones and spinal cord)! Group *Luo*-connecting point of the 3 lower *Yang*: ST, G.B., BL.

Ren-2   **Location:** on the midline, at the upper border of the pubic symphysis, in the skin crease that forms when bending forward; level with KID-11, SP-12, ST-30.
Notes: local point for the urogenital region.

Ren-4   **Location:** 2 cun superior to the upper border of the pubic symphysis.
Notes: internal meeting point of the 3 lower *Yin* meridians (SP, LIV, KID), front-*Mu* point of the Small Intestine; tonifies Essence (*Jing*), *Qi*, *Yang*, Blood (*Xue*) and *Yin*; better than Ren-6 for the treatment of deficiency patterns.

Ren-6   **Location:** 1.5 cun inferior to the umbilicus.
Notes: 'Sea of *Qi*' – tonifies the Kidneys, original *Qi* and *Yang Qi*; nourishing point.

SP-9   **Location:** with the knee flexed, in the depression inferior to the medial condyle of the tibia, at the same level as G.B.-34.
Notes: *He*-sea point; eliminates Dampness and Heat, regulates the Water passages; for retention of urine and incontinence.

SP-10   **Location:** with the knee flexed, 2 cun superior to the upper patellar border, medial to the vastus medialis.
Notes: 'Sea of Blood (*Xue*)'; nourishes and cools the Blood (*Xue*), moves *Qi* and Blood (*Xue*), has an effect on the urogenital region.

ST-31   **Location:** at the level of the perineum, on a line connecting the anterior superior iliac spine and the lateral upper border of the patella.
Notes: local point; strengthens the *Qi* and Blood (*Xue*).

ST-32   **Location:** 6 cun superior to the patella, on the rectus femoris muscle.
Notes: meeting point of the arteries and veins.

ST-36   **Location:** 0.5 cun lateral to the anterior crest of the tibia, 1.5 cun inferior to the lower border of the head of the fibula (G.B.-34).
Notes: *He*-sea point, master point of hormones, hypertension; tonifies *Qi* and Blood (*Xue*), promotes building-up of muscles.

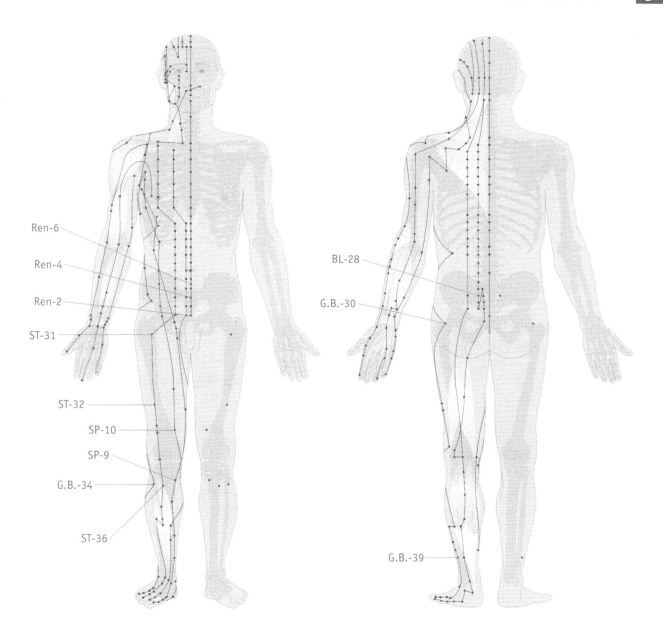

Ren-6
Ren-4
Ren-2
ST-31
ST-32
SP-10
SP-9
G.B.-34
ST-36

BL-28
G.B.-30

G.B.-39

6.15.9 Tumour pain

The point prescription has to be based on the site of the primary tumour (organ), the affected meridians, and the accompanying signs and symptoms ('Rule of Three' after Alexander Meng).

TCM

TCM interprets tumour pain as *Qi* stagnation or as *Qi* and Blood (*Xue*) stagnation; therefore bloodletting at the points LU-5 and BL-40 [BL-54 Bi] is often part of the basic point prescription.

Individual point combination

Ear acupuncture can also be applied based on the 'Rule of Three' after Meng. It has been proven beneficial to use either intradermal needles or pressballs.

Xi-cleft points of the affected organs

For example, LU-6 (bronchial carcinoma), ST-34 (stomach carcinoma), S.I.-6 and L.I.-7 (carcinoma of the small and large intestine).

First and last point of the affected meridian

For example, LU-1 and LU-11 for bronchial carcinoma.

Front-*Mu* and back-*Shu* points of the affected meridian

For example, LU-1 and BL-13 for bronchial carcinoma.

For *Yang*-organ carcinoma (ST, S.I., L.I., G.B., BL)

The *He*-sea point of the affected organ is particularly effective: ST-36, ST-37, ST-39, G.B.-34, BL-40 [BL-54 Bi].

The 8 *Hui*-meeting points

(→ 5.2.3) Ren-12, Ren-17, BL-11, BL-17, LU-9, G.B.-34, G.B.-39.
Used to support the *Yin* organs, *Yang* organs, vital energy *Qi*, breath *Qi*, Blood (*Xue*), muscles, tendons, blood vessels, bones, brain, spinal cord, marrow.

Calming points (harmonizing the Heart and the Liver)

ST-36 and BL-15, HE-7, P-6, P-7, LIV-2, LIV-3.

Tumour pain, terminal stage

Opioids are indispensable.
L.I.-4, ST-36, SP-6, P-6, pressure-sensitive points, and points adjacent to the painful area.
TCM considers cancer also as a stagnation of pathogenic *Qi* (*Xie Qi*) in the *Yin* organs (Lungs, Spleen, Liver, Kidneys).

Projection zones from these *Yin* organs also occur around the large joints. The joints often show signs of involvement. Treatment of the relevant region, for example with acu-injections (injections at acupuncture points), can alleviate the tumour pain.

Axilla for the Liver

ST-19.

Elbow for the Lungs

P-2.

Inguinal groove for the Spleen

SP-12.

Popliteal crease for the Kidneys

SP-10.

Acupuncture points

BL-11 **Location:** 1.5 cun lateral to the spinous process of T1.
Notes: *Hui*-meeting point of the bones.
BL-13 **Location:** 1.5 cun lateral to the spinous process of T3.
Notes: back-*Shu* point of the Lungs.
BL-15 **Location:** 1.5 cun lateral to the spinous process of T5.
Notes: back-*Shu* point of the Heart.
BL-17 **Location:** 1.5 cun lateral to the spinous process of T7, approximately level with the inferior angle of the scapula.
Notes: *Hui*-meeting point of the Blood, back-*Shu* point of the diaphragm.
BL-40 **Location:** in the centre of the popliteal crease, between the tendons of the semitendinosus and the biceps femoris.
Notes: *He*-sea point, command point of the back; bloodletting eliminates *Qi* and Blood (*Xue*) stagnation.
G.B.-34 **Location:** with the knee flexed, in the depression anterior and inferior to the head of the fibula.
Notes: *He*-sea point of the Gall Bladder, *Hui*-meeting point of the tendons, master point of the musculature.
G.B.-39 **Location:** 3 cun superior to the lateral malleolus, on the posterior border of the fibula.
Notes: *Hui*-meeting point of the marrow (of the bones and spinal cord)! Group *Luo*-connecting point of the 3 lower *Yang*: ST, G.B., BL.

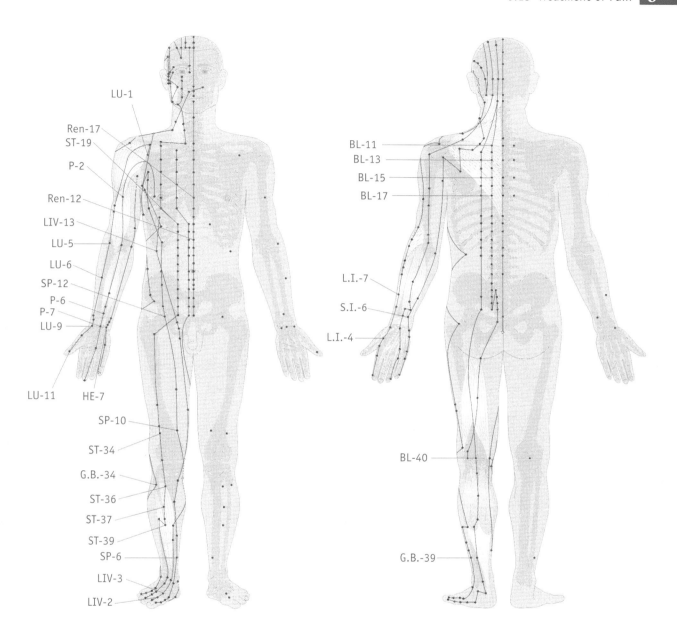

LU-1
Ren-17
ST-19
P-2
Ren-12
LIV-13
LU-5
LU-6
SP-12
P-6
P-7
LU-9
LU-11   HE-7
SP-10
ST-34
G.B.-34
ST-36
ST-37
ST-39
SP-6
LIV-3
LIV-2

BL-11
BL-13
BL-15
BL-17
L.I.-7
S.I.-6
L.I.-4
BL-40
G.B.-39

HE-7 **Location:** on the ulnar aspect of the wrist crease, on the radial aspect of the pisiform bone.
Notes: *Shu*-stream point, *Yuan*-source point, sedation point.

L.I.-4 **Location:** on the dorsum of the hand, at the highest point of the muscle bulge between the 1st and 2nd metacarpal bones.
Notes: *Yuan*-source point, metabolic point; moves *Qi*, analgesic, eliminates pathogens and toxins, combined with ST-36 tonifies the defensive *Qi* (*Wei Qi*).

L.I.-7 **Location:** on a line connecting L.I.-5 and L.I.-11, 5 cun proximal to the wrist crease (or L.I.-5).
Notes: *Xi*-cleft point.

LIV-2 **Location:** on the web between the 1st and 2nd toes, at the lateral aspect of the metatarsophalangeal joint of the 1st toe.
Notes: *Ying*-spring point, sedation point; clears Liver Fire, benefits the Heart, calms the Spirit, alleviates depression.

LIV-3 **Location:** on the dorsum of the foot, in the depression distal to the junction of the 1st and 2nd metatarsal bones.
Notes: *Shu*-stream point and *Yuan*-source point; subdues Liver *Yang*, eliminates internal Wind, promotes the smooth flow of *Qi*, calms the Spirit.

LIV-13 **Location:** on the lower border of the free end of the 11th rib.
Notes: *Hui*-meeting point of the *Zang* organs, front-*Mu* point of the Spleen, metabolic point.

LU-1 **Location:** find LU-2 first (on the lower border of the clavicle, 6 cun lateral to the anterior midline), LU-1 is located directly below in the 1st ICS. Caution: pneumothorax!
Notes: as front-*Mu* point of the Lung, combines well with its corresponding back-*Shu* point BL-13; effective if combined with LU-11 (combination of first and last point of the channel).

LU-5 **Location:** on the cubital crease, radial to the tendon of the biceps.
Notes: *He*-sea point and sedation point; bloodletting eliminates *Qi* and Blood (*Xue*) stagnation.

LU-6 **Location:** 7 cun superior to the wrist crease, on a line connecting LU-5 (on the cubital crease, radial to the tendon of the biceps) and LU-9 (on the wrist crease, radial to the radial artery).
Notes: *Xi*-cleft point.

LU-9 **Location:** on the wrist crease, radial to the radial artery.
Notes: *Hui*-meeting point and master point of the blood vessels, *Shu*-stream point, *Yuan*-source point and tonification point.

LU-11 **Location:** on the thumb, next to the radial corner of the nail.
Notes: *Jing*-well point; as terminal point effective if combined with the first point of the meridian.

P-2 **Location:** on the upper arm, 2 cun distal to the anterior axillary fold, between the two head of the biceps.
Notes: local point for the Lungs.

P-6 **Location:** 2 cun proximal to the midpoint of the palmar wrist crease, between the tendons of the flexor carpi radialis and palmaris longus.
Notes: *Luo*-connecting point and opening point of the *Yin Wei Mai*, master point for vomiting; mobilizes the Blood (*Xue*), *Qi* and Phlegm stagnation.

P-7 **Location:** on the palmar aspect of the wrist joint, between the tendons of the flexor carpi radialis and palmaris longus.
Notes: *Yuan*-source point, *Shu*-stream point, sedation point; calms the Heart, Spirit and Stomach.

Ren-12 **Location:** midway between the umbilicus and the xiphoid process.
Notes: front-*Mu* point of the Stomach, *Hui*-meeting point of the hollow organs (*Fu*).

Ren-17 **Location:** on the midline of the sternum, at the level of the 4th ICS, between the nipples (in men).
Notes: front-*Mu* point of the Pericardium, *Hui*-meeting point of the *Qi*, respiration.

S.I.-6 **Location:** in a depression just proximal and radial to the styloid process of the ulna.
Notes: *Xi*-cleft point.

SP-6 **Location:** 3 cun superior to the highest prominence of the medial malleolus, on the posterior border of the tibia.
Notes: as group *Luo*-connecting point (SP, LIV, KID), tonifies *Qi*, Blood (*Xue*) and *Yin*, nourishing point; eliminates Dampness.

SP-10 **Location:** with the knee flexed, 2 cun superior to the upper patellar border, medial to the vastus medialis.
Notes: 'Sea of Blood (*Xue*)'; nourishes and cools the Blood (*Xue*), moves *Qi* and Blood (*Xue*), eliminates Wind and Heat.

SP-12 **Location:** 3.5 cun lateral to the centre of the pubic symphysis, at the same level as Ren-2, in the inguinal groove, lateral to the femoral artery.
Notes: unblocks the meridian, tonifies *Yin*.

ST-19 **Location:** 2 cun lateral to the anterior midline, in the 7th ICS, 6 cun superior to the umbilicus, level with Ren-14.
Notes: local point for the Liver.

ST-34 **Location:** with the knee flexed, in the depression 2 cun superior to the lateral upper border of the patella.
Notes: *Xi*-cleft point.

ST-36 **Location:** 0.5 cun lateral to the anterior crest of the tibia, 1.5 cun inferior to the lower border of the head of the fibula (G.B.-34).
Notes: *He*-sea point, master point of hormones, hypertension; analgesic, nourishing, harmonizes the mind.

ST-37 **Location:** 1 cun lateral to the anterior crest of the tibia, 4 cun inferior to the lower border of the head of the fibula or 3 cun inferior to ST-36.
Notes: lower *He*-sea point of the Large Intestine.

ST-39 **Location:** 1 cun inferior to ST-38.
Notes: lower *He*-sea point of the Small Intestine.

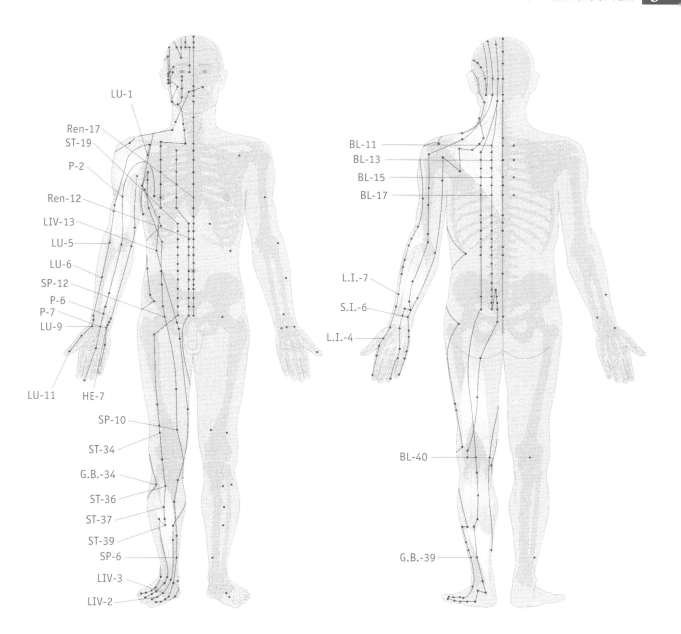

LU-1
Ren-17
ST-19
P-2
Ren-12
LIV-13
LU-5
LU-6
SP-12
P-6
P-7
LU-9
LU-11
HE-7
SP-10
ST-34
G.B.-34
ST-36
ST-37
ST-39
SP-6
LIV-3
LIV-2

BL-11
BL-13
BL-15
BL-17
L.I.-7
S.I.-6
L.I.-4
BL-40
G.B.-39

6.15.10 Treatment of pain during rehabilitation after cerebral insult, treatment based on location of pain (1)

Ideally acupuncture treatments should begin once the internal neurological condition has stabilized (approximately 10 days after the event). The general point prescription should be used here.

During the rehabilitation stage, symptomatic considerations (see table below) as well as the alleviation of joint pain are the main goals of treatment.

TCM

TCM refers to cerebral insult as *Zhong Feng* (struck by Wind) and *Zhong Zang* (*Yin* organs irritated). The impairment of voluntary movement is a symptom of Wind and/or Phlegm; both of these pathological substances 'obstruct' the meridians.
Cause: a disharmony of the Spleen causes the retention of Fluids and the accumulation of Phlegm. Stress as well as emotional and psychological strain result in Heart Fire that is too strong and in turn causes the Liver *Yang* to rise (for example triggered by anger) and internal Wind will develop. The latter stirs up the Phlegm, and this process will block the sensory orifices. Heart Fire, rising Liver Yang and Liver Wind disturb the Spirit (*Shen*).

The treatment goal is to pacify Liver Wind, cool Heart Fire, calm the Heart, eliminate the Phlegm and activate the sensory orifices.

Basic point combination

L.I.-4, L.I.-11, ST-36, SP-6, BL-40 [BL-54 Bi], P-6, G.B.-20, G.B.-21, LIV-2, Du-14 [Du-13 Bi], Du-20.
Needle with even method; 8–12 needles per treatment.

Individual point combination

Hemiparetic pain is mainly caused by lack of mobilization. Besides selecting points reflecting the accompanying signs and symptoms (see below), points focusing on the affected joints should be added.
Pain of the shoulder joint: L.I.-14, L.I.-15, T.B.-14, S.I.-9.
Elbow joint: L.I.-11, L.I.-10, HE-3, P-3.
Wrist/hand: interdigital points: S.I.-3, S.I.-5, T.B.-4, L.I.-5.

Acupuncture points

BL-40 **Location:** in the centre of the popliteal crease, between the tendons of the semitendinosus and the biceps femoris.
Notes: *He*-sea point, command point of the back; eliminates Blood (*Xue*) stagnation.

Du-14 **Location:** below the spinous process of C7.
Notes: meeting point of all *Yang* meridians.

Du-20 **Location:** on a line connecting the apices of the ears.
Notes: universal meeting point; promotes brain function, calms the Spirit, pacifies the Liver, disperses Wind.

G.B.-20 **Location:** posterior to the mastoid, between the trapezius and sternocleidomastoid on the lower border of the occiput.
Notes: main point for Wind in the head.

G.B.-21 **Location:** on the highest point of the shoulder, midway between the acromion and the spinous process of C7.
Notes: eliminates Wind-Heat, unblocks the collaterals, relaxes the tendons.

HE-3 **Location:** with the elbow fully flexed, between the medial end of the cubital crease and the medial epicondyle.
Notes: *He*-sea point and master point for depression; eliminates excess and deficiency Fire of the Heart, moves stagnation in the Heart meridian.

L.I.-4 **Location:** on the dorsum of the hand, at the highest point of the muscle bulge between the 1st and 2nd metacarpal bones.
Notes: *Yuan*-source point, metabolic point; combined with L.I.-11 eliminates Wind and Blood (*Xue*)-Heat, Blood (*Xue*) stagnation, Fire toxins, Damp-Heat and Blood (*Xue*) deficiency.

L.I.-5 **Location:** on the radial aspect of the wrist crease, in a depression between the tendons of the extensor pollicis brevis and extensor carpi radialis longus. Tip: hold the patient's wrist between 2 fingers and ask them to flex the wrist. This is the best way to locate the wrist crease. S.I.-5 is on its ulnar aspect, L.I.-5 on its radial aspect.
Notes: *Jing*-river point, Fire point; eliminates Wind-Heat, Damp-Heat and Blood-Heat locally and from the eyes, the gingiva and the throat.

L.I.-10 **Location:** on the radial aspect of the forearm, 3 cun distal to L.I.-11, on the belly of the extensor muscles.
Notes: for disorders along the pathway of the meridian, eliminates swellings, mobilizes stagnation in the Stomach and intestines.

L.I.-11 **Location:** with the arm fully flexed, at the radial end of the cubital crease.
Notes: *He*-sea point and tonification point; eliminates Damp-Heat and Wind, benefits the tendons and joints.

L.I.-14 **Location:** on the lateral aspect of the upper arm, slightly superior and anterior to the insertion of the deltoid.
Notes: local point.

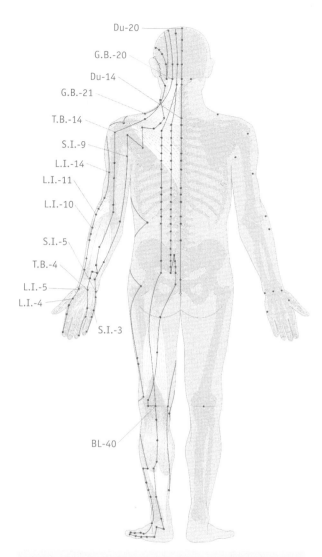

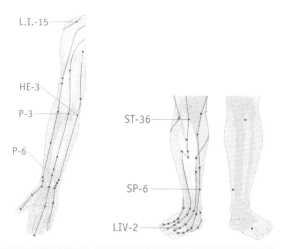

P-6 **Location:** 2 cun proximal to the midpoint of the palmar wrist crease, between the tendons of the flexor carpi radialis and palmaris longus.
Notes: *Luo*-connecting point and opening point of the *Yin Wei Mai*; mobilizes the Blood (*Xue*), *Qi* and Phlegm stagnation.

S.I.-3 **Location:** when a fist is made, on the dorsum of the hand, in the depression at the end of the most distal palmar crease.
Notes: *Shu*-stream point, tonification point and opening point of the *Du Mai*; eliminates external and internal Wind and Dampness, supports the CNS and the tendons.

S.I.-5 **Location:** on the ulnar aspect of the wrist crease, distal to the styloid process of the ulna and proximal to the triquetrum.
Notes: local point.

S.I.-9 **Location:** with the arm adducted 1 cun superior to the end of the posterior axillary fold.
Notes: local point.

SP-6 **Location:** 3 cun superior to the highest prominence of the medial malleolus, on the posterior border of the tibia.
Notes: as group *Luo*-connecting point (SP, LIV, KID), tonifies *Qi*, Blood (*Xue*) and Yin, nourishing point; eliminates Dampness.

ST-36 **Location:** 0.5 cun lateral to the anterior crest of the tibia, 1.5 cun inferior to the lower border of the head of the fibula (G.B.-34).
Notes: *He*-sea point, master point of hormones, hypertension; tonifies the Spleen, the Stomach, the *Qi*, Blood (*Xue*) and the musculature.

T.B.-4 **Location:** on the wrist crease, in the depression lateral to the tendon of the extensor digitorum longus.
Notes: *Yuan*-source point, master point for vasomotor headaches.

T.B.-14 **Location:** with the arm abducted, in the depression posterior and inferior to the acromion, between the medial and posterior fibres of the deltoid (L.I.-15 lies anterior to T.B.-14).
Notes: local point.

L.I.-15 **Location:** with the arm abducted, in the anterior of the two depressions inferior to the acromioclavicular joint, between the anterior and medial third of the deltoid (T.B.-14 is located in the posterior depression).
Notes: master point for paresis of the upper extremity.

LIV-2 **Location:** on the web between the 1st and 2nd toes, at the lateral aspect of the metatarsophalangeal joint of the 1st toe.
Notes: *Ying*-spring point, sedation point; subdues Liver Fire and Liver Wind.

P-3 **Location:** with the elbow flexed, on the cubital crease, ulnar to the tendon of the biceps (LU-5 is located radial to the tendon).
Notes: *He*-sea point; locally spasmolytic effect, opens the sensory orifices, calms the Spirit; for tremors of the arm and hand.

6.15.10 *Treatment of pain during rehabilitation after cerebral insult, treatment based on location of pain (2)*

Hip joint: G.B.-30, G.B.-31, G.B.-34.
Knee joint: ST-34, SP-9, SP-10, G.B.-34, BL-40 [BL-54 Bi].
Ankle, toes: ST-41, BL-60, KID-3, interdigital points.
Pain following an insult in the thalamic area: points with a primarily psychological effect should be used. Of particular importance are adjunctive therapies (drugs, psychotherapy). Experience has shown that this type of insult responds only moderately well to acupuncture.

Acupuncture points

BL-40 **Location:** in the centre of the popliteal crease, between the tendons of the semitendinosus and the biceps femoris.
Notes: *He*-sea point, command point of the back; eliminates Blood (*Xue*) stagnation.

BL-60 **Location:** in the depression between the Achilles tendon and the lateral malleolus.
Notes: *Jing*-river point, master point for any pain along the meridian pathway.

G.B.-30 **Location:** on a line connecting the greater trochanter and the sacral hiatus, at the junction of the lateral and medial third.

Notes: meeting point with the Bladder meridian, master point for sciatica and paresis of the legs.

G.B-31 **Location:** on the lateral aspect of the thigh; with the arms hanging down, the middle finger will indicate this point.
Notes: Wind point.

G.B.-34 **Location:** with the knee flexed, in the depression anterior and inferior to the head of the fibula.
Notes: *He*-sea point, *Hui*-meeting point of the tendons, master point of the musculature.

KID-3 **Location:** between the highest prominence of the medial malleolus and the Achilles tendon.
Notes: *Shu*-stream point and *Yuan*-source point; tonifies the Kidneys, supports Essence (*Jing*), Kidney *Yang* and Kidney *Yin*.

SP-9 **Location:** with the knee flexed, in the depression inferior to the medial condyle of the tibia, at the same level as G.B.-34.
Notes: *He*-sea point; regulates the Fluids and Dampness, tonifies Spleen *Qi*.

SP-10 **Location:** with the knee flexed, 2 cun superior to the upper patellar border, medial to the vastus medialis.
Notes: 'Sea of Blood (*Xue*)'; nourishes and cools the Blood (*Xue*), moves *Qi* and Blood (*Xue*), thus eliminating Wind and Heat.

ST-34 **Location:** with the knee flexed, in the depression 2 cun superior to the lateral upper border of the patella.
Notes: *Xi*-cleft point; local point.

ST-41 **Location:** at the midpoint of the anterior aspect of the ankle, between the tendons of the extensor hallucis longus and extensor digitorum longus.
Notes: *Jing*-river point and tonification point; local point.

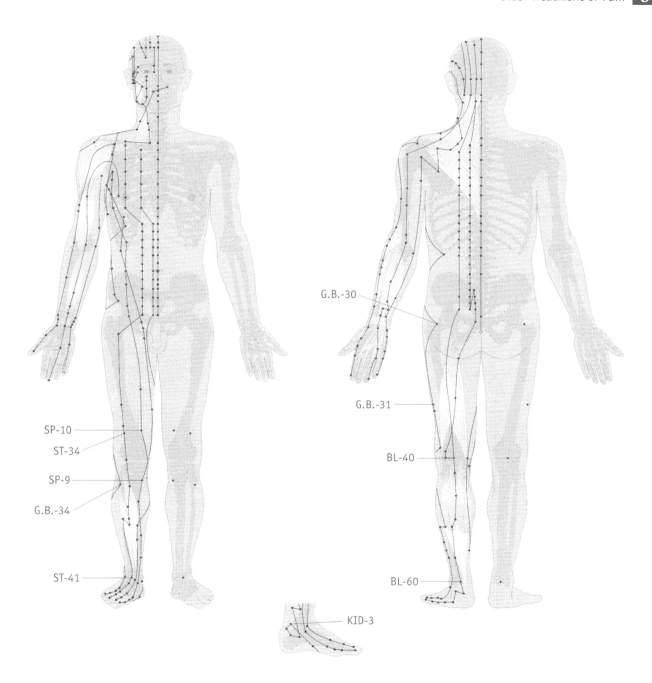

SP-10
ST-34
SP-9
G.B.-34
ST-41

G.B.-30
G.B.-31
BL-40
BL-60

KID-3

6.15.10 *Treatment of pain during rehabilitation after cerebral insult, additional points based on accompanying circumstances (3)*

Individual point combination

Wind-Heat symptoms, superficial deficiency symptoms: G.B.-20, Du-16.
Wind-Cold symptoms, superficial excess symptoms: BL-13, S.I.-3.
General Heat symptoms: L.I.-4, L.I.-11.
General symptoms of Blood (*Xue*) stasis: SP-10.
Dampness, Cold: SP-6, SP-9.
Symptoms of Phlegm: P-6, G.B.-34, BL-20, ST-36, ST-40.

Acupuncture points

BL-13 **Location:** 1.5 cun lateral to the spinous process of T3.
Notes: back-*Shu* point of the Lungs; regulates nutritive and defensive *Qi* (*Ying Qi, Wei Qi*).
BL-20 **Location:** 1.5 cun lateral to the spinous process of T12.
Notes: back-*Shu* point of the Spleen, which is responsible for the transformation of Phlegm.
Du-16 **Location:** 1 cun within the posterior hairline, in the depression inferior to the external occipital protuberance.
Notes: for disorders affecting the head and sensory organs; eliminates pathogenic Wind from the head.
G.B.-20 **Location:** posterior to the mastoid, between the trapezius and sternocleidomastoid muscles, on the lower border of the occiput.
Notes: main point for Wind in the head.
G.B.-34 **Location:** with the knee flexed, in the depression anterior and inferior to the head of the fibula.
Notes: *He*-sea point of the Gall Bladder, *Hui*-meeting point of the tendons, master point of the musculature.
L.I.-4 **Location:** on the dorsum of the hand, at the highest point of the muscle bulge between the 1st and 2nd metacarpal bones.
Notes: *Yuan*-source point, metabolic point; combined with L.I.-11 eliminates Wind-Heat, Blood (*Xue*) Heat, Blood (*Xue*) stagnation, Fire toxins, Damp-Heat and Blood (*Xue*) deficiency.

L.I.-11 **Location:** with the arm fully flexed, at the radial end of the cubital crease.
Notes: *He*-sea point and tonification point; eliminates Damp-Heat and Wind, benefits the tendons and joints.
P-6 **Location:** 2 cun proximal to the midpoint of the palmar wrist crease, between the tendons of the flexor carpi radialis and palmaris longus.
Notes: *Luo*-connecting point and opening point of the *Yin Wei Mai*; mobilizes the Blood (*Xue*), *Qi* and Phlegm stagnation.
S.I.-3 **Location:** when a fist is made, on the dorsum of the hand, in the depression at the end of the most distal palmar crease.
Notes: tonification point and opening point of the *Du Mai*; dispels external and internal Wind from the *Du Mai*, benefits the CNS and the tendons, eliminates Dampness.
SP-6 **Location:** 3 cun superior to the highest prominence of the medial malleolus, on the posterior border of the tibia.
Notes: as group *Luo*-connecting point (SP, LIV, KID), tonifies *Qi*, Blood (*Xue*) and *Yin*, nourishing point; eliminates Dampness.
SP-9 **Location:** with the knee flexed, in the depression inferior to the medial condyle of the tibia, at the same level as G.B.-34.
Notes: *He*-sea point; regulates the Fluids and Dampness, tonifies Spleen *Qi*.
SP-10 **Location:** with the knee flexed, 2 cun superior to the upper patellar border, medial to the vastus medialis.
Notes: 'Sea of Blood (*Xue*)'; nourishes and cools the Blood (*Xue*), moves *Qi* and Blood (*Xue*), thus eliminating Wind and Heat.
ST-36 **Location:** 0.5 cun lateral to the anterior crest of the tibia, 1.5 cun inferior to the lower border of the head of the fibula (G.B.-34).
Notes: *He*-sea point, master point of hormones, hypertension; tonifies the Spleen, the Stomach, the *Qi*, Blood (*Xue*) and the musculature.
ST-40 **Location:** at the midpoint of the distance between the medial malleolus and the knee joint space, 2 cun lateral to the anterior crest of the tibia.
Notes: *Luo*-connecting point (connects with SP-3). Phlegm is the product of impaired transformation due to weakness of the Spleen; also known as the 'Bisolvon' of acupuncture – demulcent.

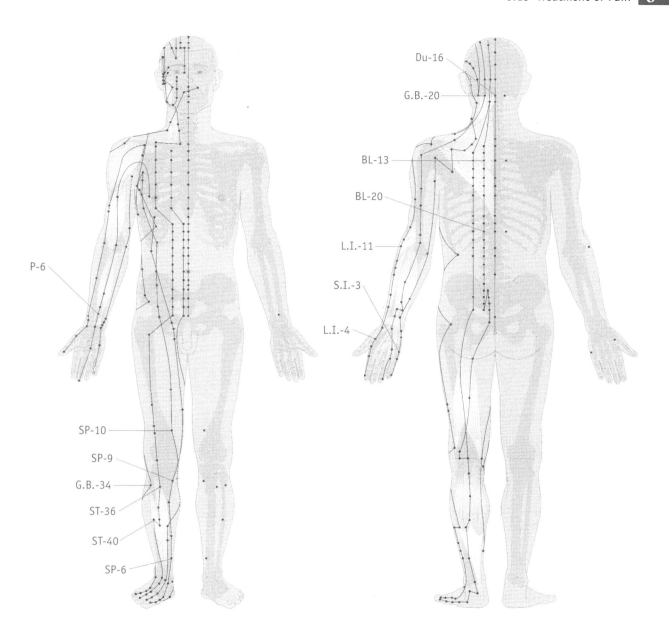

P-6

SP-10

SP-9

G.B.-34

ST-36

ST-40

SP-6

Du-16

G.B.-20

BL-13

BL-20

L.I.-11

S.I.-3

L.I.-4

6.15.10 *Treatment of pain during rehabilitation after cerebral insult, additional points based on accompanying circumstances (4)*

Individual point combination

Symptoms of *Qi* and Blood (*Xue*) deficiency

Ren-6, ST-36, SP-6, BL-18, BL-20.

Yang deficiency (*Yang Xu*)

This includes *Yang* deficiency of the Heart, Spleen, Liver and Kidneys. Kidney *Yang* deficiency tends to be dominant: aversion to cold, cold extremities, erectile dysfunction, infertility, copious urine, knee and lower back pain, vertigo, tinnitus, tiredness, lethargy.
Du-4, Ren-4, Ren-6.

Emotionally balancing points

He-7, P-7, P-6 – obtain *De Qi* sensation and retain needles for about 30 minutes or warm with moxa for 5 minutes (recommendation from Professor Chen Xinong); or, after a recommendation by Professor Lu Souyan: BL-15 (moxibustion with 3 rice grain-sized moxa threads), BL-23 (tonify, then remove the needle immediately), HE-7 (tonify, then remove the needle immediately) and SP-6 (obtain *De Qi* sensation, stimulate with reducing method and immediately remove the needle).
Kidney *Yin* deficiency: KID-3, BL-23.
Kidney *Yin* and *Yang* deficiency (e.g. during menopause): Ren-4, Ren-6, BL-31-34, BL-23, BL-26, BL-53 [BL-48 Bi].
Liver *Qi* stagnation (depression): LIV-3, LIV-13, LIV-14, G.B.-25, BL-17, BL-18, BL-19.
Stomach and Spleen deficiency (digestive disorder): Ren-12, ST-36, BL-20, BL-21, BL-22.
General deficiency: Ren-12 (ST), ST-25 (L.I.),BL-21, BL-20, ST-36, P-6.
General excess: of the Stomach: Ren-12, Ren-21, ST-36; of the Large Intestine: BL-25, ST-25, ST-37, T.B.-6.

Acupuncture points

BL-15 **Location:** 1.5 cun lateral to the spinous process of T5.
Notes: back-*Shu* point of the Heart; combined with HE-7 tonifies Heart *Qi* and *Yin*.

BL-17 **Location:** 1.5 cun lateral to the spinous process of T7, approximately level with the inferior angle of the scapula.
Notes: *Hui*-meeting point of the Blood, tonifies the Blood, moves Blood (*Xue*) stagnation; as back-*Shu* point of the diaphragm eliminates stagnation from the diaphragm.

BL-18 **Location:** 2 cun lateral to the spinous process of T9.
Notes: back-*Shu* point of the Liver; supports the Liver and Gall Bladder, eliminates Damp-Heat and Wind, moves *Qi* stagnation.

BL-19 **Location:** 1.5 cun lateral to the spinous process of T10.
Notes: back-*Shu* point of the Gall Bladder; pacifies the Stomach, relaxes the diaphragm.

BL-20 **Location:** 1.5 cun lateral to the spinous process of T11.
Notes: back-*Shu* point of the Spleen – Phlegm!

BL-21 **Location:** 1.5 cun lateral to the spinous process of T12.
Notes: back-*Shu* point and master point of the Stomach.

BL-22 **Location:** 1.5 cun lateral to the spinous process of L1.
Notes: back-*Shu* point of the Triple Burner; eliminates Dampness, opens the water passages.

BL-23 **Location:** 1.5 cun lateral to L2, level with Du-4.
Notes: back-*Shu* point of the Kidneys; tonifies the *Qi*, *Yang*, *Yin* and Essence (*Jing*) of the Kidneys.

BL-25 **Location:** 1.5 cun lateral to the lower border of the spinous process of L4.
Notes: back-*Shu* point of the Large Intestine.

BL-26 **Location:** 1.5 cun lateral to the lower border of the spinous process of L5.
Notes: back-*Shu* point of Ren-4; strengthens the lower back, eliminates obstruction from the meridian.

BL-31 **Location:** over the 1st sacral foramen.
Notes: master point for menopause.

BL-32 **Location:** over the 2nd sacral foramen.
Notes: similar to BL-31.

BL-33 **Location:** over the 3rd sacral foramen.
Notes: similar to BL-31.

BL-34 **Location:** over the 4th sacral foramen.
Notes: similar to BL-31.

BL-53 **Location:** 3 cun lateral to the posterior midline, at the level of the 2nd sacral foramen, level with BL-28.
Notes: has an effect on the urogenital region; promotes Bladder function.

continued on p. 378

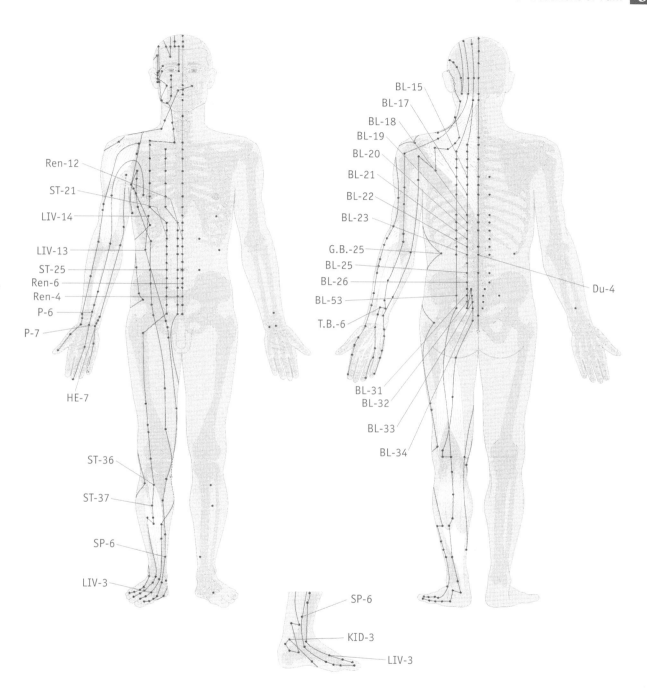

Ren-12
ST-21
LIV-14
LIV-13
ST-25
Ren-6
Ren-4
P-6
P-7
HE-7
ST-36
ST-37
SP-6
LIV-3

BL-15
BL-17
BL-18
BL-19
BL-20
BL-21
BL-22
BL-23
G.B.-25
BL-25
BL-26
BL-53
T.B.-6
Du-4

BL-31
BL-32
BL-33
BL-34

SP-6
KID-3
LIV-3

Du-4 **Location:** below the spinous process of L2.
Notes: complements the Kidney *Yin*, firms the Essence (*Jing*), strengthens the Kidney *Yang*, the lower back and the knees.

G.B.-25 **Location:** on the lower border of the free end of the 12th rib.
Notes: resolves local *Qi* stagnation; combined with LIV-13 and G.B.-24 for intercostal neuralgia and hypochondriacal pain.

HE-7 **Location:** on the ulnar aspect of the wrist crease, on the radial aspect of the pisiform bone.
Notes: *Shu*-stream point and *Yuan*-source point, sedation point; tonifies the Heart Blood, cools Heat, Fire and *Yin*, calms the Spirit and the Heart, opens the orifices of the Heart, resolves Heart *Qi* stagnation and stagnant *Qi* in the chest, improves memory and sleep.

KID-3 **Location:** between the highest prominence of the medial malleolus and the Achilles tendon.
Notes: *Shu*-stream point and *Yuan*-source point; tonifies the Kidneys, benefits the Essence (*Jing*) as well as Kidney *Yin* and *Yang*.

LIV-3 **Location:** on the dorsum of the foot, in the depression distal to the junction of the 1st and 2nd metatarsal bones.
Notes: *Shu*-stream point and *Yuan*-source point; subdues Liver *Yang*, eliminates internal Wind, promotes the smooth flow of *Qi*, calms the Spirit.

LIV-13 **Location:** on the lower border of the free end of the 11th rib.
Notes: pacifies the Liver, promotes the smooth flow of Liver *Qi*, benefits the Stomach and Spleen.

LIV-14 **Location:** on the midclavicular line, in the 6th ICS, directly below the nipple.
Notes: front-*Mu* point of the Liver; promotes the smooth flow of Liver *Qi*, harmonizes the Liver and Stomach.

P-6 **Location:** 2 cun proximal to the midpoint of the palmar wrist crease, between the tendons of the flexor carpi radialis and palmaris longus.
Notes: *Luo*-connecting point and opening point of the *Yin Wei Mai*; mobilizes the Blood (*Xue*), *Qi* and Phlegm stagnation.

P-7 **Location:** on the palmar aspect of the wrist joint, between the tendons of the flexor carpi radialis and palmaris longus.

Notes: *Yuan*-source point, *Shu*-stream point, sedation point; calms the Heart and the Spirit; local point for contractures.

Ren-4 **Location:** 2 cun superior to the upper border of the pubic symphysis.
Notes: internal meeting point of the 3 lower *Yin* meridians (SP, LIV, KID), front-*Mu* point of the Small Intestine; nourishing – tonifies Essence (*Jing*), *Qi*, *Yang*, Blood (*Xue*) and *Yin*.

Ren-6 **Location:** 1.5 cun inferior to the umbilicus.
Notes: 'Sea of *Qi*' – tonifies the Kidneys, original *Qi* and Yang *Qi*; nourishing and stabilizing point.

Ren-12 **Location:** midway between the umbilicus and the xiphoid process.
Notes: front-*Mu* point of the Stomach; combined with ST-36 also tonifies the Spleen.

SP-6 **Location:** 3 cun superior to the highest prominence of the medial malleolus, on the posterior border of the tibia.
Notes: as group *Luo*-connecting point (SP, LIV, KID), tonifies *Qi*, Blood (*Xue*) and *Yin*; nourishing point; eliminates Dampness.

ST-21 **Location:** 2 cun lateral to the midline, at the midpoint of the distance between the umbilicus and the xiphoid process level, with Ren-12.
Notes: for excess patterns! Regulates the Stomach, subdues rebellious *Qi*.

ST-25 **Location:** 2 cun lateral to the centre of the umbilicus (Ren-8).
Notes: front-*Mu* point of the Large Intestine.

ST-36 **Location:** 0.5 cun lateral to the anterior crest of the tibia, 1.5 cun inferior to the lower border of the head of the fibula (G.B.-34).
Notes: *He*-sea point, master point of hormones, hypertension; tonifies *Qi* and Blood (*Xue*).

ST-37 **Location:** 1 cun lateral to the anterior crest of the tibia, 4 cun inferior to the lower border of the head of the fibula or 3 cun inferior to ST-36.
Notes: lower *He*-sea point of the Large Intestine; combine with ST-25 for disorders of the Large Intestine.

T.B.-6 **Location:** 3 cun proximal to the midpoint of the dorsal wrist crease.
Notes: *Jing*-river point; regulates the thoracic *Qi*, mobilizes *Qi* stagnation in the Three Burners.

378

6.16 Addiction

A. Meng

Acupuncture generally achieves good results in the treatment of addiction.

TCM

In TCM, addiction does not exist as an indication, with the exception of sleep addiction due to Spleen, Heart and Kidney deficiency. Therefore, nicotine and alcohol addiction, as well as obesity, are relatively new indications.

Only a few treatment protocols and methods that have worked well in the author's experience are mentioned within the framework of this book.

Acupuncture treatment for withdrawal from hard drugs, as well as abuse of prescription drugs (e.g. tranquillizers), should take place only in specialized institutions.

6.16.1 Addiction to nicotine (1)

The success rate – defined as abstaining from cigarettes for more than 3 months – is approximately 70%. Most patients report that after the treatment there is a decreased desire for cigarettes and that the taste of cigarettes is perceived as unpleasant. The treatment should include preventive measures against possible weight gain, nervousness, restlessness and the habitual behaviour patterns. An open discussion with the patient, behavioural therapy and dietary recommendations can all help to reduce the risk of relapse.

The patient has to stop smoking completely after the 1st treatment. In general 3–6 treatments are sufficient. Besides the standard points described below, symptomatic points should be added to the point prescription from the 2nd treatment onwards. Ear acupuncture or intradermal needles are also beneficial.

Basic point combination

L.I.-4, L.I.-20, ST-36, LIV-3, Du-20.
Ear acupuncture: 101 Lungs, 100 Heart, 95 Kidneys, 97 Liver, 55 *Shen Men*.
Method: medium–strong stimulation, needle retention 20 minutes. The ear points can also be treated with intradermal needles, magnets or press balls for approximately 3 days. The patient is instructed to press these several times daily for 1–2 minutes with medium–strong pressure.

Individual point combination

Anti-nicotine point 1

Midway between LU7 and L.I.-5 **M**, this area can be very sensitive in smokers.
Method: bilateral needling with strong stimulation, needle retention 15 minutes, once daily for 4 days.

Anti-nicotine point 2

5 mm lateral to the upper end of the nasolabial groove.
Method: bilateral needling with strong stimulation, needle retention 15 minutes; needle twice during the 1st week and once during the 2nd week. In addition:

Inner restlessness

HE-7, G.B.-20.

Hunger

Ren-12, P-6.

Irritating cough

Ren-22 [Ren-21 Bi], Ren-17, Ex-HN-3 (*Yin Tang*).
Electrostimulation: L.I.-4 or ST-36.
Method: with continuous impulse between 2 and 100 Hz, medium setting, 15 minutes.
Laser acupuncture: LU-7, L.I.-5, L.I.-4.
Method: 1–2 points per treatment, 5 minutes per point.

Acupuncture points

Du-20 **Location:** on a line connecting the apices of the ears.
  Notes: universal meeting point; calms the *Shen*, pacifies the Liver, disperses Wind.
Ex-HN-3 **Location:** at the midpoint between the eyebrows.
  Notes: relaxing.
G.B.-20 **Location:** posterior to the mastoid, between the trapezius and sternocleidomastoid muscles, on the lower border of the occiput.
  Notes: eliminates Wind and Heat.
HE-7 **Location:** on the ulnar aspect of the wrist crease, on the radial aspect of the pisiform bone.
  Notes: *Shu*-stream point, *Yuan*-source point, sedation point; tonifies the Heart Blood, cools Heat, Fire and *Yin*, opens the Heart orifices, calming.
L.I.-4 **Location:** on the dorsum of the hand, at the highest point of the muscle bulge between the 1st and 2nd metacarpal bones.
  Notes: *Yuan*-source point; uplifting, has an effect on the whole respiratory tract, strengthens the dispersing function of the Lungs, eliminates Wind and Heat. Caution during pregnancy – moves *Qi*!
L.I.-5 **Location:** on the radial aspect of the wrist crease, in a depression between the tendons of the extensor pollicis brevis and extensor carpi radialis longus. Tip: hold the patient's wrist between 2 fingers and ask them to flex the wrist. This is the best way for locating the wrist crease. S.I.-5 is on its ulnar aspect, L.I.-5 on its radial aspect.
  Notes: *Jing*-river point, Fire point, eliminates Wind, Damp-Heat and Blood-Heat, locally and from the eyes, gingiva and throat.
L.I.-20 **Location:** in the nasolabial groove, level with the midpoint of the lateral border of the ala nasi.
  Notes: specific point for deficiency, stagnation and Heat patterns affecting the *Yang Ming* (L.I., ST).
LIV-3 **Location:** on the dorsum of the foot, in the depression distal to the junction of the 1st and 2nd metatarsal bones.
  Notes: *Shu*-stream point and *Yuan*-source point; subdues Liver *Yang*, eliminates internal Wind, promotes the smooth flow of *Qi*, calms the Spirit.
LU-7 **Location:** 1.5 cun proximal to the wrist crease, superior to the radial artery.
  Notes: *Luo*-connecting point, opening point of the *Ren Mai*, master point for stagnation; descends Lung *Qi* (for cough).

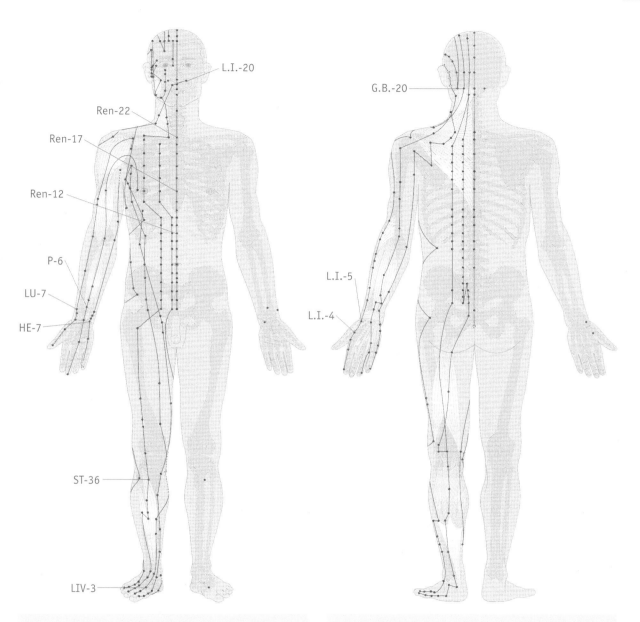

P-6 **Location:** 2 cun proximal to the midpoint of the palmar wrist crease, between the tendons of the flexor carpi radialis and palmaris longus.
Notes: *Luo*-connecting point and opening point of the *Yin Wei Mai*; has an effect on the Heart, calms the Spirit; mobilizes Blood (*Xue*), *Qi* and Phlegm stagnation.

Ren-12 **Location:** midway between the umbilicus and the xiphoid process.
Notes: front-*Mu* point of the Stomach, *Hui*-meeting point of the hollow organs (*Fu*); tonifies the Stomach and Spleen, regulates Stomach *Qi*.

Ren-17 **Location:** on the midline of the sternum, at the level of the 4th ICS, between the nipples (in men).
Notes: front-*Mu* point of the Pericardium, *Hui*-meeting point of the *Qi* and respiratory system; opens the chest.

Ren-22 **Location:** in the centre of the jugulum.
Notes: descends Lung *Qi*; for cough and Phlegm.

ST-36 **Location:** 0.5 cun lateral to the anterior crest of the tibia, 1.5 cun inferior to the lower border of the head of the fibula (G.B.-34).
Notes: *He*-sea point, master point of hormones and for hypertension; calming.

6.16.1 Addiction to nicotine (2)

Individual point combination

With bronchitis, emphysema, coronary heart disease, neurasthenia

LU-1, Ren-15, P-6; may add BL-13, BL-15, SP-6, LU-7.

With hypertension (Kidney and Liver *Yin* deficiency type)

G.B.-25, LIV-2, KID-3; may add BL-23, KID-4, Du-20.

With chronic gastritis or stomach ulcer

ST-36, P-6, LIV-13, Ren-12; may add ST-44, SP-4, BL-21, BL-20.

Acupuncture points

BL-13 **Location:** 1.5 cun lateral to the spinous process of T3.
Notes: back-*Shu* point of the Lungs.

BL-15 **Location:** 1.5 cun lateral to the spinous process of T5.
Notes: back-*Shu* point of the Heart.

BL-20 **Location:** 1.5 cun lateral to the spinous process of T11.
Notes: back-*Shu* point of the Spleen.

BL-21 **Location:** 1.5 cun lateral to the spinous process of T12.
Notes: back-*Shu* point and master point of the Stomach.

BL-23 **Location:** 1.5 cun lateral to L2, level with Du-4.
Notes: back-*Shu* point of the Kidneys; tonifies the *Qi*, *Yang*, *Yin* and Essence (*Jing*) of the Kidneys.

Du-20 **Location:** on a line connecting the apices of the ears.
Notes: universal meeting point; calms the *Shen*, pacifies the Liver, disperses Wind.

G.B.-25 **Location:** on the lower border of the free end of the 12th rib.
Notes: mobilizes *Qi* stagnation.

KID-3 **Location:** between the highest prominence of the medial malleolus and the Achilles tendon.
Notes: *Shu*-stream point and *Yuan*-source point; tonifies the Kidneys, benefits the Essence (*Jing*) as well as Kidney *Yang* and *Yin*, stabilizes the emotions.

KID-4 **Location:** on the upper border of the calcaneus, a 1/2 finger-width posterior to the medial malleolus.
Notes: *Luo*-connecting point; stabilizes the emotions.

LIV-2 **Location:** on the web between the 1st and 2nd toes, at the lateral aspect of the metatarsophalangeal joint of the 1st toe.
Notes: *Ying*-spring point, sedation point; subdues Liver Fire and Liver Wind.

LIV-13 **Location:** on the lower border of the free end of the 11th rib.
Notes: metabolic point, front-*Mu* point of the Spleen, *Hui*-meeting point of the *Zang* organs; harmonizes the Liver/Spleen, for digestive disorders due to emotions.

LU-1 **Location:** find LU-2 first (on the lower border of the clavicle, 6 cun lateral to the anterior midline); LU-1 is located directly below in the 1st ICS. Caution: pneumothorax!
Notes: front-*Mu* point of the Lungs; regulates and descends Lung *Qi*; for cough and fullness of the chest.

LU-7 **Location:** 1.5 cun proximal to the wrist crease, superior to the radial artery.
Notes: *Luo*-connecting point, opening point of the *Ren Mai*, master point for stagnation; descends Lung *Qi* (for cough).

P-6 **Location:** 2 cun proximal to the midpoint of the palmar wrist crease, between the tendons of the flexor carpi radialis and palmaris longus.
Notes: *Luo*-connecting point and opening point of the *Yin Wei Mai*; mobilizes the Blood (*Xue*), *Qi* and Phlegm stagnation.

Ren-12 **Location:** midway between the umbilicus and the xiphoid process.
Notes: front-*Mu* point of the Stomach, *Hui*-meeting point of the hollow organs (*Fu*); tonifies Stomach and Spleen, regulates Stomach *Qi*.

Ren-15 **Location:** 1 cun inferior to the xiphoid process.
Notes: calms the Spirit, benefits the original *Qi*.

SP-4 **Location:** in the depression at the junction of the base and shaft of the 1st metatarsal bone, at the junction of the red and white skin.
Notes: *Luo*-connecting point, opening point of the *Chong Mai*; tonifies the Stomach and Spleen, and therefore indirectly promotes the transformation of Phlegm.

SP-6 **Location:** 3 cun superior to the highest prominence of the medial malleolus, on the posterior border of the tibia.
Notes: as group *Luo*-connecting point (SP, LIV, KID), tonifies *Qi*, Blood (*Xue*) and *Yin*; nourishing point; eliminates Dampness.

ST-36 **Location:** 0.5 cun lateral to the anterior crest of the tibia, 1.5 cun inferior to the lower border of the head of the fibula (G.B.-34).
Notes: *He*-sea point, master point of hormones and for hypertension; calming.

ST-44 **Location:** on the interdigital fold between the 2nd and 3rd toes, near the metatarsophalangeal joint of the 2nd toe.
Notes: *Ying*-spring point; eliminates Heat from the Stomach and *Yang Ming*.

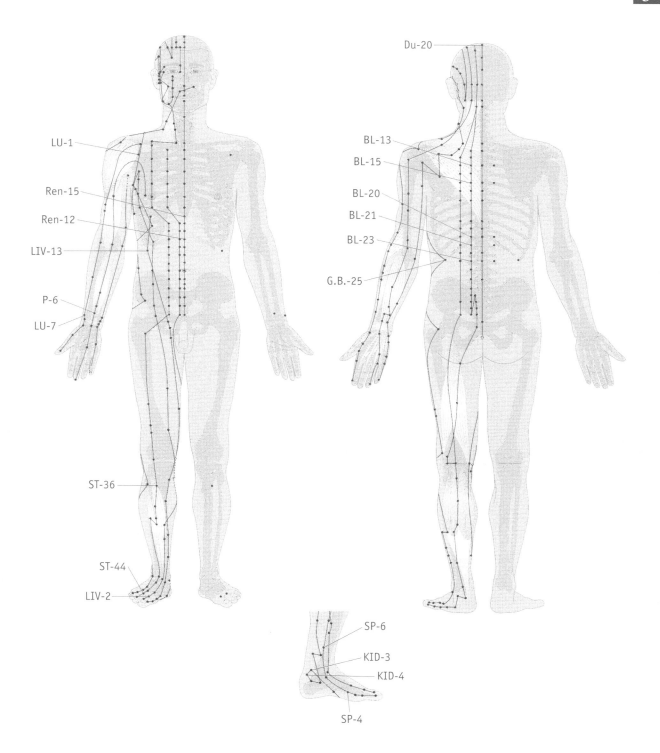

LU-1

Ren-15

Ren-12

LIV-13

P-6

LU-7

ST-36

ST-44

LIV-2

Du-20

BL-13

BL-15

BL-20

BL-21

BL-23

G.B.-25

SP-6

KID-3

KID-4

SP-4

6.16.2 Addiction to alcohol

In less severe cases, when patients themselves are keen to stop alcohol consumption, treatments can be based on the various psychovegetative symptoms.

Ear acupuncture: 55 *Shen Men*, 100 Heart, 86 Stomach, 22 endocrine system, 43 subcortex, 15 pharynx and larynx.

Method: Choose 3–4 points per treatment and needle bilaterally with medium–strong stimulation for 30–60 seconds; retain needles for 20 minutes. Alternatively, intradermal needles can be applied to sensitive ear points and retained for approximately 3 days. These should be stimulated for 5 minutes before each meal for 1–2 minutes.

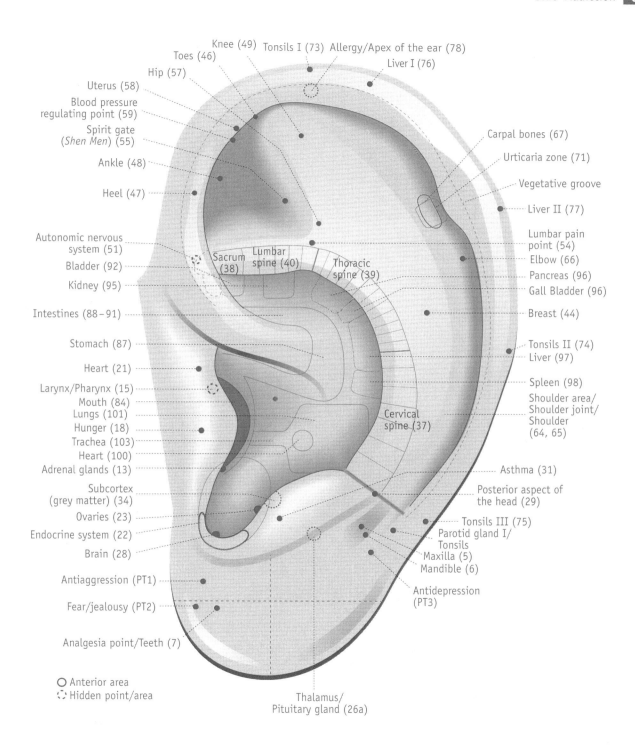

Knee (49) Tonsils I (73) Allergy/Apex of the ear (78)

Toes (46) Liver I (76)

Hip (57)

Uterus (58)

Blood pressure
regulating point (59)

Spirit gate
(*Shen Men*) (55)

Ankle (48)

Heel (47)

Carpal bones (67)

Urticaria zone (71)

Vegetative groove

Liver II (77)

Lumbar pain
point (54)

Elbow (66)

Pancreas (96)

Gall Bladder (96)

Breast (44)

Tonsils II (74)

Liver (97)

Spleen (98)

Shoulder area/
Shoulder joint/
Shoulder
(64, 65)

Asthma (31)

Posterior aspect of
the head (29)

Tonsils III (75)

Parotid gland I/
Tonsils

Maxilla (5)

Mandible (6)

Antidepression
(PT3)

Autonomic nervous
system (51)

Bladder (92)

Kidney (95)

Intestines (88–91)

Stomach (87)

Heart (21)

Larynx/Pharynx (15)

Mouth (84)

Lungs (101)

Hunger (18)

Trachea (103)

Heart (100)

Adrenal glands (13)

Subcortex
(grey matter) (34)

Ovaries (23)

Endocrine system (22)

Brain (28)

Antiaggression (PT1)

Fear/jealousy (PT2)

Analgesia point/Teeth (7)

Sacrum
(38)

Lumbar
spine (40)

Thoracic
spine (39)

Cervical
spine (37)

O Anterior area
⊙ Hidden point/area

Thalamus/
Pituitary gland (26a)

6.16.3 Obesity, adiposity (1)

Acupuncture shows good results with hyperalimentary obesity without any accompanying endocrine disorder. However, strict observation of a sensible dietary regimen is absolutely essential.

Basic point combination

ST-25, ST-36, ST-40, SP-6, BL-20, BL-21, Ren-12.
Method: medium-strength stimulation.
Ear acupuncture: 55 *Shen Men*, 87 stomach, 91 colon, 98 spleen, 84 mouth, 18 hunger point, 22 endocrine system, 96 pancreas/gall bladder.
Method: select 3–5 points per treatment and needle with medium-strength stimulation, retain needles for 30 minutes; or use intradermal needles as described above.

Individual point combination

TCM distinguishes three patterns:
- Heat retention in the Stomach
- Dampness with Spleen deficiency
- Kidney deficiency.

Heat retention in the Stomach

L.I.-11, ST-44, SP-15, T.B.-6.
For symptoms of Dampness (e.g. oedema): SP-9, SP-9.
Symptoms: eating large amounts, constipation, thirst, concentrated urine, foul breath, strong neck, heavy musculature, big stomach, tendency to arterial hypertension; **tongue body:** red; tongue coating: thick, yellow; **pulse:** forceful and rapid.

Acupuncture points

BL-20 **Location:** 1.5 cun lateral to the spinous process of T11.
Notes: back-*Shu* point of the Spleen.

BL-21 **Location:** 1.5 cun lateral to the spinous process of T12.
Notes: back-*Shu* and master point of the Stomach.

L.I.-11 **Location:** with the arm fully flexed at the radial end of the cubital crease.
Notes: *He*-sea point and tonification point; eliminates Damp-Heat.

Ren-12 **Location:** midway between the umbilicus and the xiphoid process.
Notes: front-*Mu* point of the Stomach, *Hui*-meeting point of the hollow organs (*Fu*); tonifies Stomach and Spleen, regulates Stomach *Qi*.

SP-6 **Location:** 3 cun superior to the highest prominence of the medial malleolus, on the posterior border of the tibia.
Notes: as group *Luo*-connecting point (SP, LIV, KID), tonifies *Qi*, Blood (*Xue*) and *Yin*, nourishing point; eliminates Dampness.

SP-9 **Location:** with the knee flexed in the depression inferior to the medial condyle of the tibia, at the same level as G.B.-34.
Notes: *He*-sea point; regulates the Fluids and Dampness, tonifies Spleen *Qi*.

SP-15 **Location:** on the midclavicular line, at the level of the umbilicus (Ren-8).
Notes: meeting point with the *Yin Wei Mai*; moves *Qi*, tonifies Spleen *Qi*, resolves Dampness, promotes Large Intestine functioning.

ST-25 **Location:** 2 cun lateral to the centre of the umbilicus (Ren-8).
Notes: front-*Mu* point of the Large Intestine; regulates bowel movements.

ST-36 **Location:** 0.5 cun lateral to the anterior crest of the tibia, 1.5 cun inferior to the lower border of the head of the fibula (G.B.-34).
Notes: *He*-sea point, master point of hormones and for hypertension; calming.

ST-40 **Location:** at the midpoint of the distance between the medial malleolus and the knee joint space, 2 cun lateral to the anterior crest of the tibia.
Notes: *Luo*-connecting point (connects with the Spleen meridian) – Phlegm!

ST-44 **Location:** on the interdigital fold between the 2nd and 3rd toes, near the metatarsophalangeal joint of the 2nd toe.
Notes: *Ying*-spring point; most important point to drain Stomach Fire – for ravenous appetite, halitosis, constipation.

T.B.-6 **Location:** 3 cun proximal to the midpoint of the dorsal wrist crease.
Notes: *Jing*-river point; regulates the thoracic *Qi*, mobilizes *Qi* stagnation in the Three Burners, thus also in the intestinal tract.

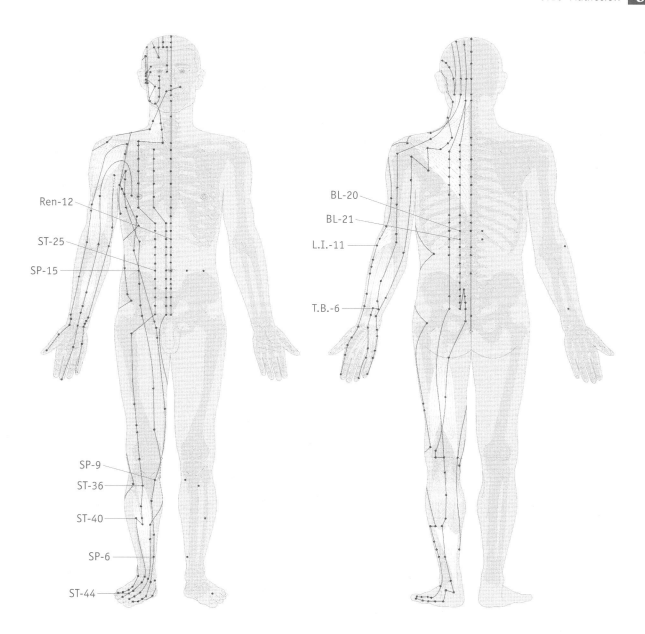

6.16.3 Obesity, adiposity (2)

Dampness retention with Spleen deficiency

ST-25, SP-9, BL-20, LIV-13, Ren-9.
Dyspnoea with exertion: P-6.
Adiposity since childhood: SP-6, BL-23.
Symptoms: eating rather less, tired, sleepy, little stamina, little thirst or thirst without desire to drink, little stools, loose stools, much flabby tissue, not very muscular, weak musculature; **tongue body:** pale, flabby, scalloped edges; **pulse:** weak.

Kidney deficiency

SP-6, BL-23, Du-4, Ren-4.
Ear acupuncture: 84 mouth, 98 spleen, 87 stomach, 95 kidneys, 22 endocrine system, 28 pituitary gland, 13 adrenal gland, may add 51 autonomic nervous system, 23 ovaries, 34 brain.
Needling or intradermal needles as described above.
Weight gain following pregnancy and birth: LIV-8, Ren-5.
Symptoms: eating normal amounts, formed to loose stools, frequent urination, lower back pain, weakness of the knees, gynaecomastia; **tongue body:** pale, flabby; pulse: deep and thin (empty Heat: stubborn, persisting headache and toothache, dull sensation in the head, tiredness, back pain, pain attacks).
Clear relationship with tiredness: **tongue body:** red; **pulse:** thin and weak (*Xi Ruo*).

Acupuncture points

BL-20 **Location:** 1.5 cun lateral to the spinous process of T11.
Notes: back-*Shu* point of the Spleen.
BL-23 **Location:** 1.5 cun lateral to L2, level with Du-4.
Notes: back-*Shu* point of the Kidneys; tonifies the *Qi*, *Yang*, *Yin* and Essence (*Jing*) of the Kidneys, hence useful for 'constitutional' obesity.
Du-4 **Location:** below the spinous process of L2.
Notes: complements Kidney *Yin*, firms the Essence (*Jing*), strengthens the Kidney *Yang*, the lower back and the knees.

LIV-8 **Location:** with the knee flexed, in the depression anterior to the medial end of the popliteal crease.
Notes: *He*-sea point.
LIV-13 **Location:** on the lower border of the free end of the 11th rib.
Notes: metabolic point and front *Mu* point of the Spleen, *Hui* meeting point of the *Zang* organs; harmonizes the Liver/Spleen; for digestive disorders due to emotions.
P-6 **Location:** 2 cun proximal to the midpoint of the palmar wrist crease, between the tendons of the flexor carpi radialis and palmaris longus.
Notes: *Luo*-connecting point and opening point of the *Yin Wei Mai*; mobilizes the Blood (*Xue*), *Qi* and Phlegm stagnation, master point for nausea.
Ren-4 **Location:** 2 cun superior to the upper border of the pubic symphysis.
Notes: internal meeting point of the 3 lower *Yin* meridians (SP, LIV, KID), front *Mu* point of the Small Intestine; nourishing – tonifies Essence (*Jing*), *Qi*, *Yang*, Blood (*Xue*) and *Yin*.
Ren-5 **Location:** 2 cun inferior to the umbilicus.
Notes: front-*Mu* point of the Triple Burner; tonifies the original *Qi*, promotes the transformation and transport in the Lower Burner, opens the water passages, influences the Bladder.
Ren-9 **Location:** 1 cun superior to the umbilicus.
Notes: promotes the transformation of Fluids and Dampness.
SP-6 **Location:** 3 cun superior to the highest prominence of the medial malleolus, on the posterior border of the tibia.
Notes: as group *Luo*-connecting point (SP, LIV, KID), tonifies *Qi*, Blood (*Xue*) and *Yin*; nourishing point; eliminates Dampness.
SP-9 **Location:** with the knee flexed in the depression inferior to the medial condyle of the tibia, at the same level as G.B.-34.
Notes: *He*-sea point; regulates the Fluids and Dampness, tonifies Spleen *Qi*.
ST-25 **Location:** 2 cun lateral to the centre of the umbilicus (Ren-8).
Notes: front-*Mu* point of the Large Intestine; regulates bowel movements.

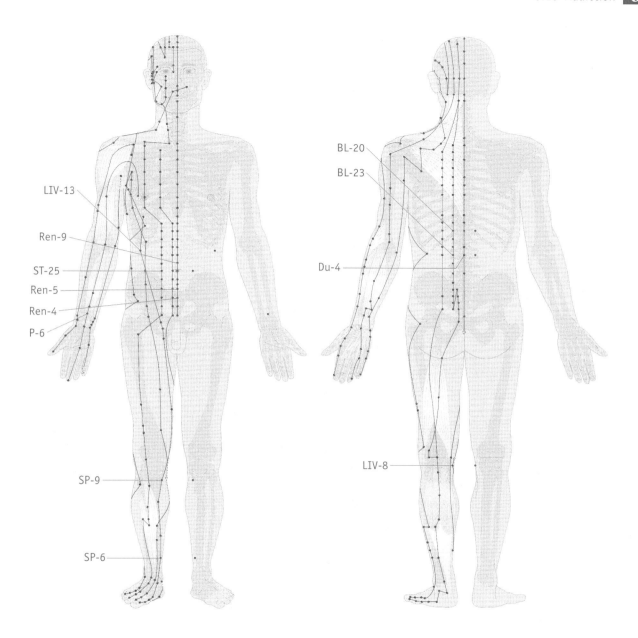

Bibliography

Arnold H-J 1976 Die Geschichte der Akupunktur in Deutschland. Haug, Heidelberg

Bachmann G 1980 Die Akupunktur – eine Ordnungstherapie, Bd 1 & 3, 3rd edn. Haug, Heidelberg

Bahr F 1991 Akupressur. Mosaik, Munich

Baldry P 1993 Acupuncture, trigger points and musculoskeletal pain, 2nd edn. Churchill Livingstone, Edinburgh

Beck R, Heydenreich A, Ots T, Pothmann R, Weinschütz T 1994 Akupunktur in der Neurologie. Hippokrates, Stuttgart

Becke H 1988 Die gefährlichen Punkte in der Schwangerschaft. Deutsche Zeitschrift für Akupunktur 31(5):110

Beijing-Shanghai-Nanjing Colleges of Traditional Chinese Medicine 1980 Essentials of Chinese acupuncture, 1st edn. Foreign Language Press, Beijing

Bensky D, Barolett R 1989 Chinese herbal medicine: formulas and strategies. Eastland Press, Seattle, WA

Bischko J 1986 Akupunktur für Fortgeschrittene, Bd III, 8th edn. Haug, Heidelberg

Bischko J 1989 Einführung in die Akupunktur, Bd 1, 15th edn. Haug, Heidelberg

Bischko J, Meng A 1988 Akupunktur für mäßig Fortgeschrittene, Bd II, 5th edn. Haug, Heidelberg

Bucek R 1984 Kurze Zusammenfassung über Laserakupunktur. Deutsche Zeitschrift für Akupunktur 27:30–36

Büssing A 1993 Akupunktur und Immunsystem. Therapeutikon 7: 542–550

Cheng R, McKibbin L, Pomeranz B, Roy B 1980 Das Verhalten des Blutplasmacortisolspiegels von Pferden nach Akupunktur und Placeboakupunktur. Der Akupunkturarzt und Auriculotherapeut 2:48–50

Cheng Xinnong 1987 Chinese acupuncture and moxibustion. Foreign Language Press, Beijing

Cheng Xinnong 1990 Chinese acupuncture and moxibustion, 2nd edn. Foreign Language Press, Beijing

Darras IC, de Vernejeul, A 1992 Isotopische Verdeutlichung der Akupunkturlinien. Deutsche Zeitschrift für Akupunktur 35(1):4–15

Deadman P, Al-Khajafi M with Baker K 1998 Manual of acupuncture. Eastland Press, Seattle, WA

Ding L 1991 Acupuncture, meridian theory and acupuncture points. Foreign Languages Press, Beijing

Dundee J W, Ghaly R G, Yang J 1990 Scientific observations on the antiemetic action of stimulation of the P6 acupuncture point. Acupuncture in Medicine 7(4):2–5

Feit R, Zmiewski P 1989 Acumoxa therapy, vols I & II. Paradigm Publications, Brookline, MA

Feucht G 1977 Die Geschichte der Akupunktur in Europa. In: Handbuch der Akupunktur und Aurikulotherapie. Haug, Heidelberg

Flaws B, Wolfe H 1983 Prince Wen Huis Cook: Chinese dietary therapy. Paradigm Publications, Brookline, MA

Focks C, Hillenbrand N 1997 Leitfaden Traditionelle Chinesische Medizin: Schwerpunkt Akupunktur, 1st edn. Urban & Fischer, Munich

Focks C, Hillenbrand N 2003 Leitfaden Traditionelle Chinesische Medizin: Schwerpunkt Akupunktur, 4th edn. Urban & Fischer, Munich

Fu W-K 1977 Die Geschichte der chinesischen Akupunktur und Moxibustion. In: Handbuch der Akupunktur und Aurikulotherapie. Haug, Heidelberg

Garten H 1994 Akupunktur bei inneren Erkrankungen. Hippokrates, Stuttgart

Gerardi A U, Dominici S, Sapia F, Morcellini M, Gaetano M A 1983 Riflessoterapia nell'allergia respiratoria. Minerva 74:2521–2531

Gleditsch J 1995 The very point technique: a needle based point detection method. Acupuncture in Medicine 13(1):20–21

Goldschmitt D, Heidbreder G 1981 Akupunkturbehandlungen bei Psoriasis. Die Medizinische Welt 32(5):158–159

Gomaa M-S 1993 Akupunktur in der Dermatologie. Aku 21:163–168

Günes A T 1989 Behandlung von Herpes zoster mit Akupunktur und Aurikulotherapie. Kongressband Teil I, Weltkongress für wissenschaftliche Akupunktur. Wien, 17–20 October 1983, 174–185; quoted in: Kubiena G 1989 Akupunktur bei Asthma, allergischen und dermatologischen Erkrankungen. Haug, Heidelberg

Haidvogel M 1990 Alternative Behandlungsmöglichkeiten atopischer Erkrankungen. Pädiatrie und Pädologie 25(6):389–396

Heine H 1988 Anatomical structure of acupoints. Journal of Traditional Chinese Medicine 8(3): 207–212

Heine H, König L 1994 Morphologische Grundlagen der Elektroakupunktur nach Voll. Deutsche Zeitschrift für Akupunkture 37(1):3–11

Huangdi Neijing Suwen: Innerer Klassiker des gelben Kaisers, elementarer Fragen (c. 300–100 BC). See Chonggung Buzhu Huangdi Suwen and translations, see Schnorrenberger, Van Nghi, Veith

Jellinger K 1984 Neuere biochemiswche Aspekte über Schmerzvermittlung und Akupunkturanalgesie. Deutsche Zeitschrift für Akupunktur 27(4):77–93

Kaada B 1984 Neurophysiologie der Vasodilatation, hervorgerufen durch transcutane Nerventstimulation (TNS). Bischko J (ed.) Handbuch der Akupunktur, Kongreßband Weltkongreß für wissenschaftliche Akupunktur. 17–20 October 1983, Vienna. Teil I, 6–22

Kampik G 1991 Propädeutik der Akupunktur, 2nd edn. Hippokrates, Stuttgart

Kaptchuk T 1992 Das große Buch der chinesischen Medizin. O W Barth, Berne

Kellner G 1966 Bau und Funktion der Haut. Deutsch Zeitschrift für Akupunktur 9(1):1–16

Kirschbaum B 1995 Die 8 außerordentlichen Gefäße. Medizinisch-Literarische Verlagsgesellschaft, Uelzen

Kitzinger E 1989 Der Akupunkturpunkt. Wilhelm Maudrich, Vienna

König G, Wancura J 1988 Praxis und Theorie der Neuen Chinesichen Akupunktur. Wilhelm Maudrich, Vienna

Krauskopf J 1993 Therapie des atopischen Ekzems mit Akupunktur. Aku 21:190–192

Kropej H 1988 Systematik der Ohrakupunktur. Haug, Heidelberg

Kubiena G 1986 Erkenntnisse aus einer Dreijahresstatistik des Ludwig Boltzmann Institutes fur Akupunktur in Wein. Deutsche Zeitschrift fur Akupunktur 29(5):113–120

Kubiena G 1989 Akupunktur bei Asthma, allergischen und dermatologischen Erkrankungen. Haug, Heidelberg

Kubiena G 1995 Kleine Klassik für die Akupunktur, new edn. Maudrich, Vienna

Kubiena G 1996 Chinesische Syndrome verstehen und verwenden. Maudrich, Vienna

Kubiena G, Meng A 1994 Die neuen Extrapunkte in der chinesischen Akupunktur: Lehrbuch, Atlas und Behandlungsprogramme mit den von der WHO empfohlenen und in China gesetzlich festgelegten 48 Extrapunkten. Maudrich, Vienna

Kubiena G, Mosch-Kang You Song 1996 Koreanische und Chinesische Handakupunktur. Maudrich, Vienna

Kubiena G, Ramakers F 2002. Bestzeitakupunktur Chronoakupunktur: Akupunktur der Meister nach der energetischen Zeit. With CD: Computerprogramm zur Feststellung des aktuellen Qi-Flusses. Maudrich, Vienna

Kubiena G, Wang Huizhu 1997 Was sind He-(Ho-)Punkte, untere He-Punkte, Shu-Punkte an den Extremitäten und Shu-Punkte auf dem Rücken? Deutsche Zeitschrift für Akupunktur 40(4):77–82

Kubiena G, Meng A, Petricek E, Petricek U 1991 Handbuch der Akupunktur. Orac, Vienna

Lai X 1993 Observation on the curative effect of acupuncture on type I allergic diseases. Journal of Traditional Chinese Medicine 13(4):243–248

Lau B H, Wong D S, Slater J M 1975 Effect of acupuncture on allergic rhinitis: clinical and laboratory evaluations. American Journal of Chinese Medicine 3(3):263–270

Lewith G T, Field J, Machin D 1983 Acupuncture compared with placebo in post-herpetic pain. Pain 17(4):361–368

Liao S J 1988 Acupuncture for poison ivy contact-dermatitis: a clinical case report. Acupuncture & Electro-therapeutics Research 13(1):31–39

Liao S J, Liao T A 1991 Acupuncture treatment for herpes simplex infection: a clinical case report. Acupuncture & Electro-therapeutics Research 16(3–4):135–142

Liu Gongwang 1998 Acupoints and meridians (1st edn 1996). Huaxia Publishing House, Beijing

Low R 1983 The secondary vessels of acupuncture – a detailed account of their energies, meridians, and control points. Thorsons Publishers, Wellingtonborough, UK

Lux G, Hagel J, Bäcker P et al. 1994 Acupuncture inhibits vagal gastric acid secretion stimulated by sham feeding in healthy subjects. Gut 35(8):1026–1029

Maciocia G 1987 Tongue diagnosis in Chinese medicine. Eastland Press, Seattle, WA

Maciocia G 1989a The foundations of Chinese medicine. Churchill Livingstone, Edinburgh

Maciocia G 1989b The practice of Chinese medicine. Churchill Livingstone, Edinburgh

Mann F 1992 Acupuncture – cure of many diseases, 2nd edn. Butterworth Heinemann, Oxford

Maresch O 1966 Das elektrische Verhalten der Haut. Deutsche Zeitschrift für Akupunktur 9(2):33–35

Matsumoto K, Birch S 1986 Extraordinary vessels. Paradigm Publications, Brookline, MA

Meng A 1976 Die Akupunktur in China von gestern und heute. In: Handbuch der Akupunktur und Aurikulotherapie. Haug, Heidelberg

Meng A 1991 Die wirklich guten Indikationen der Akupunktur und Tuina-Therapie. Deutsche Zeitschrift für Akupunkture 34:3

Meng A, Kokoschinegg P 1980 Wechselwirkung Mensch – Umwelt (Akupunkturmeridiane, die 7. Art der Empfindungsmöglichkeit beim Menschen). Free translation and comment based on an article in a Chinese daily newspaper from October 1979. Deutsche Zeitschrift für Akupunktur 23(1):14–17

Nielsen M 1986 Acupuncture and pain in dermatology. Dermatologica 17(3):143–145

Pauser G 1979 Neurophysiologie und Neurobiochemie als Grundlagen der Akupunkturanalgesie. Deutsche Zeitschrift für Akupunkture 22(5):107–109

Pauser G, Gilly H, Steinbereithner K 1977 Neurophysiologische Untersuchungen zur Wirkung der Akupunkturanalgesie. Deutsche Zeitschrift für Akupunktur 20(5)

Pomeranz B H 1977 Akupunkturwirkung durch Ausschüttung von Encephalinen und Endorphinen im Gerhirn. Lecture by D Marthaler. New Scientist 73:12

Pomeranz B H, Cheng R, Law P 1977 Acupuncture reduces electrophysiological and behavioral responses to noxious stimuli: pituitary is implicated. Experimental Neurology 54(1):172–178

Pöntinen P, Pothmann R 1993 Laser in der Akupunktur. Hippokrates, Stuttgart

Pothmann R 1992 Injektionsakupunktur. Hippokrates, Stuttgart

Pothmann R 1994 Akupunktur-Repetitorium, 2nd edn. Hippokrates, Stuttgart

Ramakers F 1996–2002 Pulse diagnosis. Personal communication, including the translation of the poem by Li Shizhen's father

Richter K, Becke H 1992 Akupunktur: Tradition – Theorie – Praxis. Ullstein Mosby, Berlin

Riederer P, Tenk H, Werner H, Bischko J, Rett A, Krisper H 1975 Manipulation of neurotransmitters by acupuncture (?). Journal of Neural Transmission 37:61–94

Riederer P, Tenk H, Werner H 1978 Biochemische Aspekte der Akupunktur. Deutsche Zeitschrift für Akupunktur 21(2):59–64

Römer A, Seybold B 2003 Akupunktur & TCM für die gynäkologische Praxis. Hippokrates, Stuttgart

Schnorrenberger C 1991 Therapie mit Akupunktur, Band II: Äußere Erkrankungen, 2nd edn. Hippokrates, Stuttgart

Schnorrenberger C 1994 Die topographisch-anatomischen Grundlagen der chinesischen Akupunktur und Ohrakupunktur, 6th edn. Hippokrates, Stuttgart

Schuler W 1993 Akupunktur in Geburtshilfe und Frauenheilkunde, 2nd edn. Hippokrates, Stuttgart

391

Solinas H, Mainville L, Auteroche B 1998 Atlas of Chinese acupuncture, meridians and collaterals. Publishing Canada Inc., Sillery, Quebec

Sommer B 1994 Akupunktur. In: Augustin M, Schmiedel V (eds) Praxisleitfaden Naturheilkunde, 2nd edn. Jungjohann Verlagsgesellschaft, Neckarsulm

Stiefvater H 1973 Praxis der Akupunktur. Haug, Heidelberg

Stux G, Stiller N, Pomeranz P 1993 Akupunktur – Lehrbuch und Atlas, 4th edn. Springer, Berlin

Wagner H, Wolkenstein E 1995 Akupunktur als adjuvante Therapie bei Morbus Crohn-Patienten und Therapiekontrolle mittels Decoderdermographie. Deutsche Zeitschrift für Akupunkture 38(5):114

Wiseman N, Ellis A 1985 Fundamentals of Chinese medicine. Paradigm Publications, Brookline, MA

Wogralik W et al. 1985 Platz der Reflextherapie bei Therapie von Krankheiten des Immunsystems. Lecture at the 4th Conference on Reflexology, Leningrad, 11–14 December 1984. Conference report: Umlauf R 1985. Deutsche Zeitschrift für Akupunkture 28(2):44

Zeitler H 1981 Akupunkturtherapie mit Kardinalpunkten. Haug, Heidelberg

Zeitler H 1983 Meridiane, ihre Punkte und Indikationen. Friedrich Vieweg, Brunswick, Germany

G.B.-21 (*Jian Jing*)	140	KID-23 (*Shen Feng*)	130	P-5 (*Jian Shi*)	130
G.B.-22 (*Yuan Ye*)	140	KID-24 (*Ling Xu*)	130	P-6 (*Nei Guan*)	132
G.B.-23 (*Zhe Jin*)	140	KID-25 (*Shen Cang*)	130	P-7 (*Da Ling*)	132
G.B.-24 (*Ri Yue*)	140	KID-26 (*Yu Zhong*)	130	P-8 (*Lao Gong*)	132
G.B.-25 (*Jing Men*)	140	KID-27 (*Shu Fu*)	130	P-9 (*Zhang Chong*)	132
G.B.-26 (*Dai Mai*)	140				
G.B.-27 (*Wu Shu*)	140	L.I.-1 (*Shang Yang*)	100	Ren-1 (*Hui Yin*)	150
G.B.-28 (*Wei Dao*)	140	L.I.-2 (*Er Jian*)	100	Ren-2 (*Qu Gu*)	150
G.B.-29 (*Ju Liao*)	140	L.I.-3 (*San Jian*)	100	Ren-3 (*Zhong Ji*)	150
G.B.-30 (*Huan Tiao*)	140	L.I.-4 (*He Gu*)	100	Ren-4 (*Guan Yuan*)	150
G.B.-31 (*Feng Shi*)	142	L.I.-5 (*Yang Xi*)	100	Ren-5 (*Shi Men*)	150
G.B.-32 (*Zhong Du*)	142	L.I.-6 (*Pian Li*)	100	Ren-6 (*Qi Hai*)	150
G.B.-33 (*Xi Yang Guan*)	142	L.I.-7 (*Wen Tiu*)	100	Ren-7 (*Yin Jiao*)	150
G.B.-34 (*Yang Ling Quan*)	142	L.I.-8 (*Xia Lian*)	100	Ren-8 (*Shen Que*)	150
G.B.-35 (*Yang Jiao*)	142	L.I.-9 (*Shang Lian*)	100	Ren-9 (*Shui Fen*)	150
G.B.-36 (*Wai Qiu*)	142	L.I.-10 (*Shou San Li*)	102	Ren-10 (*Xia Wan*)	150
G.B.-37 (*Guang Ming*)	142	L.I.-11 (*Qu Chi*)	102	Ren-11 (*Jian Li*)	150
G.B.-38 (*Yang Fu*)	142	L.I.-12 (*Zhou Liao*)	102	Ren-12 (*Zhong Wan*)	150
G.B.-39 (*Xuan Zhong*)	142	L.I.-13 (*Shou Wu Li*)	102	Ren-13 (*Shang Wan*)	150
G.B.-40 (*Qiu Xu*)	142	L.I.-14 (*Bi Nao*)	102	Ren-14 (*Ju Que*)	152
G.B.-41 (*Zu Lin Qi*)	142	L.I.-15 (*Jian Yu*)	102	Ren-15 (*Jiu Wei*)	152
G.B.-42 (*Di Wu Hui*)	144	L.I.-16 (*Ju Gu*)	102	Ren-16 (*Zhong Ting*)	152
G.B.-43 (*Xia Xi*)	144	L.I.-17 (*Tian Ding*)	102	Ren-17 (*Dan Zhong [Shao Zhong]*)	152
G.B.-44 (*Zu Qiao Yin*)	144	L.I.-18 (*Fu Tu*)	102	Ren-18 (*Yu Tang*)	152
		L.I.-19 (*He Liao/Kou He Liao*)	102	Ren-19 (*Zi Gong*)	152
HE-1 (*Jian Quan*)	112	L.I.-20 (*Ying Xiang*)	102	Ren-20 (*Hua Gai*)	152
HE-2 (*Qing Ling*)	112			Ren-21 (*Xuan Ji*)	152
HE-3 (*Shao Hai*)	112	LIV-1 (*Da Dun*)	144	Ren-22 (*Tian Tu*)	152
HE-4 (*Ling Dao*)	112	LIV-2 (*Xing Jian*)	144	Ren-23 (*Lian Quan*)	152
HE-5 (*Tong Li*)	112	LIV-3 (*Tai Chong*)	144	Ren-24 (*Cheng Jiang*)	152
HE-6 (*Yin Xi*)	112	LIV-4 (*Zhong Feng*)	144		
HE-7 (*Shen Men*)	114	LIV-5 (*Li Gou*)	144	S.I.-1 (*Shao Ze*)	114
HE-8 (*Shao Fu*)	114	LIV-6 (*Zhong Du*)	144	S.I.-2 (*Qian Gu*)	114
HE-9 (*Shao Chong*)	114	LIV-7 (*Xi Guan*)	144	S.I.-3 (*Hou Xi*)	114
		LIV-8 (*Qu Quan*)	144	S.I.-4 (*Wan Gu*)	114
KID-1 (*Yong Quan*)	126	LIV-9 (*Yin Bao*)	144	S.I.-5 (*Yang Gu*)	114
KID-2 (*Ran Gu*)	126	LIV-10 (*Zu Wu Li*)	144	S.I.-6 (*Yang Lao*)	114
KID-3 (*Tai Xi*)	126	LIV-11 (*Yin Lian*)	144	S.I.-7 (*Zhi Zheng*)	114
KID-4 (*Da Zhong*)	126	LIV-12 (*Ji Mai*)	146	S.I.-8 (*Xiao Hai*)	114
KID-5 (*Shui Quan*)	126	LIV-13 (*Zhang Men*)	146	S.I.-9 (*Jian Zhen*)	114
KID-6 (*Zhao Hai*)	126	LIV-14 (*Qi Men*)	146	S.I.-10 (*Nao Shu*)	114
KID-7 (*Fu Liu*)	126	LU-1 (*Zhong Fu*)	98	S.I.-11 (*Tian Zong*)	114
KID-8 (*Jiao Xin*)	126	LU-2 (*Yun Men*)	98	S.I.-12 (*Bing Feng*)	116
KID-9 (*Zhu Bin*)	128	LU-3 (*Tian Fu*)	98	S.I.-13 (*Qu Yuan*)	116
KID-10 (*Yin Gu*)	128	LU-4 (*Xia Bai*)	98	S.I.-14 (*Jian Wai Shu*)	116
KID-11 (*Heng Gu*)	128	LU-5 (*Chi Ze*)	98	S.I.-15 (*Jian Zhong Shu*)	116
KID-12 (*Da He*)	128	LU-6 (*Kong Zui*)	98	S.I.-16 (*Tian Chuang*)	116
KID-13 (*Qi Xue*)	128	LU-7 (*Lie Que*)	98	S.I.-17 (*Tian Rong*)	116
KID-14 (*Si Man*)	128	LU-8 (*Jing Qu*)	98	S.I.-18 (*Quan Liao*)	116
KID-15 (*Zhang Zhu*)	128	LU-9 (*Tai Yuan*)	98	S.I.-19 (*Ting Gong*)	116
KID-16 (*Huang Shu*)	128	LU-10 (*Yu Ji*)	98		
KID-17 (*Shang Qu*)	128	LU-11 (*Shao Shang*)	98	SP-1 (*Yin Bai*)	110
KID-18 (*Shi Guan*)	128			SP-2 (*Da Du*)	110
KID-19 (*Yin Du*)	128	P-1 (*Tian Chi*)	130	SP-3 (*Tai Bai*)	110
KID-20 (*Fu Tong Gu*)	130	P-2 (*Tian Quan*)	130	SP-4 (*Gong Sun*)	110
KID-21 (*You Men*)	130	P-3 (*Qu Ze*)	130	SP-5 (*Shang Qiu*)	110
KID-22 (*Bu Lang*)	130	P-4 (*Xi Men*)	130	SP-6 (*San Yin Jiao*)	110

SP-7 (*Lou Gu*)	110	ST-14 (*Ku Fang*)	104	ST-43 (*Xian Gu*)	108
SP-8 (*Di Ji*)	110	ST-15 (*Wu Yi*)	104	ST-44 (*Nei Ting*)	108
SP-9 (*Yin Ling Quan*)	110	ST-16 (*Ying Chuang*)	104	ST-45 (*Li Dui*)	108
SP-10 (*Xue Hai*)	110	ST-17 (*Ru Zhong*)	104		
SP-11 (*Ji Men*)	110	ST-18 (*Ru Gen*)	106	T.B.-1 (*Guan Chong*)	132
SP-12 (*Chong Men*)	112	ST-19 (*Bu Rong*)	106	T.B.-2 (*Ye Men*)	132
SP-13 (*Fu She*)	112	ST-20 (*Cheng Man*)	106	T.B.-3 (*Zhong Zhu*)	132
SP-14 (*Fu Jie*)	112	ST-21 (*Liang Men*)	106	T.B.-4 (*Yang Chi*)	132
SP-15 (*Da Heng*)	112	ST-22 (*Guan Men*)	106	T.B.-5 (*Wai Guan*)	132
SP-16 (*Fu Ai*)	112	ST-23 (*Tai Yi*)	106	T.B.-6 (*Zhi Gou*)	132
SP-17 (*Shi Dou*)	112	ST-24 (*Hua Rou Men*)	106	T.B.-7 (*Hui Zong*)	132
SP-18 (*Tian Xi*)	112	ST-25 (*Tian Shu*)	106	T.B.-8 (*San Yang Luo*)	134
SP-19 (*Xiong Xiang*)	112	ST-26 (*Wai Ting*)	106	T.B.-9 (*Si Du*)	134
SP-20 (*Zhou Rong*)	112	ST-27 (*Da Ju*)	106	T.B.-10 (*Tian Jing*)	134
SP-21 (*Da Bao*)	112	ST-28 (*Shui Dao*)	106	T.B.-11 (*Qing Leng Yuan*)	134
		ST-29 (*Gui Tai*)	106	T.B.-12 (*Xiao Luo*)	134
ST-1 (*Cheng Qi*)	104	ST-30 (*Qi Chong*)	106	T.B.-13 (*Nao Hui*)	134
ST-2 (*Si Bai*)	104	ST-31 (*Bi Guan*)	106	T.B.-14 (*Jian Liao*)	134
ST-3 (*Ju Liao*)	104	ST-32 (*Fu Tu*)	106	T.B.-15 (*Tian Liao*)	134
ST-4 (*Di Cang*)	104	ST-33 (*Yin Shi*)	108	T.B.-16 (*Tian You*)	134
ST-5 (*Da Ying*)	104	ST-34 (*Liang Qiu*)	108	T.B.-17 (*Yi Feng*)	136
ST-6 (*Jia Che*)	104	ST-35 (*Du Bi*)	108	T.B.-18 (*Qi Mai, Ti Mai, Zi Mai*)	136
ST-7 (*Xia Guan*)	104	ST-36 (*Zu San Li*)	108	T.B.-19 (*Lu Xi*)	136
ST-8 (*Tou Wei*)	104	ST-37 (*Shang Ju Xu*)	108	T.B.-20 (*Jiao Sun*)	136
ST-9 (*Ren Ying*)	104	ST-38 (*Tiao Kou*)	108	T.B.-21 (*Er Men*)	136
ST-10 (*Shui Tu*)	104	ST-39 (*Xia Ju Xu*)	108	T.B.-22 (*Er He Liao*)	136
ST-11 (*Qi She*)	104	ST-40 (*Feng Long*)	108	T.B.-23 (*Si Zhu Kong*)	136
ST-12 (*Que Pen*)	104	ST-41 (*Jie Xi*)	108		
ST-13 (*Qi Hu*)	104	ST-42 (*Chong Yang*)	108		

Acupuncture points (pinyin name)

Index

Note: page numbers in *italics* indicate figures or tables.

Index